T0295054

Piermattei's Atlas of

Surgical Approaches to the Bones and Joints

of the Dog and Cat

Piermattei's Atlas of

Surgical Approaches to the Bones and Joints

of the Dog and Cat

FIFTH EDITION

Kenneth A. Johnson, MVSc, PhD, FACVSc

Diplomate, American College of Veterinary Surgeons
Diplomate, European College of Veterinary Surgeons
Professor and Director of Orthopaedic Surgery
Associate Dean of Veterinary Clinical Sciences
The University of Sydney
Sydney, Australia

Illustrations by F. Dennis Giddings, AMI

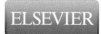

3251 Riverport Lane
St. Louis, Missouri 63043

PIERMATTEI'S ATLAS OF SURGICAL APPROACHES TO THE BONES   ISBN: 978-1-4377-1634-4
AND JOINTS OF THE DOG AND CAT

Copyright © 2014, 2004, 1993, 1979, 1966 by Saunders, an imprint of Elsevier Inc.

No part of this publication may be reproduced or transmitted in any form or by any means, electronic or mechanical, including photocopying, recording, or any information storage and retrieval system, without permission in writing from the publisher. Details on how to seek permission, further information about the Publisher's permissions policies and our arrangements with organizations such as the Copyright Clearance Center and the Copyright Licensing Agency, can be found at our website: www.elsevier.com/permissions.

This book and the individual contributions contained in it are protected under copyright by the Publisher (other than as may be noted herein).

Notices

Knowledge and best practice in this field are constantly changing. As new research and experience broaden our understanding, changes in research methods, professional practices, or medical treatment may become necessary.

Practitioners and researchers must always rely on their own experience and knowledge in evaluating and using any information, methods, compounds, or experiments described herein. In using such information or methods they should be mindful of their own safety and the safety of others, including parties for whom they have a professional responsibility.

With respect to any drug or pharmaceutical products identified, readers are advised to check the most current information provided (i) on procedures featured or (ii) by the manufacturer of each product to be administered, to verify the recommended dose or formula, the method and duration of administration, and contraindications. It is the responsibility of practitioners, relying on their own experience and knowledge of their patients, to make diagnoses, to determine dosages and the best treatment for each individual patient, and to take all appropriate safety precautions.

To the fullest extent of the law, neither the Publisher nor the authors, contributors, or editors, assume any liability for any injury and/or damage to persons or property as a matter of products liability, negligence or otherwise, or from any use or operation of any methods, products, instructions, or ideas contained in the material herein.

International Standard Book Number: 978-1-4377-1634-4

Vice President and Publisher: Linda Duncan
Content Strategy Director: Penny Rudolph
Content Development Specialist: Brandi Graham
Publishing Services Manager: Catherine Jackson
Senior Project Manager: David Stein
Designer: Teresa McBryan

Printed in India

Last digit is the print number: 9   8   7

Working together
to grow libraries in
developing countries

www.elsevier.com • www.bookaid.org

Dedicated to those colleagues
who pioneered the anatomic approach to surgery
and made this volume possible,
especially Wade O. Brinker
and R. Bruce Hohn.

Preface

One of the first things to notice about this new fifth edition of the *Atlas* is the change in name to *Piermattei's Atlas of Surgical Approaches to the Bones and Joints of the Dog and Cat*. This change is formal recognition of just one facet of the immense and pioneering contributions of Donald L. Piermattei to veterinary orthopedics. As the originator and senior author of the first four editions of this iconic book, he created the solid foundations describing the anatomic surgical approaches to the bones and joints in dogs and cats for orthopedic surgery.

Since publication of the first edition, this book has grown in size, with more approaches being added thanks to the contributions of colleagues who have published descriptions of new approaches. In this fifth edition, we have added several new approaches specifically for the cat in recognition of the subtle, yet important, anatomic differences in this species. Also we have modified and updated some previously existing approaches to improve the anatomic detail. Furthermore, some minimally invasive approaches to the shaft of the tibia, humerus, and femur have been introduced to facilitate the move toward minimally invasive osteosynthesis of diaphyseal fractures.

The marvellous clarity of anatomic detail in the drawings added and revised in this edition was once again produced by Dennis Giddings. His skill and anatomic knowledge have contributed immeasurably to the quality of this edition, and I am immensely grateful to him for his collaboration. Regrettably, Dennis and I have never met in person; all of our interactions have been through the Internet. Nevertheless, he still managed to interpret and decipher my instructions, sketches, and thoughts to produce excellent new illustrations.

Donald Piermattei has been a very significant mentor and guiding star in my professional career in veterinary orthopedics. I feel truly honored to have been asked by Don to take on the care and revision of his *Atlas*. So I hope that he feels a genuine pride and pleasure in what Dennis and I, together with Elsevier Publishers, have produced in this new edition. I am reminded that very few of us have the talent and foresight to make great achievement alone. Thus you will see that the dedication to the late Wade O. Brinker and R. Bruce Hohn has endured. It is so important to recognize the gifts of knowledge and wisdom that were so freely given by our mentors. In this context the words of Bernard of Chartres are most apposite.

"If I have seen further, it is by standing on the shoulders of giants."

Kenneth A. Johnson,
MVSc, PhD, FACVSc, DACVS, DECVS
Sydney, Australia

Contents

SECTION 7
The Hindlimb

SECTION 1

General Considerations

- Attributes of an Acceptable Approach to a Bone or Joint
- Factors to Consider When Choosing an Approach
- Aseptic Technique
- Surgical Principles
- Anatomy

Attributes of an Acceptable Approach to a Bone or Joint

The bones and joints must be exposed in a manner that ensures the preservation of the anatomic and physiologic functions of the area invaded. Major blood vessels, nerves, ligaments, and tendons must be avoided or protected. Maximal use must be made of muscle separation, with incision of muscles being avoided whenever possible. Transection of muscle bellies must be kept at an absolute minimum; tenotomy or osteotomy of the muscles at their origin or insertion is much preferred. Skin incisions must be made in such a manner that the vascular supply to the wound margins is not impaired and so that underlying implants such as bone plates do not create tension on the skin closure. No pedicles or sharp angles should exist in the incision because these points commonly undergo avascular necrosis and may produce wound breakdown, infection, or excessive scar formation. A cosmetically acceptable scar should be one goal of the surgery.

In general, the procedure should not add unnecessary trauma to that which the injured area has already sustained. Although the incision may be longer, an adequately large exposure is, in the final analysis, less traumatic than a smaller exposure. With the smaller approach, the surgeon tends to exert excessive pressure when retracting muscles, which directly injures the muscle and also impairs circulation to the area.

Factors to Consider When Choosing an Approach

THE AREA TO BE EXPOSED

The problem of choosing the best approach is easily solved in some instances. For example, there is only one logical way to expose the midshaft of the femur (see Approach to the Shaft of the Femur, Plate 77), and therefore the decision is easily made. Other regions do not lend themselves to such clear-cut answers. In some instances, the choice is purely a matter of the surgeon's personal preference. The hip joint perhaps illustrates this best, there being many choices for exposure of this general region. Ultimately, it rests with the surgeon to evaluate all approaches and to adapt those most suitable.

The exposure required for bone plating is generally more extensive than for bone-pinning techniques. In this instance, it may be useful or necessary to combine two or more of the approaches illustrated. This is discussed further in the section "The Type of Fracture or Luxation."

MINIMALLY INVASIVE EXPOSURE OF BONES AND JOINTS

With the trend in fracture surgery toward "biological fracture repair," there is a much greater recognition of the importance of preservation of soft-tissue attachments, bone blood supply, and fracture hematoma, all of which have a critical role in the early phase of bone healing. This evolution has been facilitated by the greater availability of preoperative computed tomography imaging for fracture planning, intraoperative fluoroscopic imaging, indirect fracture reduction techniques, and new fracture fixation implants.

Perfect anatomic reduction of intra-articular fractures is possible with the aid of intraoperative fluoroscopic imaging, and therefore a complete open approach to the joint might not be required. This allows insertion of Kirschner wires and lag screws through small "stab incisions" to complete the fracture stabilization. Moreover, indirect reduction techniques can be applied to diaphyseal fractures to obtain overall alignment without the need for anatomic fracture reduction. For diaphyseal fracture stabilization, the technique of minimally invasive plate osteosynthesis can be applied. Small skin incisions are made in the proximal and distal metaphyseal regions of the bone, without exposing the fracture site directly. Afterward the two incisions are connected by a longitudinal epiperiosteal tunnel, so that the bone plate can be slid through the tunnel, across the fracture site (e.g., see Minimally Invasive Approach to the Shaft of the Humerus, Plate 36).

The minimally invasive approach to fracture repair is more technically demanding than traditional open reduction and internal fixation. The surgeon should have additional training and experience to perform it well. The availability of intraoperative fluoroscopic imaging is important for the evaluation of the fracture reduction and implant position. However, surgeons should be ready to convert from a minimally invasive approach to an open approach if the procedure becomes too difficult. Timely conversion to an open approach is important if the surgeon is to avoid excessive exposure of surgical personnel and the patient to radiation, undue damage to the soft tissues, inadequate fracture alignment, and technical mistakes in implant placement resulting in poor fixation.

BREED, SIZE, AND CONFORMATION OF THE ANIMAL

The region of the hip may also be used to illustrate the relationship of the patient's physique to the problem. We are speaking here not only of the size, but also of the body conformation and the degree of obesity of the patient. Chondrodystrophoid breeds are a particular challenge. The shapes and contours of many muscles in the limbs are distorted, and close attention is required to ensure that you end up where you really want to be.

The obese patient is also a serious problem for the surgeon, for it is difficult to identify muscles when their fascial sheaths are obscured by fat. The only help for this problem is to dissect fat off the deep fascia with the skin to allow better visualization of the underlying muscles. A longer skin incision may be required to achieve adequate exposure at the level of the bones.

THE TYPE OF FRACTURE OR LUXATION

Multiple injuries require multiple approaches or perhaps a combination of methods. By scanning the approaches to various areas of a bone, one can easily note those that lend themselves to combining. An example might be a combination of one of the approaches to the hip or pelvis with the Approach to the Shaft of the Femur (Plate 77). The most likely alternative approaches are listed for each procedure.

ASSOCIATED SOFT-TISSUE DAMAGE OR INFECTION

When a choice of approaches exists, the extent and location of associated injuries can influence the choice of approach. Bruising and hematoma formation make the identification of fascial sheaths and muscle bellies more difficult. Furthermore, fractures and luxations result in changes in orientation and position of the muscles in the region. An attempt is always made to avoid exposing bone through an existing skin wound or sinus tract. The reason for this is to prevent the transfer of infected or contaminated material to the bone and the surrounding deep structures. The same reasoning is applied to open fractures of more than a few hours' duration. When there is no alternative to approaching through such an area, the traumatic wound must be meticulously débrided and lavaged. It is then prepared again for surgery and redraped, and fresh gloves and instruments are used for the fracture repair.

Aseptic Technique

The keystone on which success or failure of open bone and joint surgery rests is meticulous devotion to the ritual of aseptic technique. True enough, gentle handling of tissues and an anatomically sound approach are of utmost importance, but they go for naught in the presence of wound infection or osteomyelitis. The incidence of these sequelae can be reduced to less than 3% by attention to rigid asepsis and the proper use of antibiotic drugs. In clean cases, where no contamination or infection is suspected, an appropriate dose of a bactericidal antibiotic (e.g., a beta-lactam such as a cephalosporin or amoxicillin with clavulanic acid) is administered intravenously at the time of anesthesia and repeated in 90 minutes. It must be understood that to be effective at the time of surgery, the antibiotic drug must be administered preoperatively with sufficient time to allow effective serum levels of the drug to be present. Antibiotic medications are not administered postoperatively unless contamination or infection is suspected, or serious tissue damage is noted during surgery. In such cases, antibiotic medications are continued for at least 7 days postoperatively. Choice of antibiotic drug used long term should be based on culture and sensitivity of samples taken during surgery.

A detailed discussion of the methods of sterilization of packs, gowns, and other supplies is beyond the scope of this book. In general, autoclaving at 250°F and 15-lb pressure and with a contact time of 12 to 15 minutes is the most practical way of sterilizing instruments and cloth materials such as drapes and gowns. Sterilizer indicators[1] that undergo a color change when exposed to proper sterilization conditions should be used in every pack. Total time in the autoclave is different from contact time; total time is that which is sufficient for steam penetration of the largest pack for the minimum contact time of 12 to 15 minutes. Sterilizer indicators are the only means of establishing the correct total time. Ethylene oxide is also a very useful sterilization method because it allows sterilization of items that would be damaged by heat and therefore allows the use of electric drills and other hardware store items in surgery.

Proper skin preparation, positioning, and draping of the patient are critical elements of aseptic technique that are commonly neglected. For all procedures on limbs, including the hip or shoulder region, a stockinette draping procedure is advised. Draping the whole limb in a sterile, double-thickness cotton stockinette allows the limb to be handled by the surgeon and manipulated in any way necessary. When reducing fractures, the need for alignment of the total limb in all planes is obvious. When reducing luxations, the whole limb can be used to supply additional leverage or torque to aid in reduction.

The limb is clipped circumferentially from the inguinal or axillary area with a #40 blade and electric clippers to some distance distal to the proposed skin incision. For approaches to the hip or shoulder, the clipping extends proximally to the midline of the back. When the approach is below the elbow or stifle, the clipping usually starts just above the toes and extends proximally only to the elbow or stifle region. Adhesive tape is applied to the toes or foot to form a stirrup from which the leg can be suspended. The remaining unclipped area is covered with gauze or a latex or plastic glove and adhesive tape (Figure 1A and B).

The patient is next placed on the surgery table with the clipped leg uppermost and the leg suspended by adhesive tape attached to the stirrup and to an infusion stand or a hook in the ceiling (Figure 2). Abduction of the limb to a 45- to 60-degree angle from midline is adequate to allow skin disinfection and draping.

---

[1]Comply Thermalog Steam Chemical Indicator, 3M, St. Paul, Minn.

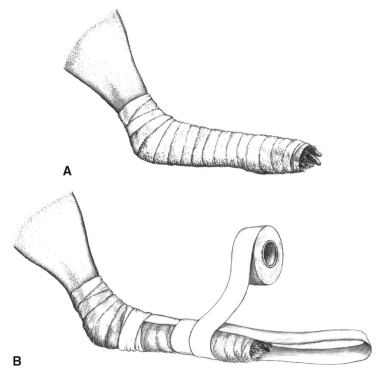

A

B

■ **Figure 1.**
A, The unclipped portion of the lower limb is covered with roller gauze bandage or a latex or plastic glove from the toes proximally to the clipped area. **B,** Adhesive tape is used to make a stirrup and to cover the gauze or glove.

Povidone-iodine[2] ("organic iodine") or chlorhexidine[3] preparations have proved most efficacious for disinfection of the patient's skin. Using sterile gauze sponges immersed in surgical scrub preparation diluted 50% with sterile saline solution or water, the patient's skin is scrubbed, starting in the area of the incision and working outward to the limits of the clipped area. After 1 minute of scrubbing, the suds are wiped off with dry, sterile sponges. Again, the wiping starts in the area of the incision and proceeds toward the periphery of the clipped area. This cycle is repeated 5 times, and after the final rinse the whole area is sprayed or wiped with povidone-iodine or chlorhexidine solution, or 70% to 80% isopropyl alcohol, which is allowed to remain and dry on the skin. Povidone-iodine and chlorhexidine surgical scrubs are also highly effective for the scrubbing of the surgeon's hands.

The patient is now ready for draping as soon as the surgeon or assistant is gowned and gloved. Four sterile towels are first placed around the leg at the inguinal or axillary region (Figure 3). The circulating assistant now grasps the leg on the unprepped area and cuts the suspending tape while holding the leg in position. The surgeon grasps the foot through a sterile towel that has been partially rolled (Figure 4A) and then wraps the towel around the unprepped area while holding the limb up and away from the table. The towel is folded over the toes and secured with towel clamps (Figure 4B). Now the rolled stockinette is placed over the foot (Figure 4C) and unrolled down the leg, taking care not to touch any unprepped areas in the process. When the stockinette meets the towels, the two are joined together and attached to the skin with towel forceps (Figure 5A). A method for the hip or shoulder region is shown in Figure 5B and C. (The cotton gauze stockinette is previously prepared and

[2]Betadine surgical scrub and Betadine antiseptic solution, Purdue-Frederick Co., Norwalk, Conn.
[3]Nolvasan surgical scrub, Fort Dodge Laboratories, Fort Dodge, Iowa; Hibiclens skin cleanser, Stuart Pharmaceuticals, Wilmington, Del.

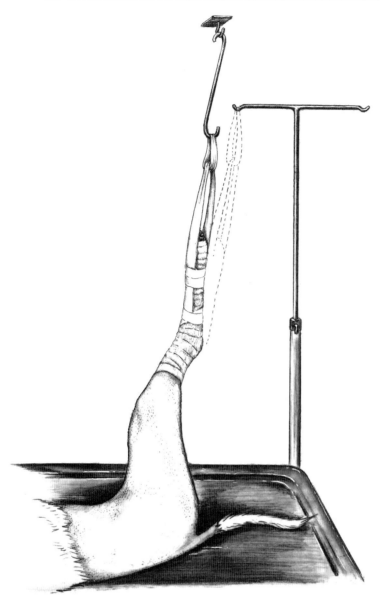

■ **Figure 2.**

Suspension of the clipped limb preparatory to skin disinfection. An infusion stand or a hook in the ceiling is used. Adhesive tape can be run directly to the infusion stand from the tape stirrup or to an elongated S-shaped metal rod interposed between the ceiling and the foot.

■ **Figure 3.**

Pattern for laying towels around the inguinal or axillary region.

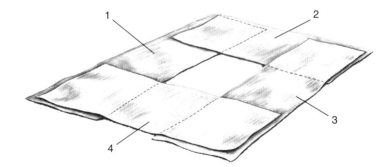

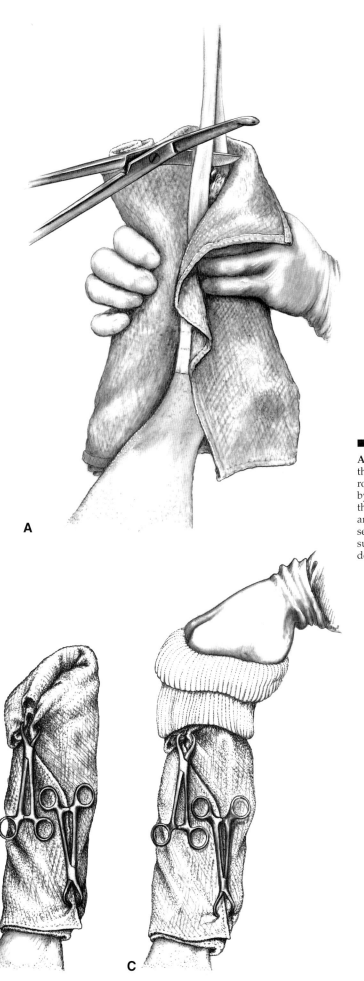

■ **Figure 4.**

A, The surgeon grasps the suspended foot through a sterile towel that has been folded and rolled. The suspending tape is cut close to the foot by the technician. **B,** The towel is wrapped around the foot, taking care to cover all of the unprepped area. After the towel is folded over the toes, it is secured to the limb with towel clamps. **C,** The surgeon grasps the foot through a sterile, double-thickness, rolled stockinette.

A

B   C

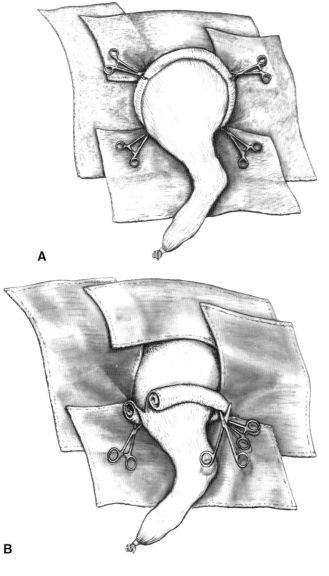

A

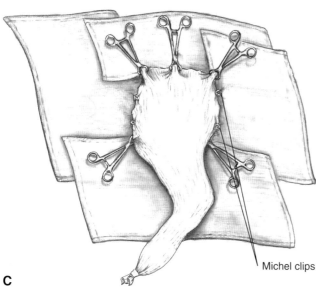

B

■ **Figure 5.**

A, Four towels are attached to the stockinette and skin with towel forceps. **B,** When the stockinette must be rolled proximally to the midline over the hip or shoulder region, the distal towel forceps are attached to the medial half of the rolled stockinette, and the lateral half of the roll is cut close to the forceps. **C,** The lateral half of the rolled stockinette is rolled proximally and clipped to skin and towels proximal to the hip or shoulder. Michel skin clips can be used to supplement the towel forceps.

Michel clips

C

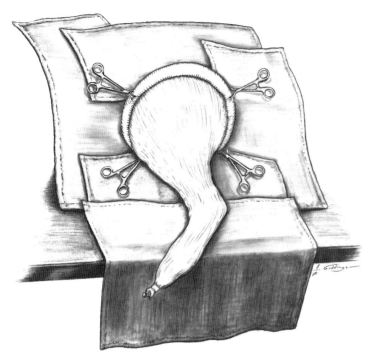

■ **Figure 6.**
When the four towels do not cover the surgical table, a fifth towel is used to allow the stockinetted limb to rest on the table preparatory to final draping.

sterilized. Cut the stockinette twice as long as the leg, using a suitable diameter for the thigh or brachium. Pull half the stockinette inside the other half and tie or tape the cut ends together to make an elongated bag. Roll the uncut end toward the closed end as if rolling a stocking. Wrapping and sterilizing complete the preparation. Alternatively, a presterilized impervious stockinette[4] can be used.)

The leg can now be allowed to rest on the table, atop the sterile towels. If the towel under the leg does not cover the table top, a fifth towel is added (Figure 6). The patient and table are next covered with a large fenestrated drape with the stockinette-draped limb protruding through the fenestration. The large drape is accordion folded to allow easy opening (Figures 7 and 8). Alternative methods of applying the large drape are available. Four large sheets can be placed around the limb as in Figure 9, or the split-sheet method shown in Figure 10 can be used. The choice of cotton muslin drapes or of impregnated paper materials is a matter of personal preference. In any case, the large drape should adequately cover the table and the patient. For smaller dogs and cats, this means a drape of 48 × 48 inches (120 × 120 cm) minimum, and for larger breeds, 48 × 72 inches (120 × 180 cm) minimum.

The stockinette is cut over the proposed skin incision. After the skin is incised, the cut edges are folded under and are attached to the stockinette with 16-mm Michel skin clips (Figure 11A) or by suturing (Figure 11B). Skin towels can be attached if preferred. Adhesive plastic drapes[5] have some qualities that make them useful in certain situations, although their cost has somewhat limited their use in veterinary surgery. Because they are both impervious to moisture and transparent, they are useful around areas that are difficult to prepare, such as the feet and the perineal region, and where visualization of a large area is essential during surgery, as in corrective osteotomies. Unfortunately, these drapes do not adhere well to

---

[4]Ortho Dog Leggings, General Econopak, Philadelphia.
[5]Barrier Sterile Surgical Incise Drapes, Surgikos Inc., Arlington, Tex.

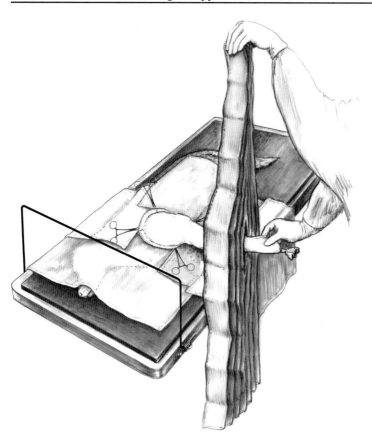

■ **Figure 7.**

A fenestrated and accordion-folded outer drape is positioned on the stockinetted limb by the surgeon.

■ **Figure 8.**

The left half of the accordion-folded drape has been spread, and the right half is positioned to complete the draping procedure.

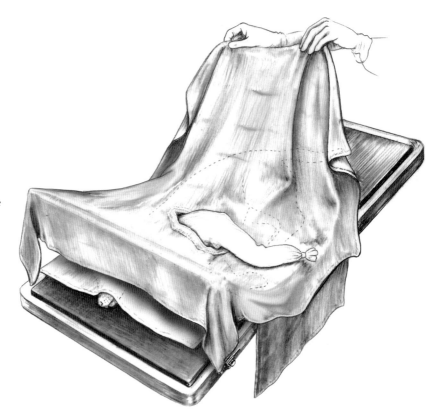

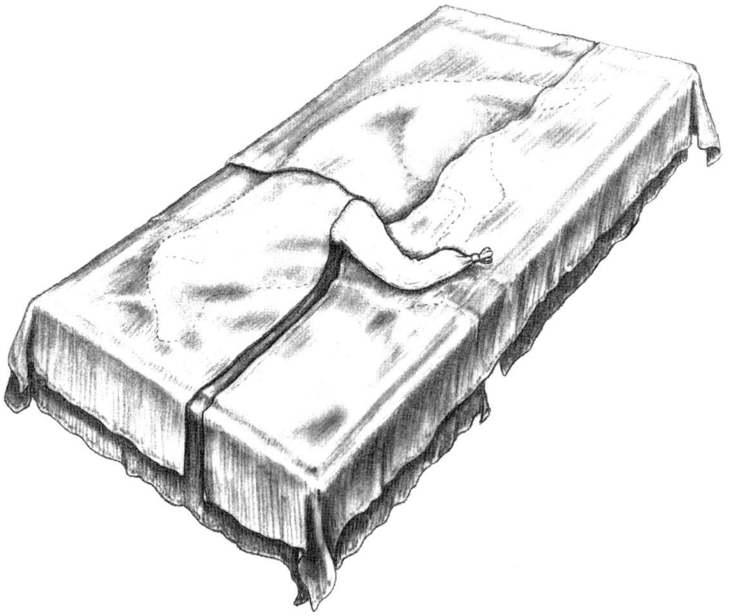

■ **Figure 9.**
Four large sheets, used in a manner similar to the initial towels, can be used as an outer drape.

animal skin, even when it is well clipped and scrubbed. Additional adhesive[6] must be sprayed on the skin to create good adhesion (Figure 12A), but even then there is considerable loosening of the plastic from the skin if there is much movement of the area during surgery. When used with a stockinette for limb draping, the stockinette is applied as usual, and then a rather large hole is cut in the stockinette to expose a generous area of skin for adhesion of the drape. Alternatively, the stockinette is unrolled only partway proximally and the plastic drape is used to cover the rest of the area proximal to the four towels. In the hip and shoulder regions, the stockinette can be attached to the towels medially but not laterally, leaving an open area laterally for the adhesive drape (Figure 12B).

Preparation and draping of the lower limbs present some special problems in aseptic technique. If the surgery is to be in the area of the carpus or tarsus, the limb is clipped distally to the proximal phalanges, and the toes are wrapped in adhesive tape to allow suspension of the limb for scrubbing. Because the toes are not prepped, they must be covered intraoperatively in such a way as to prevent strikethrough of fluids and contamination of the surgical field. As the technician cuts the suspending tape, the surgeon supports the limb by grasping the foot through a sterile towel (Figure 13A) and then placing a stockinette on the limb as described previously (Figure 13B). A sterile surgical glove is then used to cover the toes and part of the metacarpus (metatarsus) (Figure 13C). The glove is secured to the foot with a wrapping of sterile elastic bandage material. Adhesive plastic drapes can be substituted for stockinette quite effectively because they eliminate the need for placing the surgical glove to prevent strikethrough.

If the surgical field extends into the midportion of the metacarpus (metatarsus), the entire foot must be prepared because there is no way to isolate the field from the rest of the foot. Following clipping, the limb is suspended by a Backhaus towel forceps clamped through a toenail (Figure 14). During scrubbing, particular attention should be paid to the pads because they are very difficult to cleanse and disinfect adequately. The limb and foot are then covered with stockinette as before, but there is now no need for the surgical glove because the entire

---

[6]Aerozoin, Grafco, Hauppauge, NY.

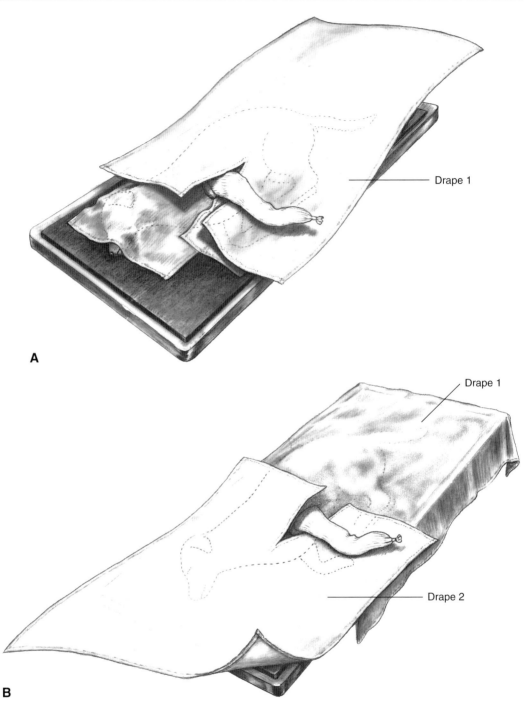

■ **Figure 10.**

A, The split-sheet method for an outer drape. Drape 1 is split for a distance of 18 to 24 inches perpendicular to the short end, and the limb is placed on top of one half of the sheet. **B,** Drape 2 is applied in a similar manner so that an 18- to 24-inch overlap of the two sheets occurs.

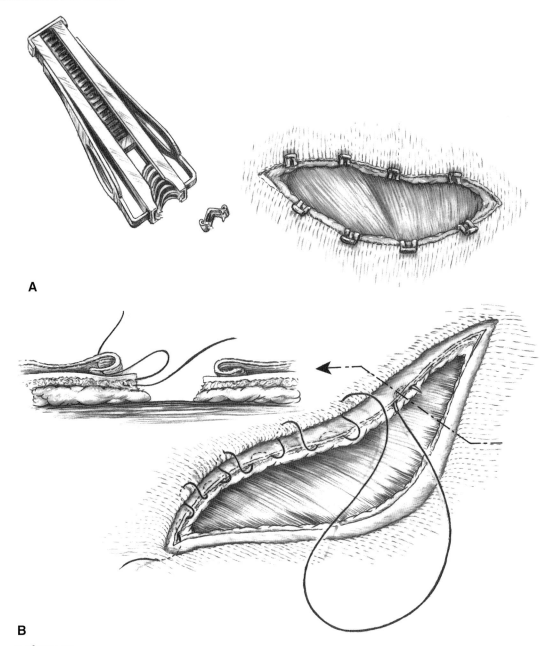

■ Figure 11.

A, A skin incision has been made after cutting the stockinette along the proposed line of incision. The stockinette is then clipped to the skin with 16-mm Michel wound clips. **B,** The stockinette can be sutured in place. Note that the suture is placed in the dermis, not the skin, and then through the rolled edge of the stockinette. A taper-point needle is preferred.

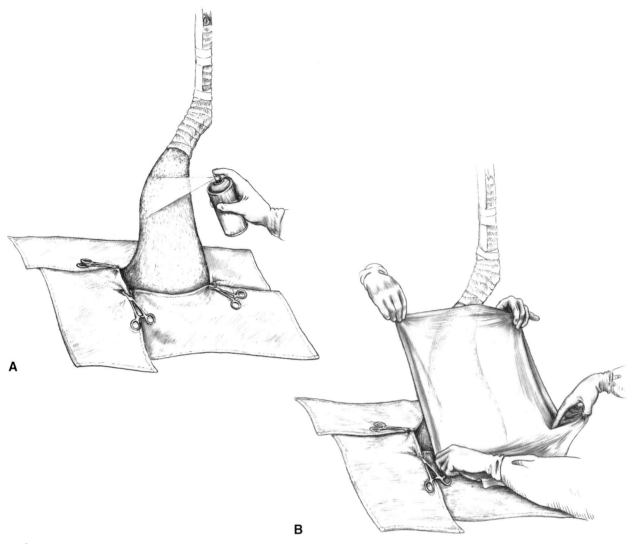

■ Figure 12.

Placing a transparent plastic adhesive drape. **A,** Sterile adhesive material is sprayed over the prepped area in the region where the adhesive drape will be applied. **B,** After removing the paper backing, the adhesive plastic drape is placed on the prepared skin and pressed in place to adhere it to the skin. A stockinette will be placed over the limb distal to the plastic drape.

foot is prepped. Alternatively, adhesive plastic drapes can be substituted for stockinette. For incisions on the trunk, neck, and head, the draping technique is considerably simplified. After skin preparation, the area of the incision is delineated by laying four sterile towels around the area, which are then attached to the skin with towel forceps. The large drape, similar in size to that described previously, is simply placed over the area and opened. Skin towels are clipped or sewn to the skin after the skin incision is completed. When using disposable paper drapes, it is often convenient to clip the drape directly to the incised skin and thus dispense with skin towels.

It is a point worth stressing that adequate draping simplifies the workload of the surgeon by eliminating the need to worry about where a hand or instrument may come to rest in an unguarded moment. If the drape is large enough, any area within a reasonable distance from the incision is "safe." The longer the procedure, the more important draping and all other

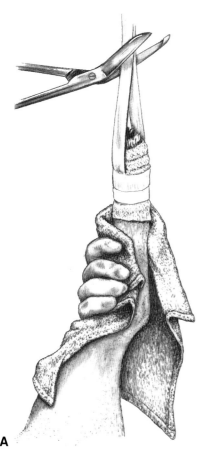

■ Figure 13.

Draping the foot when the region of the toes has not been prepped. **A,** The surgeon grasps the suspended foot through a sterile towel. The suspending tape is cut close to the foot by the technician. **B,** The stockinette is unrolled proximally while the limb is supported by the opposite hand. **C,** A sterile glove is placed on the foot to cover the unprepped portion and is secured in place with sterile elastic bandage material (Vetrap, 3M Animal Care Products, St. Paul, Minn). Bandage material, glove, and stockinette are incised over the area of the skin incision.

A

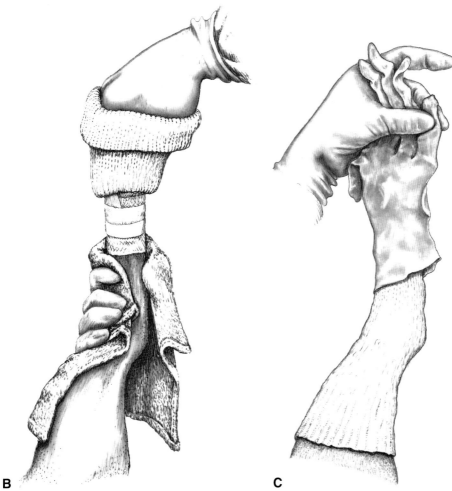

B

C

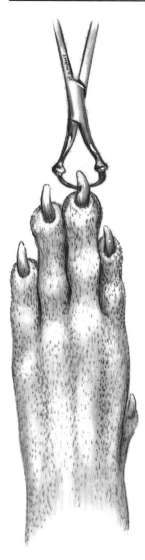

■ Figure 14.

When the entire foot is to be prepped, the foot is suspended with a Backhaus towel forceps placed into a toenail.

aspects of asepsis become. Procedures lasting longer than 1 hour are significantly more prone to wound infections than are shorter operations.

Surgical Principles

Assuming that aseptic technique is scrupulously practiced, the success or failure of an open approach rests on the surgeon's skill in handling tissues atraumatically. Although many of the methods herein described are well known to the experienced surgeon, it is hoped that this review will be useful to the practicing surgeon, in addition to serving as an introduction to this subject for the student.

INCISING AND RETRACTING SKIN AND SUBCUTANEOUS TISSUES

The skin and dermal fascia are incised cleanly and completely before an attempt is made to pick up bleeding vessels. The incision will gape widely when the fascia is completely cut,

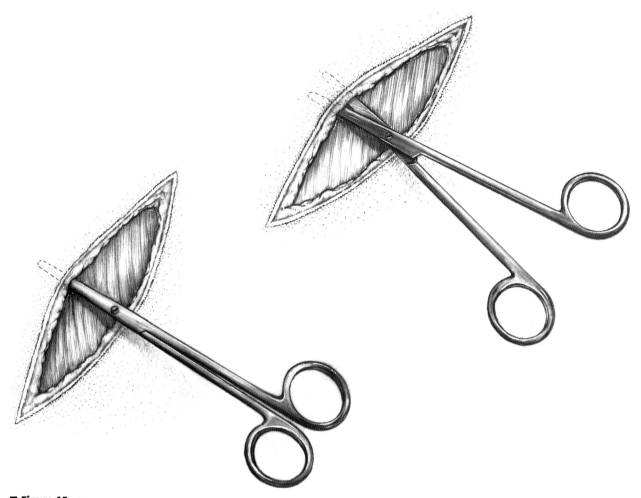

■ **Figure 15.**
Undermining skin and subcutaneous fascia and fat by using Metzenbaum scissors and blunt dissection technique.

and subsequent eversion of the cut edges facilitates the clamping of bleeders. Meticulous hemostasis is necessary for optimal skin healing. The use of an electrosurgical apparatus for coagulating smaller bleeders is invaluable as a time saver and as a way of achieving a dry surgical field. Regrettably, this technique is not often enough used by veterinary surgeons.

In most cases, subcutaneous fat is incised on the same line as the skin. The fat is incised down to the deep fascial layer, which lies directly on the muscles. It is usually necessary to bluntly separate fat from fascia by the undermining technique shown in Figure 15. This method allows the skin to be widely retracted with minimal interference with its blood supply and exposes the fascia to allow the visualization necessary for the proposed fascial incision.

Hemostatic (crushing) clamps should never be applied to the cut edges of the skin, and even Allis forceps are best fastened to subcutaneous fascia to avoid possible trauma. The use of retractors is highly encouraged as a means of avoiding tissue damage. Useful examples of these are shown in Figure 16. The Gelpi self-retaining retractor is virtually a third hand for the surgeon working alone. Hohmann and Meyerding laminectomy retractors are particularly valuable in the region of the pelvis and hip joint. When selecting rake-type retractors

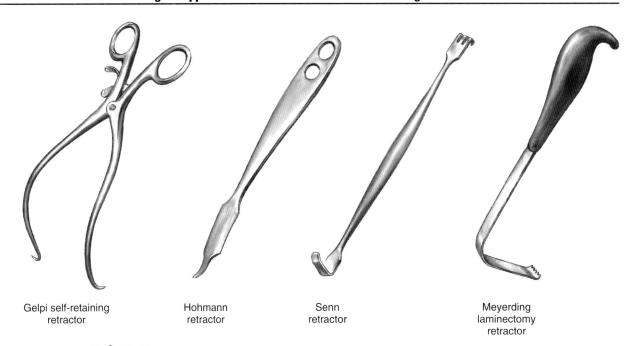

Gelpi self-retaining
retractor

Hohmann
retractor

Senn
retractor

Meyerding
laminectomy
retractor

■ **Figure 16.**

These retractors are representative of types useful in small animal orthopedic surgery.

such as the Volkmann, Senn, or Mathieu, those with sharp teeth are preferred over those with rounded teeth. The points on the latter tend to slip more, resulting in more trauma than the sharp points produce.

Deep fascia may be loosely adherent to the musculature and may actually slide freely over the muscles, as with the fascia lata, or it may be tightly adherent to the deep structures and difficult to separate from the muscle sheaths. The latter condition is particularly true distal to the elbow and the stifle joint.

A method of incising movable fascia to avoid damaging deep structures is depicted in Figure 17. Tightly adherent fascia is incised with the scalpel, with care being taken to make the incisions directly over muscle separations whenever possible. Fascia is rarely retracted by itself but is usually retracted with the muscles exposed by the fascial incision.

MUSCLE SEPARATION, ELEVATION, AND RETRACTION

Muscles are separated and elevated from the bone to obtain exposure of the bone. The incision of muscles, particularly by transection, is avoided wherever possible, and tenotomy is held to a minimum. Nothing contributes more to an early return of function than the intelligent and gentle handling of muscles.

Muscles are held against the bone by the deep fascia that surrounds the trunk and limbs like a tube. When this fascia is incised, muscles are relatively free except at their origins and insertions. The space between muscles, called the intermuscular septum, is occupied by rather loose fascial tissue. Bellies of adjacent muscles rarely adhere to one another. Therefore, to separate muscles after the incision of the deep fascia, it is necessary to divide only the intermuscular septa. This is accomplished as shown in Figure 18.

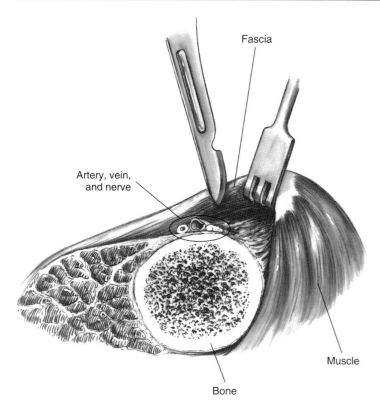

Fascia

Artery, vein,
and nerve

Muscle

Bone

■ **Figure 17.**
Method of incising deep fascia. The muscle sheath is
grasped with forceps and lifted to elevate the fascia
from deeper structures.

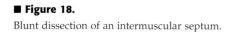

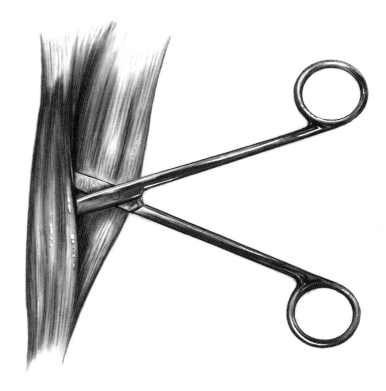

■ **Figure 18.**
Blunt dissection of an intermuscular septum.

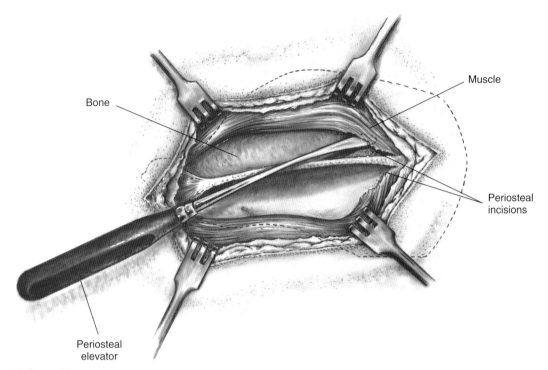

■ **Figure 19.**

Subperiosteal elevation of a muscle.

Once the muscles have been separated from one another, they must be elevated and retracted. In some cases, muscles are easily elevated from underlying bone because there are no extensive periosteal attachments in the area. As an example, the bellies of the vastus lateralis and vastus intermedius muscles are easily separated from the shaft of the femur in the dog (see Approach to the Shaft of the Femur, Plate 77) by bluntly separating the loose periosteal attachments of the muscular fascia in a manner similar to that shown in Figure 18.

In areas where the muscle is more firmly adherent to the bone, the muscle must be elevated in a different manner. Subperiosteal elevation allows muscle to be freed from bone at its origin or insertion without disturbing the muscle fibers. The periosteum is incised and undermined with a periosteal elevator (Figure 19). A narrow, slightly curved, sharp elevator such as the Langenbeck or AO pattern works well. Because the periosteum of the dog is rather thin and firmly attached in the area of muscular attachments, its elevation is difficult in skeletally mature animals. In immature animals, the periosteum is tough and thick enough to allow incision and elevation of the intact periosteum.

One form of muscular attachment to bone that is of interest is the fleshy attachment, in which muscular fascia is attached to the periosteum over a large area, as is well illustrated by the origin of the middle gluteal muscle on the iliac wing and crest. Fleshy attachments are elevated by the incision of the fascial connection with the periosteum. The periosteal elevator, scalpel blade, or bone chisel is held almost flat against the bone, and the muscle is separated with a "shaving" action. It is important that this elevation be done in the correct direction relative to the direction of the muscle fibers. The elevation should proceed in the same direction as the fibers because this allows muscle fibers to be peeled off the periosteum of the mature dog with less fraying and tearing than does elevation in the opposite direction

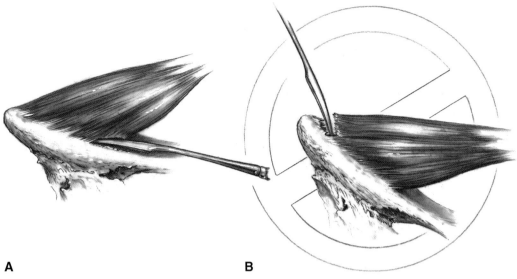

A   B

■ **Figure 20.**

Elevation of muscle from bone in a mature animal. **A,** When the elevating instrument and the muscle fibers form a V relative to each other, the muscle peels cleanly from the periosteum. **B,** When the elevating instrument and muscle fibers form an X relative to each other, the muscle fibers are cut irregularly before they peel away from the bone.

(Figure 20). Such areas cannot be sutured back to the bone but will reattach by fibrosis if the primary tendinous origin or insertion is left intact or sutured.

In some cases muscles are freed by incising their tendon or aponeurosis of origin or insertion on the bone. This technique is called tenotomy. In some cases sufficient stump is left attached to the bone so that sutures can be placed to reunite the tendon (see Part E of Plate 26 and Figure 21). Because in some cases the tendons may be too short for convenient suturing, they are sometimes cut close to the bone and reattached directly to the bone with sutures (Figure 22). In other cases, the tendon or aponeurosis is severed close to the bone and no attempt is made at suturing. The best example of this is the elevation of the lumbar muscles from the lumbar vertebrae in Approach to the Thoracolumbar Vertebrae through a Dorsal Incision (Plate 18).

Finally, the bony insertion of the tendon can be osteotomized to allow reflection of the tendon and muscle (see Plate 84). Osteotomies can be performed with power oscillating or reciprocating saws, hand saws, Gigli wire saws, or osteotomes. Saline irrigation while sawing helps to prevent thermal necrosis of bone that could result in delayed union or nonunion of an osteotomy. Although these bone fragments might be reattached in many ways, some of the most useful are shown in Figures 23 and 24.

After the muscles have been elevated, they are retracted and held with muscle retractors. The retractors shown in Figure 16 are quite adequate, although there are many other types available. At least one self-retaining and one handheld retractor are necessary for adequate exposure. A person operating without an assistant could well use two self-retaining retractors.

In the course of separating and elevating muscles, many large blood vessels and major nerve trunks will be encountered in the fascial planes between muscles. These structures must obviously be preserved at all costs. The anatomy of the area should be kept firmly in mind or reviewed if necessary before each procedure. See the section "Anatomy" for more discussion on this subject.

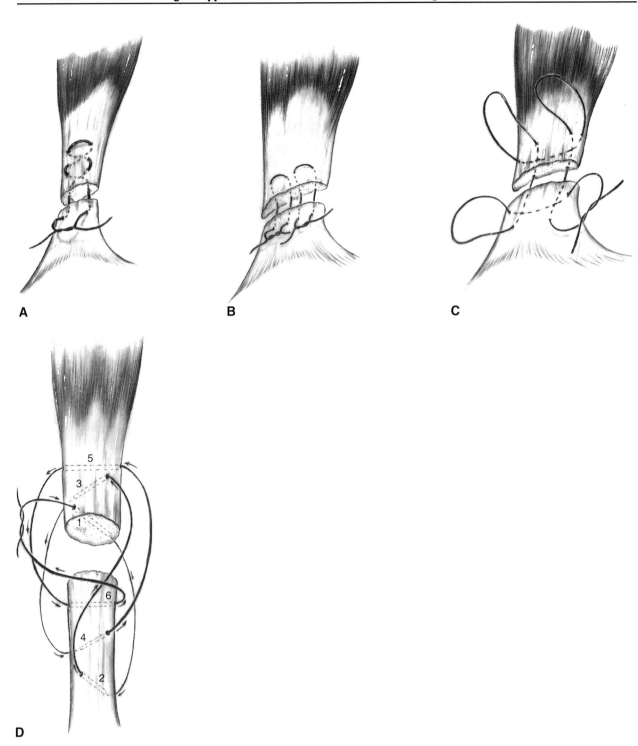

A

B

C

D

■ Figure 21.

Tendon and ligament suture patterns. **A,** Modified Bunnell-Mayer suture pattern used in a small tendon cut close to the bone. **B,** Horizontal mattress suture pattern used in a large, flat tendon. **C,** The locking-loop (Kessler) suture creates a very secure closure of either tendon or ligament. **D,** The pulley suture is easy to place in small tendons (or ligaments) and has very good holding power. The initial needle passes 1 and 2 are placed in a near-far pattern. Passes 3 and 4 are rotated 120 degrees from 1 and 2 and are placed midway between the near and far positions. Passes 5 and 6 are rotated 120 degrees from 3 and 4 and are placed in the far-near pattern. (After Berg RJ, Egger EL: In vitro comparison of the three loop pulley and locking loop suture patterns for repair of canine weightbearing tendons and collateral ligaments, *Vet Surg* 15:107-110, 1986.)

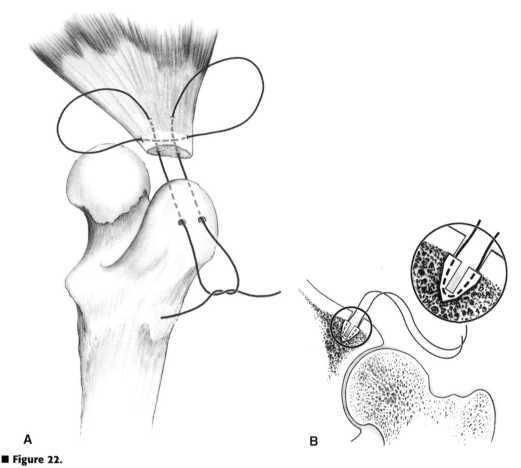

■ Figure 22.

A, A large tendon cut at its insertion is reattached with a locking-loop suture passed through holes drilled in the bone. **B,** A bone anchor can also be used for reattachment of joint capsule, ligament, or tendon to bone.

Whenever possible the nerve or vessel is retracted with an adjoining muscle; this technique takes advantage of the muscle as padding and also prevents undue stretching of the nerve or vessel. On occasion these structures must be retracted by themselves to achieve adequate exposure of underlying structures. In such a case, the vessel or nerve is carefully freed from its enveloping fascia by blunt dissection. A mosquito hemostat is very useful for this dissection because its use avoids the accidental severing of structures that is possible with dissection scissors. When the vessel or nerve has been sufficiently loosened, $\frac{1}{4}$-inch Penrose tubing is passed around the structure and is then used to maintain traction. This practice is considerably less traumatic than retraction with a metal instrument.

CLOSURE

Suture materials have been dramatically improved in their handling qualities and performance in recent years. Catgut has been virtually replaced by synthetic absorbable materials, and the monofilaments have emerged as the nonabsorbable materials of choice. Selection of suture materials and patterns seems to be a highly personal matter with surgeons, and one would have a difficult time arriving at a consensus, but the following selections have served the authors well.

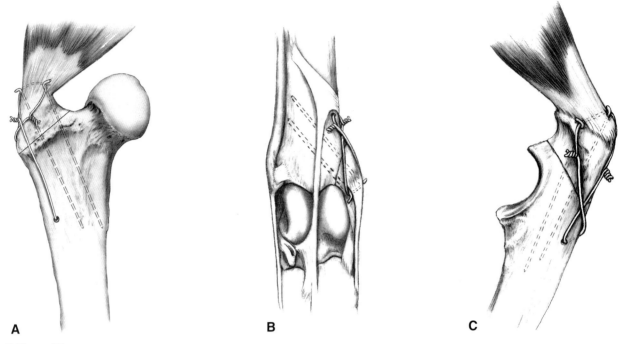

■ **Figure 23.**

Examples of two pins or Kirschner wires and tension band wire used to reattach osteotomized bone that is subject to tension forces. **A,** Greater trochanter. **B,** Medial malleolus. **C,** Olecranon.

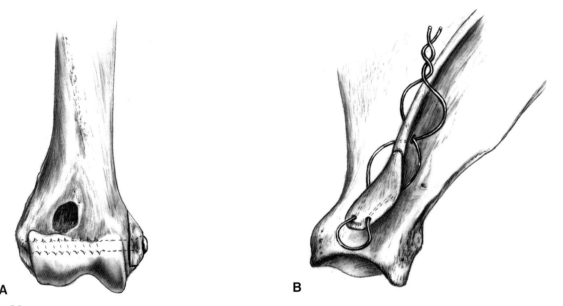

■ **Figure 24.**

Other methods of securing osteotomized bone. **A,** A lag screw placed through the medial humeral condyle. No screw threads cross the osteotomy line. **B,** Wire fixation of an osteotomized acromion process on the scapular spine.

Suture Material. *Nonabsorbable.* Any material that is to be buried must be sterilized by steam or ethylene oxide. Chemical sterilization or dispensing from cassettes is not reliable. Monofilament materials such as nylon and polypropylene have a lower infection rate and less local reaction associated with them than do braided materials and are the choice for most applications in which long-lasting strength is important and for skin closure.
Absorbable. Two styles of synthetic materials are available. The first are the braided materials characterized by polyglactin (Vicryl[7]) and polyglycolic acid (Dexon[8]). They have pleasant handling qualities and a half-life of about 14 days in situ, and they elicit less local reaction than does catgut. The second synthetic material is polydioxanone (PDS[9]), which is a monofilament material with an in situ half-life of about 50 days. Although its handling qualities are not as good as those of the braided materials, it is a very versatile suture that will maintain its strength long enough for healing in almost any situation. It can therefore replace nonabsorbable material in many cases and thereby decrease the infection rate associated with nonabsorbable materials, especially in the larger sizes.

Joint Capsule. This tissue supports sutures well. Interrupted stitches are generally used because of their reliability and safety. Suture material selection for joint capsule closure is the subject of a wide variety of opinions. Some general rules are as follows:
• When the closure can be made without tension and the capsule is not important in stabilizing the joint, use continuous sutures of small gauge (2-0 to 4-0) absorbable material or an interrupted pattern with nonabsorbable materials.
• If the capsule must be closed under tension or is being imbricated to add stability, use interrupted sutures of nonabsorbable material in sizes 3-0 to 1. The choice of material is not critical; however, monofilament materials such as nylon or polypropylene are not as prone to becoming infected as are the braided materials. It is important with any nonabsorbable material that the suture not penetrate the synovial membrane in an area that would allow the suture to rub on articular cartilage. Such contact will cause erosion of the cartilage. Lembert and mattress patterns allow slight imbrication, whereas the simple interrupted pattern allows edge-to-edge apposition.

Muscle. Sutures tend to cut and pull through this relatively soft tissue. A horizontal mattress pattern offers the best resistance against being pulled out should it be necessary to suture fleshy portions of muscles. The external fascial sheath of the muscle is the strongest part of muscle tissue and thus is most important in supporting sutures.

Tendons and Ligaments. Although tendons are dense and strong because of the longitudinal and parallel arrangement of their fibers, most suture patterns tend to cut through them. A selection of the most-used patterns is shown in Figure 21. Monofilament material works best in these tissues, because it glides through tissue easily and allows all slack to be removed from the pattern before tying.
Osteotomized bone with tendon or ligaments attached must be securely fixed in place for rapid fracture healing to occur. Because of muscle pull, there is a tendency for these bone fragments to be unstable and for delayed union to occur, with a resulting delay in the limb's return to function. Also, thermal necrosis of bone created by sawing without irrigation, or use of dull blades, can contribute to delayed union of an osteotomy. The tension band wire

[7]Ethicon Inc., Somerville, NJ.
[8]Davis and Geck, Wayne, NJ.
[9]Ethicon Inc., Somerville, NJ.

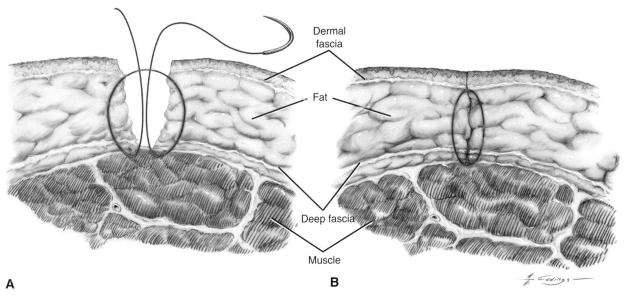

■ Figure 25.
Method of placing sutures in subcutis. **A,** Simple stitch engages dermal fascia, fat, and muscular or deep fascia. **B,** When the stitch is pulled tight, it apposes all subcutaneous tissues, eliminates dead space, and thereby prevents the formation of serum pockets.

technique illustrated in Figure 23 is a very effective way of overcoming these muscular forces. Lag screw fixation or simple wire sutures can also be used in certain situations, as illustrated in Figure 24.

Deep Fascia. No special precautions need to be taken here because this tissue holds sutures well. Simple interrupted or simple running patterns work equally well. The use of synthetic absorbable material combined with good knot-tying technique makes continuous patterns completely practical here.

Subcutaneous Fascia and Dermal Fat. Proper closure of this layer is important for two reasons: (1) the space created by incising and undermining the fat fills with serum unless the space is obliterated, and (2) closure of the fascia can relieve most of the tension on skin sutures. Simple interrupted or continuous patterns are used. The method of placing a buried knot at commencement of the simple continuous suture pattern is illustrated in Figure 25.

Skin. Simple interrupted sutures are the usual choice in the closure of skin, although many prefer the vertical mattress or cruciate patterns. Interrupted sutures are preferred by most, although continuous intradermal closures using synthetic absorbable sutures have worked well in the hands of the author.

Anatomy

Plates 1 through 5 are included here to provide ready reference to the major muscles, vessels, and nerves of the forelimbs and hindlimbs. These plates are not intended to substitute for detailed study of a suitable anatomy text. For this the following books are highly recommended, although many others are suitable:

Crouch JE: *Text-atlas of cat anatomy,* Philadelphia, 1969, Lea & Febiger.

Evans HE, de Lahunta A: *Miller's anatomy of the dog,* ed 4, Philadelphia, 2012, WB Saunders.

An experienced surgeon who uses open approaches on a daily basis soon has the anatomy of each one well in mind, but the surgeon who is exposed only occasionally to a given region often will find difficulty in performing in it. A major problem for all, but more so for the less experienced, is the distortion of normal anatomy due to trauma. Subcutaneous tissues and muscles become hemorrhagic and swollen, making identification difficult. In addition, points of origin and insertion of muscles and tendons are often displaced because of fractures. A good grasp of regional anatomy is absolutely essential in these situations.

Do not be apologetic about reviewing the anatomy of a region before surgery. Consider it not an admission of ignorance but instead the badge of a dedicated and conscientious surgeon who has the welfare of the patient uppermost in mind.

PLATE 1
Subcutaneous Musculature of the Canine Forequarter

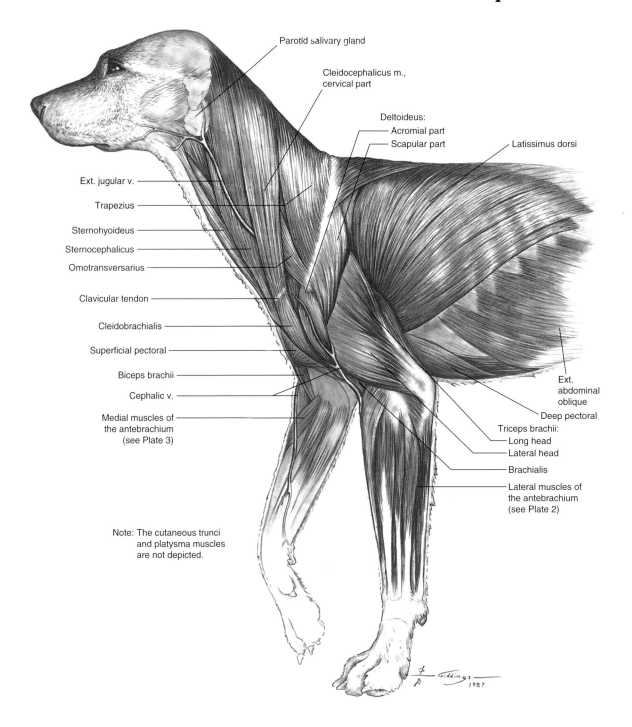

Parotid salivary gland

Cleidocephalicus m.,
cervical part

Deltoideus:
Acromial part
Scapular part

Latissimus dorsi

Ext. jugular v.

Trapezius

Sternohyoideus

Sternocephalicus

Omotransversarius

Clavicular tendon

Cleidobrachialis

Superficial pectoral

Biceps brachii

Cephalic v.

Medial muscles of
the antebrachium
(see Plate 3)

Ext.
abdominal
oblique

Deep pectoral

Triceps brachii:
Long head
Lateral head

Brachialis

Lateral muscles of
the antebrachium
(see Plate 2)

Note: The cutaneous trunci
and platysma muscles
are not depicted.

Giddings
1987

PLATE 2
Deep Musculature of the Canine Thoracic Limb, Lateral View

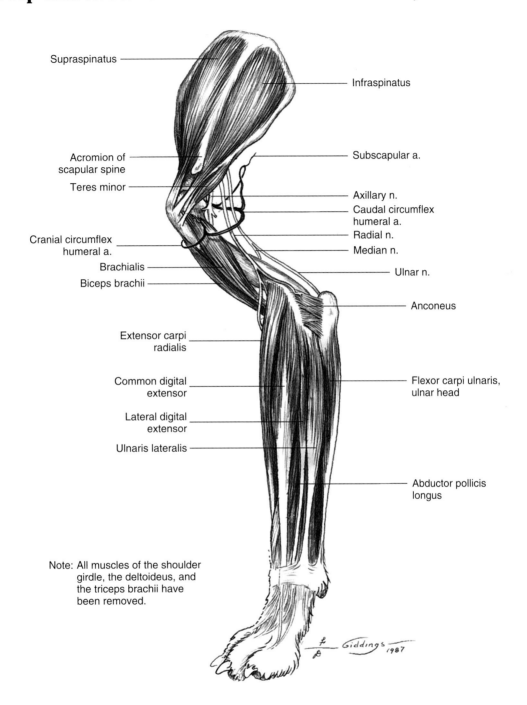

Supraspinatus

Infraspinatus

Acromion of
scapular spine

Subscapular a.

Teres minor

Axillary n.

Caudal circumflex
humeral a.

Cranial circumflex
humeral a.

Radial n.

Median n.

Brachialis

Biceps brachii

Ulnar n.

Anconeus

Extensor carpi
radialis

Common digital
extensor

Flexor carpi ulnaris,
ulnar head

Lateral digital
extensor

Ulnaris lateralis

Abductor pollicis
longus

Note: All muscles of the shoulder
girdle, the deltoideus, and
the triceps brachii have
been removed.

Giddings
1987

PLATE 3

Deep Musculature of the Canine Thoracic Limb, Medial View

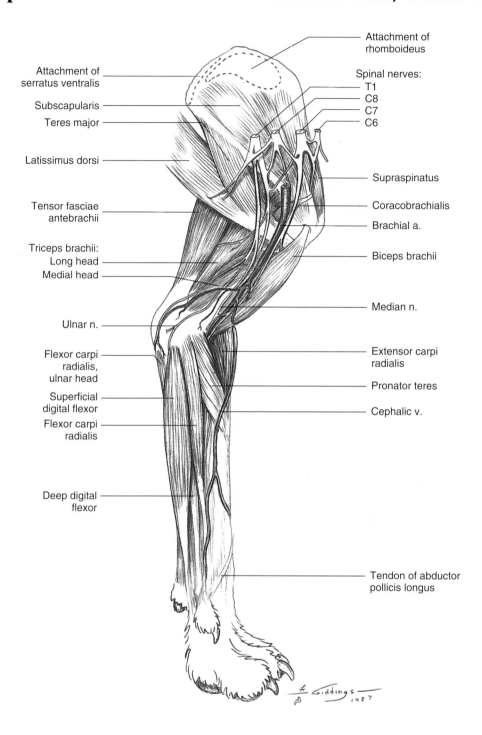

Attachment of
rhomboideus

Attachment of
serratus ventralis

Spinal nerves:
T1
C8
C7
C6

Subscapularis

Teres major

Latissimus dorsi

Supraspinatus

Coracobrachialis

Brachial a.

Tensor fasciae
antebrachii

Biceps brachii

Triceps brachii:
Long head
Medial head

Median n.

Ulnar n.

Flexor carpi
radialis,
ulnar head

Extensor carpi
radialis

Pronator teres

Superficial
digital flexor

Cephalic v.

Flexor carpi
radialis

Deep digital
flexor

Tendon of abductor
pollicis longus

PLATE 4
Subcutaneous Musculature of the Canine Hindquarter

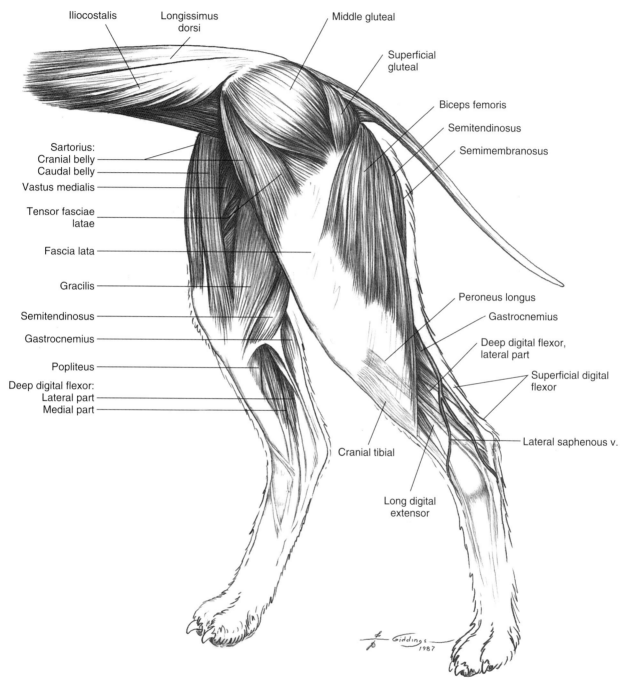

Iliocostalis

Longissimus dorsi

Middle gluteal

Superficial gluteal

Biceps femoris

Semitendinosus

Semimembranosus

Sartorius:
Cranial belly
Caudal belly

Vastus medialis

Tensor fasciae latae

Fascia lata

Gracilis

Semitendinosus

Gastrocnemius

Popliteus

Deep digital flexor:
Lateral part
Medial part

Peroneus longus

Gastrocnemius

Deep digital flexor, lateral part

Superficial digital flexor

Lateral saphenous v.

Cranial tibial

Long digital extensor

Note: Cutaneous muscles have been removed.

PLATE 5
Deep Musculature of the Canine Hindquarter

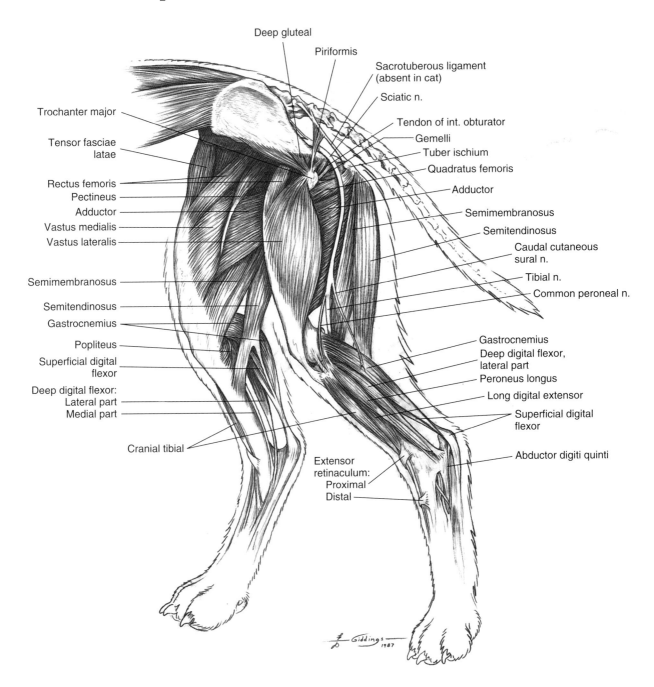

Deep gluteal

Piriformis

Sacrotuberous ligament (absent in cat)

Sciatic n.

Tendon of int. obturator

Gemelli

Tuber ischium

Quadratus femoris

Adductor

Semimembranosus

Semitendinosus

Caudal cutaneous sural n.

Tibial n.

Common peroneal n.

Trochanter major

Tensor fasciae latae

Rectus femoris

Pectineus

Adductor

Vastus medialis

Vastus lateralis

Semimembranosus

Semitendinosus

Gastrocnemius

Popliteus

Superficial digital flexor

Deep digital flexor: Lateral part Medial part

Cranial tibial

Gastrocnemius

Deep digital flexor, lateral part

Peroneus longus

Long digital extensor

Superficial digital flexor

Abductor digiti quinti

Extensor retinaculum: Proximal Distal

Giddings 1987

Note: Muscles removed on the lateral side include the middle and deep gluteals, tensor fasciae latae, and biceps femoris. Muscles removed from the medial side include the sartorius and gracilis.

SECTION 2

The Head

Approach to the Rostral Shaft of the Mandible

Based on a Procedure of Rudy[40]

INDICATION

Open reduction of fractures of the rostral shaft of the mandible.

PATIENT POSITIONING

Dorsal recumbency with the head extended.

DESCRIPTION OF THE PROCEDURE

A. The skin incision is made slightly lateral to the ventral midline of the mandible from the level of the canine tooth to the level of the molar teeth.
   The flat and very thin platysma muscle will be incised with the subcutaneous fascia and is then retracted with the fascia and skin.
B. Dorsal retraction of the platysma and skin exposes the shaft of the mandible. Subperiosteal elevation of the mylohyoideus muscle can be used to increase the exposure of the medial side of the bone.

ADDITIONAL EXPOSURE

Exposure of the entire shaft of the mandible is obtained by extending the approach more caudally (Plate 7).

CLOSURE

Elevated muscles are sutured to fascia on the surface of the mandible. The platysma and subcutaneous fascia are closed in one layer.

PLATE 6
Approach to the Rostral Shaft of the Mandible

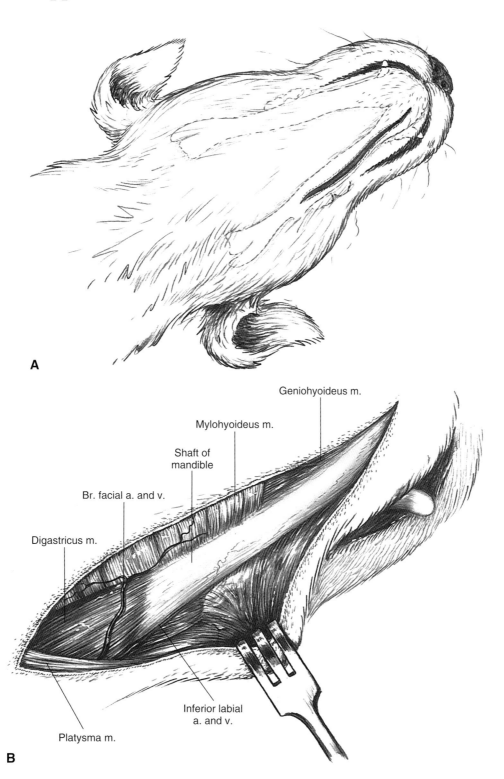

A

Geniohyoideus m.

Mylohyoideus m.

Shaft of mandible

Br. facial a. and v.

Digastricus m.

Inferior labial a. and v.

Platysma m.

B

Approach to the Caudal Shaft and Ramus of the Mandible

INDICATION

Open reduction of fractures in this region.

PATIENT POSITIONING

Dorsal recumbency with the head extended.

DESCRIPTION OF THE PROCEDURE

A. The incision is centered on the ventral surface of the mandible, commencing at the angular process of the mandible and extending cranially approximately one half the length of the mandible.

B. The platysma muscle is incised with the skin to reveal the superficial portion of the masseter muscle laterally and the digastricus muscle lying ventromedially over the shaft of the mandible. An incision is made in the intermuscular septum between the masseter and the digastricus muscles. Lateral to this incision is the large facial vein and accompanying nerve trunks. The periosteal insertion of the digastricus muscle on the shaft of the mandible is incised and elevated.

C. Lateral retraction of the masseter and subperiosteal elevation of part of its insertion in the masseteric fossa allow good exposure of the lateral side of the shaft and ventral part of the ramus, and medial retraction of the digastricus and deeper-lying mylohyoideus muscle gives exposure of the medial side of the shaft. The mylohyoideus and rostral insertion of the masseter muscle both can be elevated for more exposure of the ventral border of the mandible.

ADDITIONAL EXPOSURE

Ventral exposure of the entire shaft and ramus of the mandible is obtained by combining with the approaches described in Plates 6 and 8.

CLOSURE

The intermuscular septum between the digastricus and masseter muscles is closed, with care being taken not to impinge the facial vessels. Platysma muscle is included with subcutaneous fascia in a separate layer.

PLATE 7
Approach to the Caudal Shaft and Ramus of the Mandible

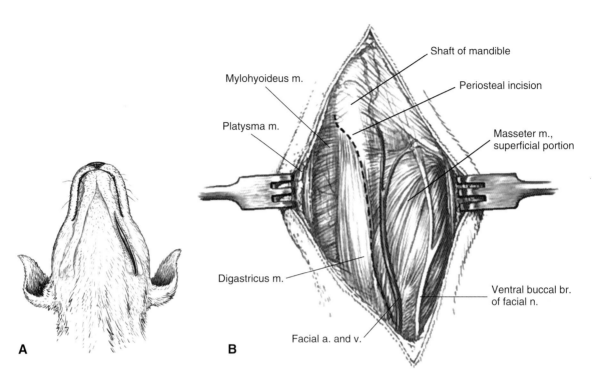

Mylohyoideus m.

Platysma m.

Digastricus m.

Facial a. and v.

Shaft of mandible

Periosteal incision

Masseter m.,
superficial portion

Ventral buccal br.
of facial n.

A

B

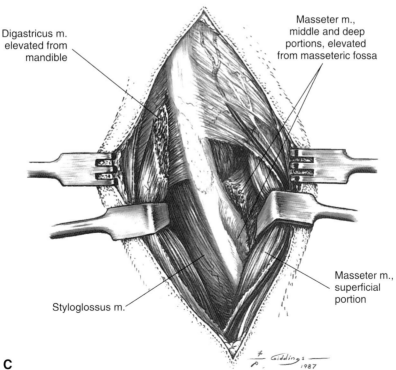

Digastricus m.
elevated from
mandible

Masseter m.,
middle and deep
portions, elevated
from masseteric fossa

Styloglossus m.

Masseter m.,
superficial
portion

C

Approach to the Ramus of the Mandible

INDICATION

Open reduction of fractures.

PATIENT POSITIONING

Lateral recumbency with the affected side uppermost.

DESCRIPTION OF THE PROCEDURE

A. The skin incision starts dorsally over the temporomandibular joint and extends rostroventrad to end over the mandibular shaft at the level of the last molar.
B. The incision is deepened through subcutaneous tissue and platysma muscle. The dorsal and ventral buccal branches of the facial nerve and the parotid gland and duct are identified and preserved. An incision is made across the fibers of the superficial layers of the masseter muscle, roughly paralleling the caudal border of the mandible.
C. After cutting through the superficial layer of the masseter muscle, the middle and deep layers can be elevated from their insertion on the caudal and ventral parts of the masseteric fossa. Careful dorsal dissection and retraction allow exposure of the ramus to the level of the temporomandibular joint.

ADDITIONAL EXPOSURE

Separate exposure of the temporomandibular joint is obtained by the approach described in Plate 9. The parotid duct and branches of the facial nerve must be preserved.

CLOSURE

The middle and deep layers of the masseter muscle fall back against the mandible when the superficial layer incision is closed. Mattress sutures are placed in the strong aponeurosis covering the superficial layer of the masseter muscle. Platysma muscle and skin are closed in separate layers.

PLATE 8

Approach to the Ramus of the Mandible

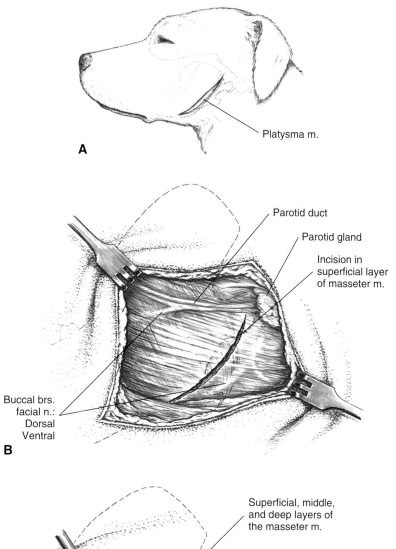

Platysma m.

A

Parotid duct

Parotid gland

Incision in
superficial layer
of masseter m.

Buccal brs.
facial n.:
Dorsal
Ventral

B

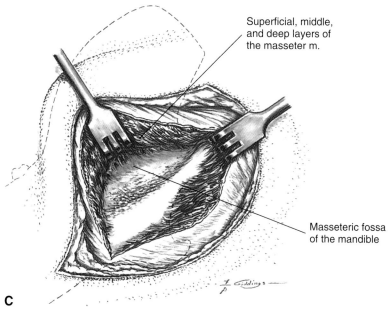

Superficial, middle,
and deep layers of
the masseter m.

Masseteric fossa
of the mandible

C

Approach to the Temporomandibular Joint

INDICATIONS

1. Open reduction of luxations.
2. Open reduction of fractures.

PATIENT POSITIONING

Lateral recumbency with the affected side uppermost.

DESCRIPTION OF THE PROCEDURE

A. The skin incision follows the ventral border of the zygomatic arch and crosses the temporomandibular joint caudally.
B. The platysma muscle, directly under the skin, is incised on the same line. A periosteal incision is made along the origin of the masseter muscle on the zygomatic arch.
C. Subperiosteal elevation of the masseter muscle exposes the joint. The mandibular condyle and interior of the joint are brought into view by wide incision of the joint capsule.

ADDITIONAL EXPOSURE

Separate and greater exposure of the ramus is obtained by the approach described in Plate 8. The parotid duct and branches of the facial nerve must be preserved.

CLOSURE

The masseter muscle is sutured to fascia on the dorsal edge of the zygomatic arch. Platysma and skin are closed in separate layers.

PLATE 9

Approach to the Temporomandibular Joint

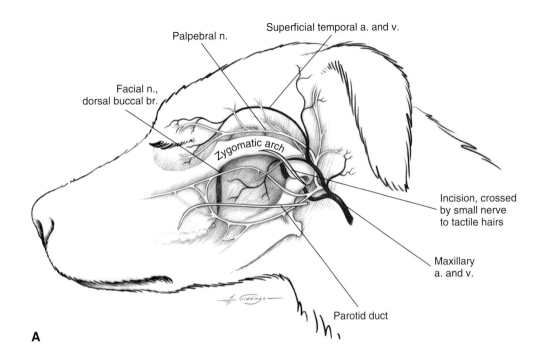

Palpebral n.

Superficial temporal a. and v.

Facial n.,
dorsal buccal br.

Zygomatic arch

Incision, crossed
by small nerve
to tactile hairs

Maxillary
a. and v.

Parotid duct

A

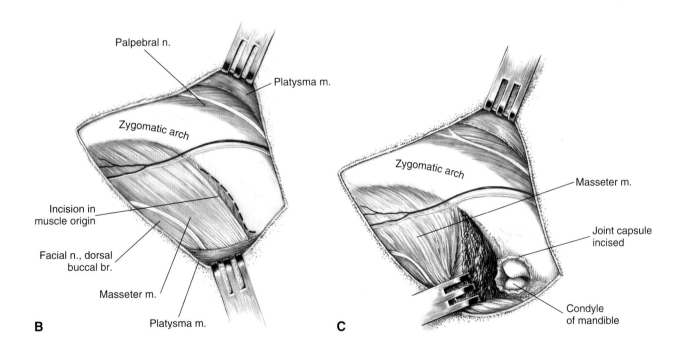

Palpebral n.

Platysma m.

Zygomatic arch

Incision in
muscle origin

Facial n., dorsal
buccal br.

Masseter m.

Platysma m.

B

Zygomatic arch

Masseter m.

Joint capsule
incised

Condyle
of mandible

C

Approach to the Dorsolateral Surface of the Skull

Based on a Procedure of Hoerlein, Few, and Petty[18]

INDICATIONS

1. Open reduction of fractures of the frontal and parietal bones and the dorsal parts of the sphenoid and temporal bones.
2. Exposure of cerebral hemispheres.

PATIENT POSITIONING

Ventral recumbency with the head supported (see Plate 10, Part A).

DESCRIPTION OF THE PROCEDURE

A. The midline skin incision extends from the external occipital protuberance to the level of the eyes. Alternate incisions are also shown and are superior for reaching the more basilar area of the skull.
B. As the subcutaneous fascia is incised and retracted, three muscles are immediately encountered: rostrally the frontalis and interscutularis, the fibers of which run transversely; caudally the occipitalis, with its fibers running parallel to the midline. These muscles are incised on the midline and retracted with the skin.
C. The temporalis muscle is covered by a layer of dense fascia, which is incised on the lateral side of the sagittal and frontal crests. The incision is then deepened to include the periosteum. One or both sides are incised, depending on the type of exposure desired.
D. The temporalis is elevated from the skull subperiosteally and retracted laterally. For bilateral exposure, both muscles are elevated and retracted.

CLOSURE

The temporal fascia is joined at the midline along the sagittal crest. Because the incisions curve laterally to follow the frontal crests, the temporal fascia is sutured to the loose fascia lying between the frontal crests. The frontalis, interscutularis, and occipitalis muscles are closed on the midline.

PLATE 10
Approach to the Dorsolateral Surface of the Skull

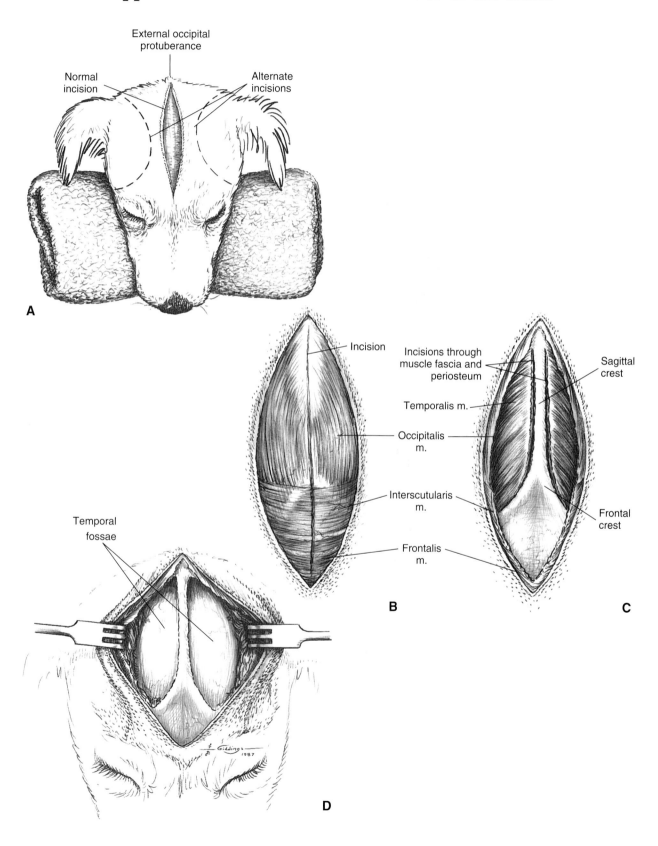

Approach to the Caudal Surface of the Skull

Based on a Procedure of Hoerlein, Few, and Petty[18]

INDICATIONS

1. Open reduction of fractures of the occipital bone.
2. Exposure of the caudal portion of the cerebellum and the cranial portion of the brain stem.

PATIENT POSITIONING

Ventral recumbency with the neck flexed and the head supported (see Plate 10, Part A).

DESCRIPTION OF THE PROCEDURE

A. The midline portion of the skin incision extends caudally from the external occipital protuberance to the spinous process of the axis (C2). The transverse incision follows the nuchal crest of the occiput and ends just short of the base of the ears.
   The subcutaneous fascia is incised in the same lines as the skin and is undermined with the skin to allow lateral retraction of each skin flap. The platysma muscle will be incised and retracted with subcutaneous fascia.
B. The first muscles seen upon retraction of the skin are the cervicoscutularis and superficial cervicoauricularis. Originating on the exposed area of the cervical midline and passing cranially toward the ears, these muscles resemble a chevron with the point situated caudally. The muscles are incised on the midline and each muscle belly allowed to retract. The temporal muscles, the external occipital protuberance, and the dorsal cervical muscles inserting on the occiput can now be visualized.
C. The splenius capitis and rhomboideus muscles are transected close to their origin on the nuchal line of the occiput. The use of electrocautery for this cutting is very helpful in minimizing hemorrhage. Enough tissue is left on the occiput to allow resuturing of the muscles. The midline incision runs from the external occipital protuberance to the spinous process of the axis (C2).
D. Muscle elevation continues laterally and ventrally to expose the occipital bone, the foramen magnum, and the dorsal arch of the atlas (C1).

CLOSURE

The cervical muscles are attached to the occiput by using mattress sutures that engage the fibrous muscle insertions remaining on the bone. The external sheath of the temporal muscles may also be used to securely anchor these sutures.

COMMENTS

The caudal brain stem and cranial spinal cord may be exposed by elevating the muscles from the atlas and performing a dorsal laminectomy on this vertebra.

PLATE 11

Approach to the Caudal Surface of the Skull

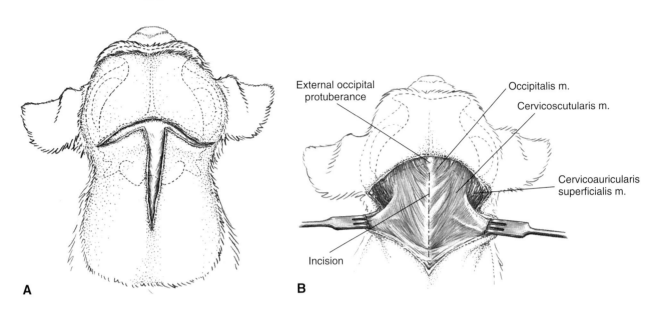

A

External occipital
protuberance

Occipitalis m.

Cervicoscutularis m.

Cervicoauricularis
superficialis m.

Incision

B

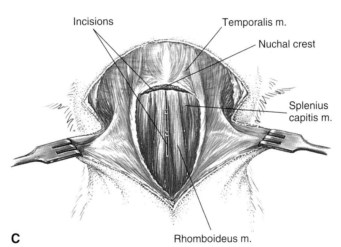

Incisions

Temporalis m.

Nuchal crest

Splenius
capitis m.

Rhomboideus m.

C

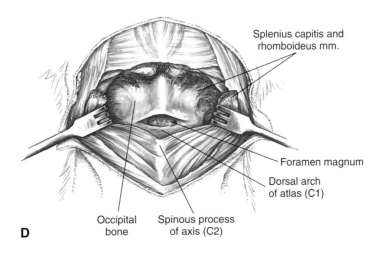

Splenius capitis and
rhomboideus mm.

Foramen magnum

Dorsal arch
of atlas (C1)

Occipital
bone

Spinous process
of axis (C2)

D

SECTION 3

The Vertebral Column

- Approach to Cervical Vertebrae 1 and 2 Through a Ventral Incision

- Approach to Cervical Vertebrae 1 and 2 Through a Dorsal Incision

- Approach to Cervical Vertebrae and Intervertebral Disks 2-7 Through a Ventral Incision

- Approach to the Midcervical Vertebrae Through a Dorsal Incision

- Approach to Cervical Vertebrae 3-6 Through a Lateral Incision

- Approach to the Caudal Cervical and Cranial Thoracic Vertebrae Through a Dorsal Incision

- Approach to the Thoracolumbar Vertebrae Through a Dorsal Incision

- Approach to the Thoracolumbar Intervertebral Disks Through a Dorsolateral Incision

- Approach to the Thoracolumbar Intervertebral Disks Through a Lateral Incision

- Approach to Lumbar Vertebra 7 and the Sacrum Through a Dorsal Incision

- Approach to the Lumbosacral Intervertebral Disk and Foramen Through a Lateral Transilial Osteotomy

- Approach to Lumbar Vertebrae 6 and 7 and the Sacrum Through a Ventral Abdominal Incision

- Approach to the Caudal Vertebrae Through a Dorsal Incision

Approach to Cervical Vertebrae 1 and 2 Through a Ventral Incision

Based on a Procedure of Sorjonen and Shires[47]

INDICATIONS

1. Treatment of fractures of the ventral aspect of cervical vertebrae 1 and 2.
2. Vertebrae C1-C2 arthrodesis for atlantoaxial instability.

PATIENT POSITIONING

The animal is placed in the supine position with a sandbag under the neck to cause marked extension of the cranial cervical vertebrae. Placing the animal in a V-shaped trough will elevate the shoulder region and increase the extension of the cervical spine (see Plate 12A).

DESCRIPTION OF THE PROCEDURE

A. The skin incision begins on the midline between the angles of the mandible and ends in the midcervical region.
B. The incision is deepened through the subcutis and between the paired bellies of the sternohyoideus muscles to expose the trachea.
C. Retraction of the sternohyoideus muscles exposes the larynx and its muscles. The right sternothyroideus muscle is isolated and detached from its insertion on the thyroid process of the larynx. The thyroid gland should be protected during this dissection.

PLATE 12

Approach to Cervical Vertebrae 1 and 2 Through a Ventral Incision

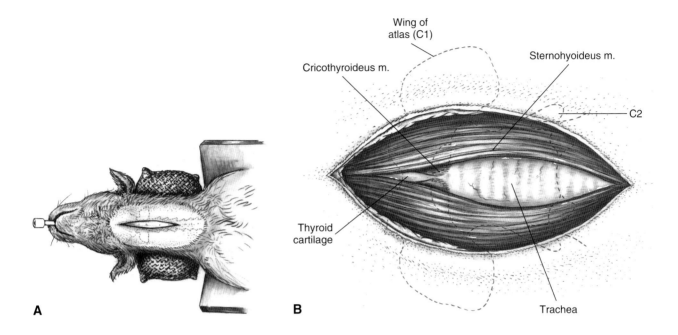

A

B

Wing of atlas (C1)

Cricothyroideus m.

Sternohyoideus m.

C2

Thyroid cartilage

Trachea

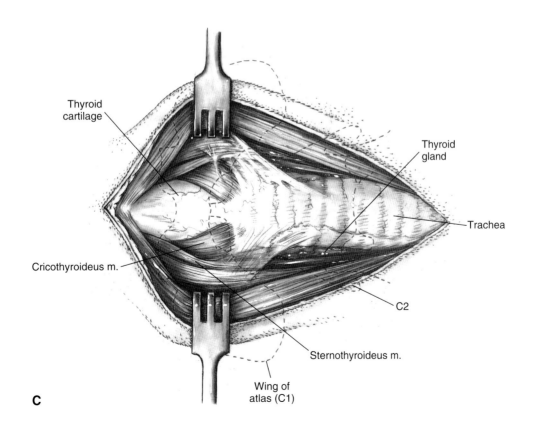

C

Thyroid cartilage

Thyroid gland

Trachea

Cricothyroideus m.

C2

Sternothyroideus m.

Wing of atlas (C1)

Approach to Cervical Vertebrae 1 and 2 Through a Ventral Incision *continued*

D. Retraction of the larynx and trachea to the left side (medially) is preceded by ligation or cautery of several small vessels running between the carotid artery/internal jugular vein and the thyroid gland or trachea. The recurrent laryngeal nerve must be protected during this dissection and retraction. Muscle retraction to the right side (laterally) also includes the carotid artery, the internal jugular vein, and the vagosympathetic trunk. The longus colli muscles are now exposed. The ventral tubercle of C1 is located by palpation, and the longus colli muscle fibers are transected close to the tubercle.

E. Elevation of muscle fibers from the ventral arch of C1 and the body of C2 proceeds laterally until the articulations are exposed.

ADDITIONAL EXPOSURE

This approach can be extended caudally (see Plate 14) to obtain ventral exposure of the entire cervical spine.

CLOSURE

Neither the deep fascia in the region of the trachea nor the longus colli muscles are sutured. The sternothyroideus muscle is reattached to the thyroid process by sutures, and the sternohyoideus muscles and subcutis are closed on the midline in layers.

PLATE 12

Approach to Cervical Vertebrae 1 and 2 Through a Ventral Incision *continued*

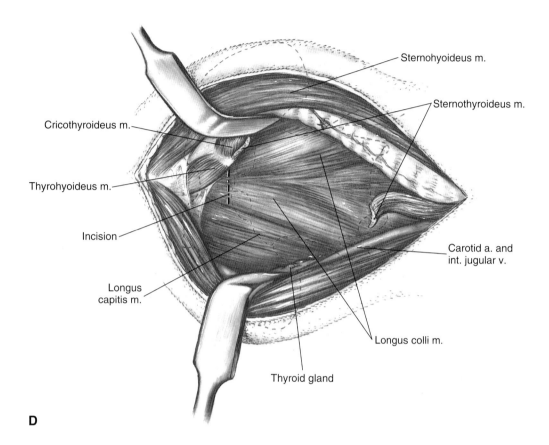

Sternohyoideus m.

Sternothyroideus m.

Cricothyroideus m.

Thyrohyoideus m.

Incision

Longus capitis m.

Carotid a. and int. jugular v.

Longus colli m.

Thyroid gland

D

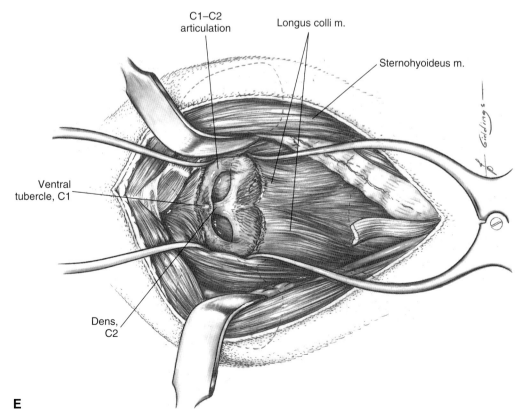

C1–C2 articulation

Longus colli m.

Sternohyoideus m.

Ventral tubercle, C1

Dens, C2

E

Approach to Cervical Vertebrae 1 and 2 Through a Dorsal Incision

Based on a Procedure of Funkquist[15]

INDICATIONS

1. Open reduction and stabilization of atlantoaxial luxation.
2. Open reduction of fractures of vertebrae C1 and C2.

PATIENT POSITIONING

Dorsal recumbency with the neck slightly flexed and supported by a sandbag bolster or folded towel (see Plate 13A).

DESCRIPTION OF THE PROCEDURE

A. The skin incision is made on the dorsal midline starting at the level of the occipital protuberance, extending caudally to the level of the third or fourth cervical vertebra.
B. Skin is undermined and retracted and subcutaneous fascia incised on the midline to expose the occipitalis, cervicoscutularis, and cervicoauricularis superficialis muscles. Caudal and lateral to these muscles are the thin fibers of the platysma muscle. These muscles are incised on the midline fibrous raphe to allow elevation and lateral retraction of these muscles.

PLATE 13
Approach to Cervical Vertebrae 1 and 2 Through a Dorsal Incision

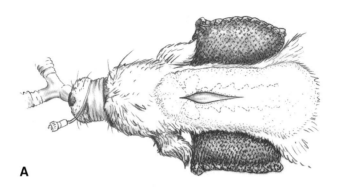

A

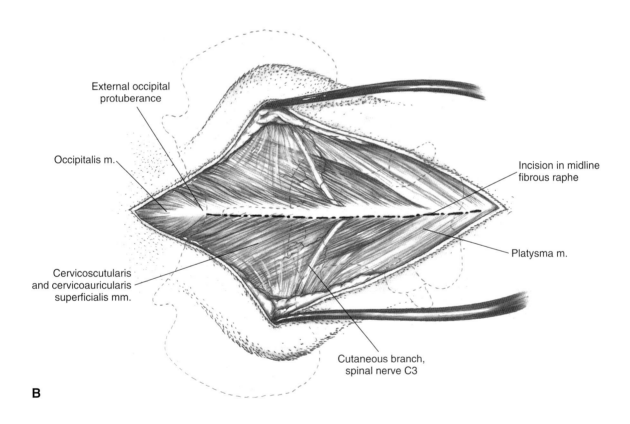

External occipital
protuberance

Occipitalis m.

Cervicoscutularis
and cervicoauricularis
superficialis mm.

Incision in midline
fibrous raphe

Platysma m.

Cutaneous branch,
spinal nerve C3

B

Approach to Cervical Vertebrae 1 and 2 Through a Dorsal Incision *continued*

C. Deepening the midline incision will allow separation of the paired bellies of the biventer cervicis superficially and the deeper rectus capitis attached to the dorsal spine of C2. The insertion of the rectus capitis muscle is incised along the lateral border of the spine of C2 to allow its elevation from the bone by combined sharp and blunt dissection.

D. As the dissection is carried deeper onto the lamina of C2, care should be taken to avoid the vertebral artery, which courses through the muscles slightly ventrolateral to the articular processes. The interarcuate (yellow) ligament covering the foramina between C1 and C2 is carefully incised to expose the spinal cord and the root of spinal nerve C1. The dorsal atlanto-occipital membrane of the foramen magnum may also be incised to expose the cranial rim of the dorsal arch of C1.

ADDITIONAL EXPOSURE

This approach can be extended caudally (see Plates 15 and 17) to obtain dorsal exposure of the entire cervical spine.

CLOSURE

Each muscle layer is closed on the midline to its opposite member.

COMMENTS

This exposure may be done bilaterally, using the same technique, where exposure of the entire dorsal aspect of the vertebrae is desirable.

PLATE 13

Approach to Cervical Vertebrae 1 and 2 Through a Dorsal Incision *continued*

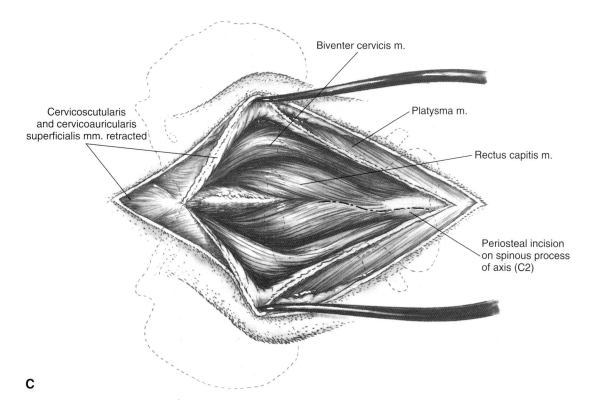

Biventer cervicis m.

Platysma m.

Rectus capitis m.

Cervicoscutularis and cervicoauricularis superficialis mm. retracted

Periosteal incision on spinous process of axis (C2)

C

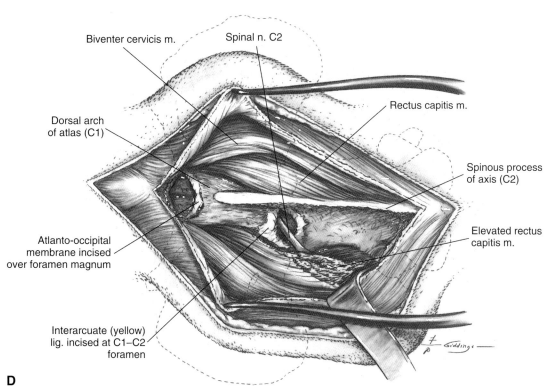

Biventer cervicis m.

Spinal n. C2

Rectus capitis m.

Dorsal arch of atlas (C1)

Spinous process of axis (C2)

Atlanto-occipital membrane incised over foramen magnum

Elevated rectus capitis m.

Interarcuate (yellow) lig. incised at C1–C2 foramen

D

Approach to Cervical Vertebrae and Intervertebral Disks 2-7 Through a Ventral Incision

Based on a Procedure of Olsson[33]

INDICATIONS

1. Fenestration and curettage of intervertebral disks C2-C7.
2. Decompression of cervical spinal cord by ventral slot of intervertebral disks C2-C7.
3. Distraction and fusion of intervertebral disks C5-C6 and C6-C7 for caudal cervical spondylomyelopathy.
4. Open reduction and ventral stabilization of fractures and luxations of C2-C7.

PATIENT POSITIONING

The animal, with tracheal catheter in place, is secured in the supine position. Passage of an esophageal stethoscope will facilitate subsequent identification of the esophagus during the approach. A sandbag is placed under the neck to cause definite extension of the cervical vertebral column. It is often useful to elevate the body by positioning the animal's trunk in a V-shaped trough to gain more extension of the cervical spine (see Plate 14A). However, extreme cervical hyperextension should be avoided because it can exacerbate intervertebral disk protrusion, causing spinal cord compression and injury.

DESCRIPTION OF THE PROCEDURE

A. The skin incision extends from the manubrium to the larynx.
B. Continuing the skin incision through the subcutaneous tissues, small transverse bundles of the sphincter colli superficialis muscle are identified and transected in the ventral midline. Retraction of the subcutaneous tissues exposes the mastoid part of the sternocephalicus muscles arising from the manubrium. Underlying the sternocephalicus muscles are the sternohyoideus muscles.

PLATE 14

Approach to Cervical Vertebrae and Intervertebral Disks 2-7 Through a Ventral Incision

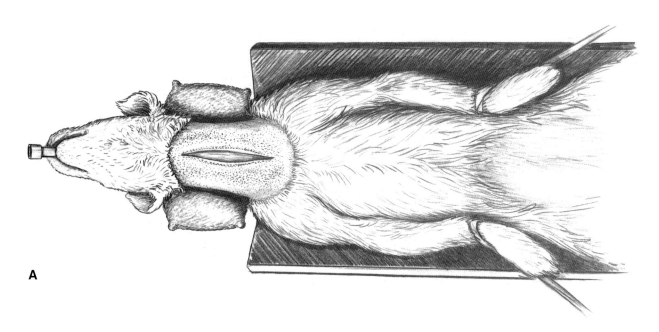

A

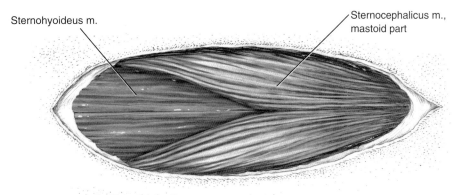

Sternohyoideus m.

Sternocephalicus m., mastoid part

B

Approach to Cervical Vertebrae and Intervertebral Disks 2-7 Through a Ventral Incision *continued*

C. The incision is deepened by midline separation of the paired bellies of the mastoid part of the sternocephalicus muscles and the underlying sternohyoideus muscles. With separation of the median raphe between the paired sternohyoideus muscles, the caudal thyroid vein is found in the fascia overlying the trachea. The caudal thyroid vein should be preserved, and lateral branches of the vein arising from the adjacent right sternohyoideus muscle are divided and cauterized as necessary.

D. Lateral retraction of these muscles exposes the trachea, esophagus, deep cervical fascia, carotid sheath, and internal jugular vein. At this stage of the approach, the location of the esophagus is readily determined by palpation of the esophageal stethoscope that is within the esophageal lumen.

PLATE 14

Approach to Cervical Vertebrae and Intervertebral Disks 2-7 Through a Ventral Incision *continued*

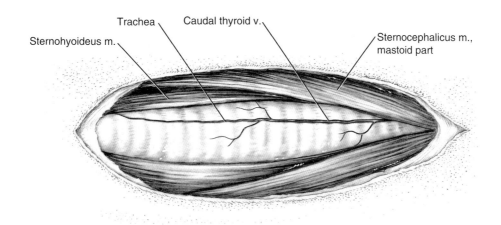

Trachea — Caudal thyroid v.

Sternohyoideus m.

Sternocephalicus m., mastoid part

C

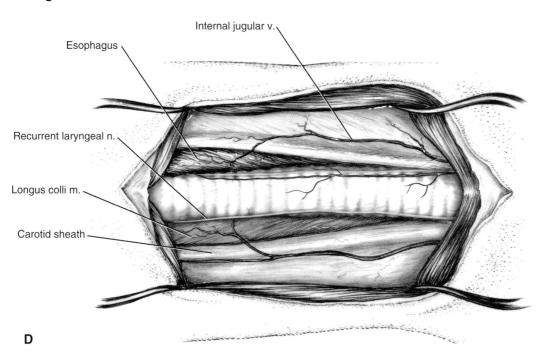

Internal jugular v.

Esophagus

Recurrent laryngeal n.

Longus colli m.

Carotid sheath

D

Approach to Cervical Vertebrae and Intervertebral Disks 2-7 Through a Ventral Incision *continued*

E. Left lateral retraction of the trachea and esophagus using nontoothed retractors allows blunt dissection close to the trachea through the deep cervical fascia to the longus colli muscle, which covers the ventral surfaces of the cervical vertebrae. Care should be taken not to injure the recurrent laryngeal nerve or the esophagus during this dissection. The right carotid sheath containing the right carotid artery, the vagosympathetic nerve trunk, and the internal jugular vein is usually retracted to the right side of midline, but alternatively it can be moved to the left, along with the trachea. The midline ventral crest of the vertebrae can be palpated through the longus colli muscle. A short transverse incision is made through the longus colli tendon of insertion just caudal to the crest.

F. Separation of longus colli muscle fibers overlying each ventral crest exposes the disk.

PLATE 14

Approach to Cervical Vertebrae and Intervertebral Disks 2-7 Through a Ventral Incision *continued*

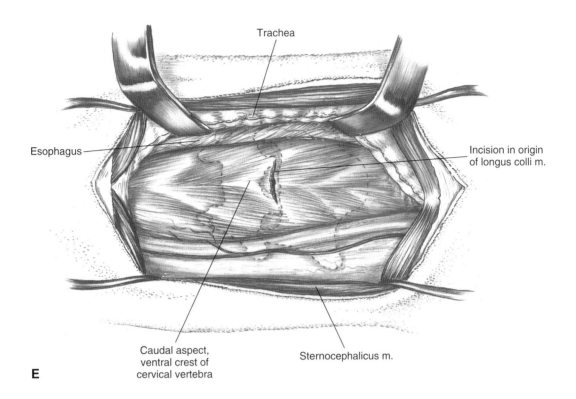

Trachea

Esophagus

Incision in origin
of longus colli m.

Caudal aspect,
ventral crest of
cervical vertebra

Sternocephalicus m.

E

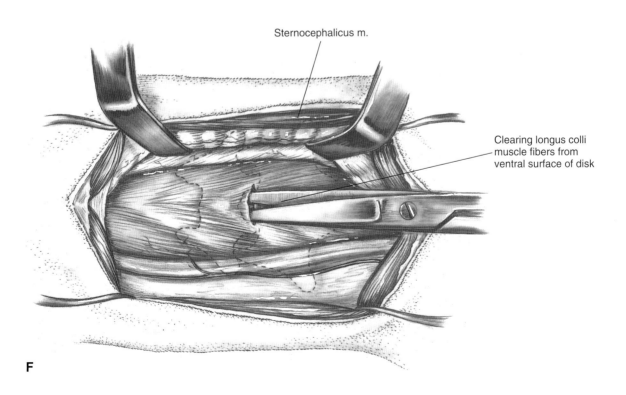

Sternocephalicus m.

Clearing longus colli
muscle fibers from
ventral surface of disk

F

Approach to Cervical Vertebrae and Intervertebral Disks 2-7 Through a Ventral Incision *continued*

G. By working caudally from the prominence, the tendon is gently scraped from the bone until the ventral longitudinal ligament is exposed. The exact location of the intervertebral space can be identified by exploration with a 22-gauge needle, which is walked off the crest caudally until it penetrates the ventral longitudinal ligament and the annulus fibrosus of the disk.

H. Fenestration is accomplished by a stab incision through the ventral longitudinal ligament and the annulus fibrosus. This opening into the disk may have to be enlarged for disk curettage.

ADDITIONAL EXPOSURE

This approach can be extended cranially (see Plate 12) to obtain ventral exposure of the entire cervical spine.

CLOSURE

The deep fascia is not sutured. The sternohyoideus and mastoid parts of the sternocephalicus muscle are closed along the midline, and the subcutaneous fascia is likewise united.

COMMENTS

Care must be used in the retraction of tissues to avoid damage to the carotid sheath; the esophagus and trachea; and the right recurrent laryngeal nerve, which lies on the right dorsolateral aspect of the trachea. The location of a specific intervertebral space is determined by first identifying the caudal borders of the wings of the atlas by palpation. The ventral midline crest that lies on a line directly between the wings is the ventral tubercle of the atlas (C1). Other vertebrae can then be numbered by counting caudally from C1. Alternatively, the large transverse processes of C6 are easily palpated. The C5-C6 disk is between and slightly cranial to the cranial edges of the processes.

PLATE 14

Approach to Cervical Vertebrae and Intervertebral Disks 2-7 Through a Ventral Incision *continued*

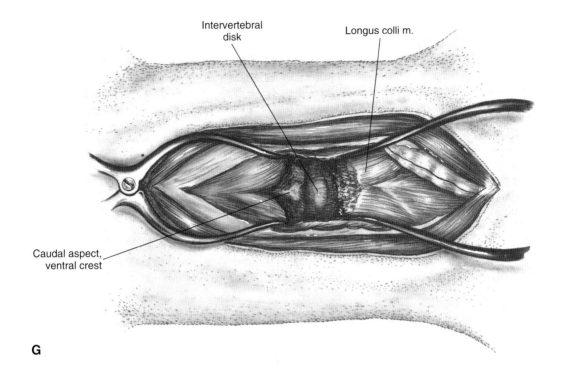

Intervertebral disk

Longus colli m.

Caudal aspect, ventral crest

G

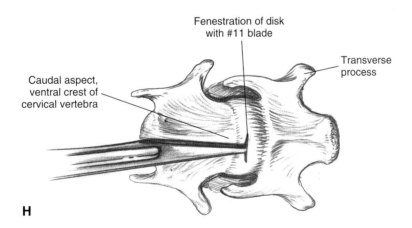

Fenestration of disk with #11 blade

Transverse process

Caudal aspect, ventral crest of cervical vertebra

H

Approach to the Midcervical Vertebrae Through a Dorsal Incision

Based on a Procedure of Funkquist[15]

INDICATIONS

1. Open reduction of fractures and luxations of vertebrae C2-C5.
2. Dorsal laminectomy of vertebrae C2-C5.

PATIENT POSITIONING

The animal is positioned in sternal recumbency, with a sandbag placed under the neck to elevate it and to cause flexion of the cervical spine. A tracheal catheter is imperative to maintain a patent airway in this position (see Plate 15A).

DESCRIPTION OF THE PROCEDURE

A. The midline skin incision extends from the external occipital protuberance to the first thoracic vertebra.
B. As the subcutaneous fascia is incised and the skin margins retracted, the almost transparent fibrous aponeurosis of the platysma muscle comes into view.
   An incision is now made through the median fibrous raphe. This incision is deepened until the nuchal ligament (missing in the cat) is exposed.

PLATE 15

Approach to the Midcervical Vertebrae Through a Dorsal Incision

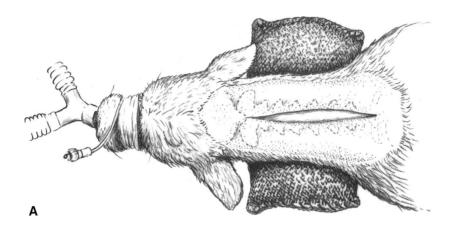

A

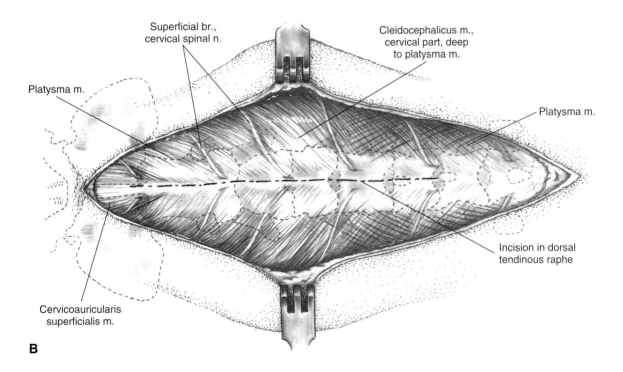

Superficial br.,
cervical spinal n.

Cleidocephalicus m.,
cervical part, deep
to platysma m.

Platysma m.

Platysma m.

Incision in dorsal
tendinous raphe

Cervicoauricularis
superficialis m.

B

Approach to the Midcervical Vertebrae Through a Dorsal Incision *continued*

C. The dorsolateral cervical muscles separated by this incision are retracted laterally to expose the nuchal ligament. The spinous processes can now be palpated under the ligament.

An incision is made in the rectus capitis, spinalis et semispinalis cervicis, and multifidus muscles along one side of the nuchal ligament. The incision is deepened along the lateral side of the spinous processes to the vertebral laminae.

D. Elevation with a periosteal elevator and retraction of the muscles from the vertebrae are done first on the side that was incised. The insertion of the nuchal ligament is now elevated from the spinous process of the axis, and the ligament is retracted with the muscles on the side opposite the incision. The ligament remains firmly attached to the muscles of one side and cranially to the axis.

Lateral elevation of muscles from the laminae should be limited to the lateral aspect of the articular processes to avoid branches of the vertebral artery coursing ventrolaterally to the processes.

ADDITIONAL EXPOSURE

This approach can be extended cranially and caudally (see Plates 13 and 17) to obtain dorsal exposure of the entire cervical spine.

CLOSURE

The nuchal ligament is secured to the axis by two sutures of nonabsorbable material. These sutures are passed through holes drilled transversely through the spinous process of the axis.

The external fascia of the deep muscles can now be sutured to the nuchal ligament. The median fibrous raphe is closed next, followed by the subcutaneous fascia.

COMMENTS

If the spinous process of the axis has been removed in the course of laminectomy, the nuchal ligament is secured to the rectus capitis muscle by mattress sutures that bite deeply into this muscle.

PLATE 15

Approach to the Midcervical Vertebrae Through a Dorsal Incision *continued*

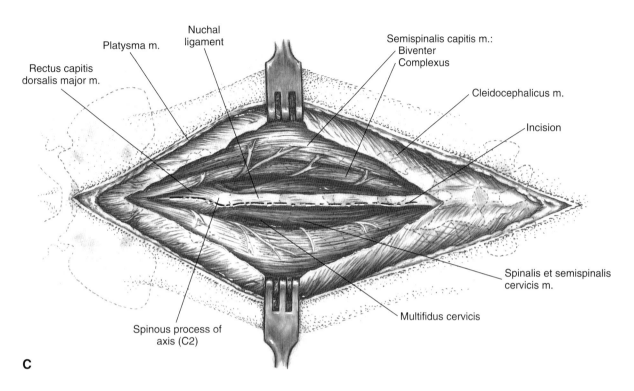

Rectus capitis dorsalis major m.

Platysma m.

Nuchal ligament

Semispinalis capitis m.:
Biventer
Complexus

Cleidocephalicus m.

Incision

Spinalis et semispinalis cervicis m.

Multifidus cervicis

Spinous process of axis (C2)

C

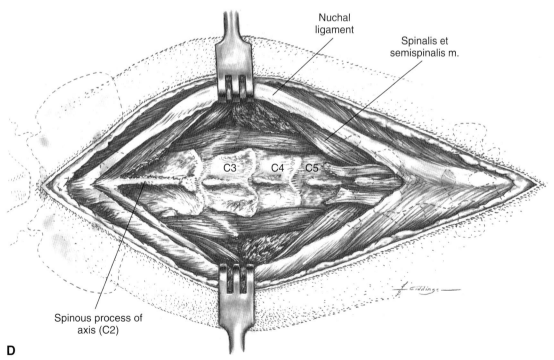

Nuchal ligament

Spinalis et semispinalis m.

C3   C4   C5

Spinous process of axis (C2)

D

Approach to Cervical Vertebrae 3-6 Through a Lateral Incision

Based on the Procedures of Lipsitz and Bailey[26] and Rossmeisl, Lanz, Inzana, and Bergman[39]

INDICATIONS

1. Hemilaminectomy at C3-C4, C4-C5, or C5-C6 for removal of lateral or intraforaminal disk extrusion or resection of spinal cord tumors.
2. Hemilaminectomy at C3-C4, C4-C5, or C5-C6 for resection of ventral and dorsal spinal nerve roots affected by neoplasia.

PATIENT POSITIONING

Lateral recumbency with uppermost forelimb retracted caudally (see Plate 16A).

DESCRIPTION OF THE PROCEDURE

A.   An incision is made through the skin and underlying platysma muscle from the cranial border of the scapula to the wing of the atlas.

B.   The incised wound margins are retracted to expose the brachiocephalicus and trapezius muscles. Separate between these muscles in a dorsal to ventral, oblique direction. The superficial cervical artery and vein, which emerge from between these two muscles, are retracted caudally and ligated. Underlying these vessels are the superficial cervical lymph nodes. The brachiocephalicus muscle is transected at the level of the articular facets.

C.   Retraction of the transected brachiocephalicus muscle exposes the splenius muscle dorsocranially and also the serratus ventralis muscle that runs obliquely from under the cranial border of the scapula in a cranioventral direction. Cranial nerve XI (accessory nerve) crosses the serratus ventralis muscle to innervate the trapezius muscle.

PLATE 16
Approach to Cervical Vertebrae 3-6 Through a Lateral Incision

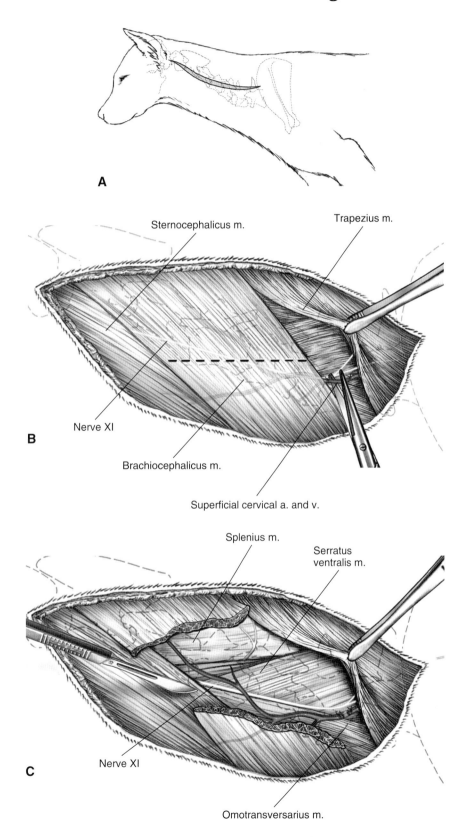

A

Sternocephalicus m.

Trapezius m.

Nerve XI

Brachiocephalicus m.

Superficial cervical a. and v.

B

Splenius m.

Serratus
ventralis m.

Nerve XI

Omotransversarius m.

C

Approach to Cervical Vertebrae 3-6 Through a Lateral Incision *continued*

D.   As an alternative, exposure of the C5-C7 vertebral segments can be achieved without transection of the brachiocephalicus muscle, by further extension of the separation between the brachiocephalicus and trapezius muscles in an oblique direction. The brachiocephalicus muscle is retracted cranioventrally, rather than being transected. Exposure of C6-C7 is increased further by simultaneous abduction and caudal retraction of the scapula, without the need to incise the muscular attachments on the cranial border of the scapula.

In the C3-C5 region, the brachiocephalicus muscle is incised longitudinally in the direction of the muscle fibers, instead of being transected. Using a grid technique, the divided brachiocephalicus muscle is separated to expose the underlying splenius and serratus ventralis muscles.

E.   The dorsal border of the serratus ventralis muscle is elevated all the way caudally to its origin on the scapula. It may then be reflected ventrally to fully expose the underlying splenius muscle. Vascular bundles between the deep surface of the serratus ventralis and splenius muscles are ligated and divided.

F.   Reflection of the serratus ventralis continues to its insertions on the lateral processes of the vertebrae, exposing the longissimus cervicis and longissimus capitis muscles. These muscles are elevated and retracted ventrally. For orientation, the prominent transverse process of C6 is located by palpation.

PLATE 16

Approach to Cervical Vertebrae 3-6 Through a Lateral Incision *continued*

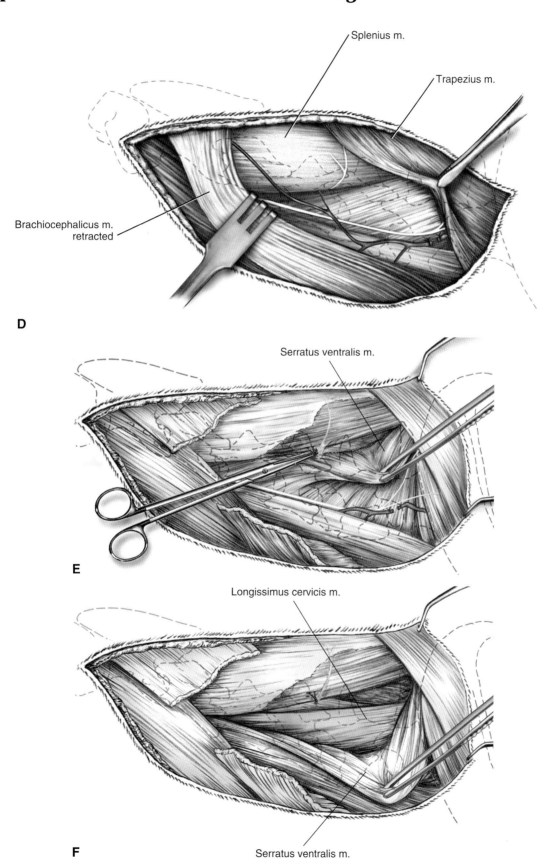

Splenius m.

Trapezius m.

Brachiocephalicus m.
retracted

D

Serratus ventralis m.

E

Longissimus cervicis m.

F

Serratus ventralis m.

Approach to Cervical Vertebrae 3-6 Through a Lateral Incision *continued*

G, H. The splenius muscle is retracted dorsally to expose the underlying semispinalis complexus muscle. The articular facets of C3-C4, C4-C5, and C5-C6 can be palpated at the junction between the semispinalis muscle and the two longissimus muscles. The tendinous origins of the semispinalis complexus and multifidus cervicis muscles are incised from the articular facets with scissors or electrocautery. These two muscles are then elevated from the dorsal lamina of the cervical vertebrae to the base of the spinous process using a periosteal elevator.

ADDITIONAL EXPOSURE

The C6-C7 intervertebral disk space and vertebrae are not readily accessible because of the overlying scapular and forelimb musculature. However, caudal extension of the lateral approach for hemilaminectomy of the caudal cervical vertebrae and exposure of the nerve roots is possible in conjunction with forelimb amputation in cases of brachial plexus neoplasia.

Cranial extension of the lateral approach beyond the C3-C4 intervertebral disk is prevented by the large dorsal branch of the third spinal nerve that exits from the C2-C3 foramen.

CLOSURE

The serratus ventralis muscle is sutured to the splenius muscle using a simple continuous pattern. The transected brachiocephalicus muscle is apposed with mattress pattern sutures. Closure of subcutaneous tissues and skin is routine.

PLATE 16

Approach to Cervical Vertebrae 3-6 Through a Lateral Incision *continued*

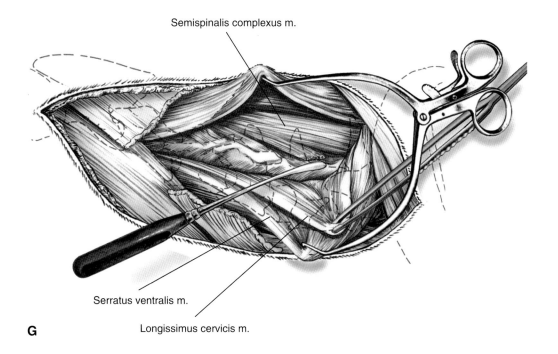

Semispinalis complexus m.

Serratus ventralis m.

Longissimus cervicis m.

G

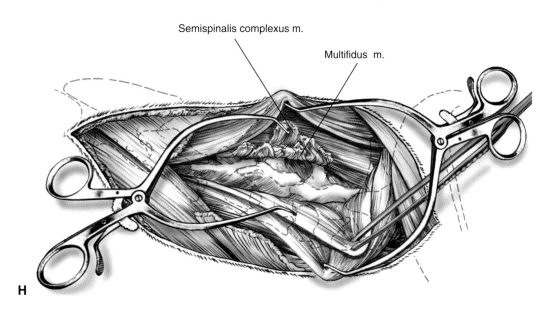

Semispinalis complexus m.

Multifidus m.

H

Approach to the Caudal Cervical and Cranial Thoracic Vertebrae Through a Dorsal Incision

Based on a Procedure of Parker[35]

INDICATIONS

1. Dorsal laminectomy for decompression of the spinal cord for ruptured intervertebral disk, spinal canal malformation and stenosis, synovial cyst, or vertebral fractures of C5-T3.
2. Resection of tumors of the spinal cord or vertebral lamina and dorsal spines of C5-T3.

PATIENT POSITIONING

With the animal in sternal recumbency, the forelegs are crossed under the chest and tied to the opposite sides of the table (see Plate 17A). Sandbags are useful for preventing shifting of position and for positioning the head, which can lie on the table.

DESCRIPTION OF THE PROCEDURE

A. A skin incision is made on the dorsal midline from the midcervical to the cranial thoracic region, approximately C4-T6.
B. The dorsal midline tendinous raphe is seen after incision of subcutaneous tissues on the midline. At this point a decision must be made as to which side of the midline will be chosen for the dissection. This may be dictated by pathology present or may be the choice of the surgeon. An incision is made in the tendinous raphe slightly toward the side selected (right side is illustrated).

PLATE 17

Approach to the Caudal Cervical and Cranial Thoracic Vertebrae Through a Dorsal Incision

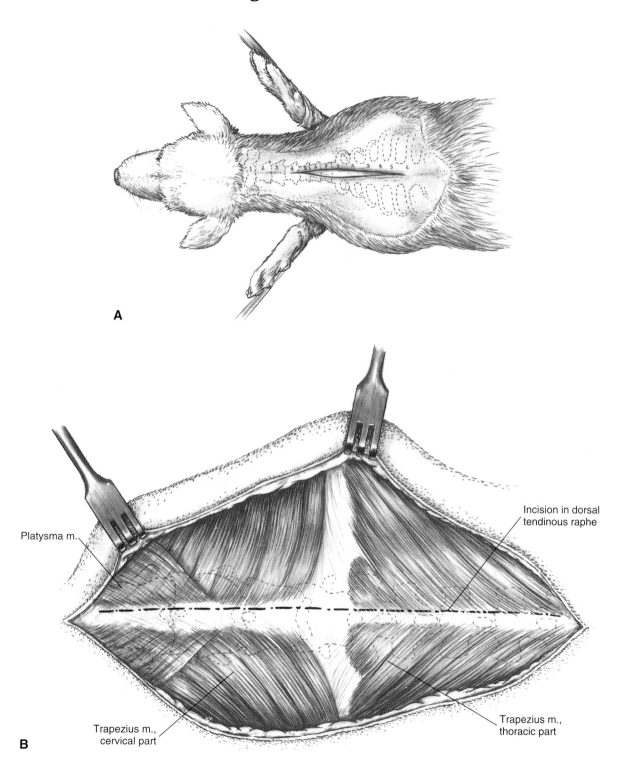

A

B

Platysma m.

Incision in dorsal tendinous raphe

Trapezius m., cervical part

Trapezius m., thoracic part

Approach to the Caudal Cervical and Cranial Thoracic Vertebrae Through a Dorsal Incision *continued*

C. Trapezius and rhomboideus muscles can be retracted to reveal the medial surface of the subscapularis muscle, the splenius muscle cranially, and the serratus dorsalis muscle caudally. The right scapula can now be retracted laterally. Incisions are now made in the origin of the splenius and the serratus dorsalis muscles on the tendinous raphe. A portion of the cranial serratus muscle may originate from fascia of the splenius.

PLATE 17

Approach to the Caudal Cervical and Cranial Thoracic Vertebrae Through a Dorsal Incision *continued*

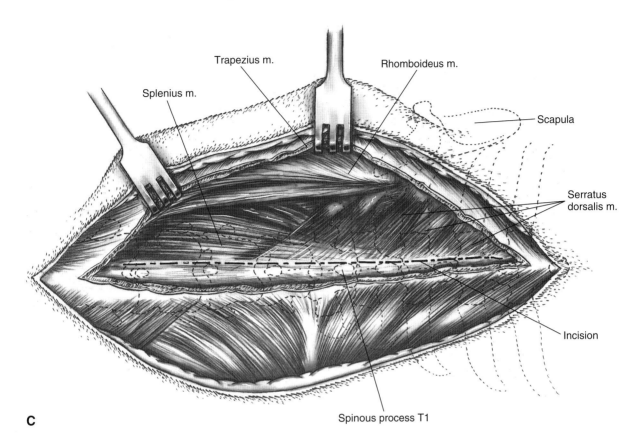

C

Approach to the Caudal Cervical and Cranial Thoracic Vertebrae Through a Dorsal Incision *continued*

D. Lateral retraction of the splenius and serratus dorsalis muscles exposes the nuchal ligament, the dorsal thoracic spines, and the underlying long spinal muscles. These muscles, the longissimus thoracis et lumborum, the spinalis et semispinalis thoracis, and the spinalis cervicis, are separated from the midline by a combination of sharp and blunt dissection. As this dissection proceeds ventrally along the lateral surfaces of the dorsal vertebral spines, the dorsal laminae of the vertebrae will come into view.

E. Continued dissection of the long spinal muscles and the multifidus muscle will completely expose the dorsal laminae and pedicles of the vertebrae. The surgeon must be aware of the danger of incising or tearing the vertebral artery ventral to the articular processes. This artery can be damaged when elevating muscle bellies from C7 and T1. Once torn, ligation is difficult and pressure must be used for hemostasis. The large interarcuate space between C7 and T1 can be palpated and the yellow ligament incised to expose the spinal cord. The size of this space makes it an ideal starting point for dorsal laminectomy, as does the space between C6 and C7.

ADDITIONAL EXPOSURE

This approach can be extended cranially and caudally (see Plates 13, 15, and 18) to obtain dorsal exposure of the entire cervical and cranial thoracic vertebrae.

CLOSURE

All muscle bellies are attached to the midline tendinous raphe or nuchal ligament in layers. The considerable subcutaneous tissues merit special care in closure to prevent seroma formation.

COMMENTS

To perform a dorsal laminectomy, the dorsal spines of the affected vertebrae must be removed. This creates some apparent difficulty with the thoracic vertebrae because the nuchal ligament originates on the spines of T1-T3. However, these spines can be cut with no ill effects because the nuchal ligament is somewhat continuous with the supraspinous ligament. This gives the effect of lengthening the nuchal ligament's origin caudal to the dorsal spine of T3.

PLATE 17

Approach to the Caudal Cervical and Cranial Thoracic Vertebrae Through a Dorsal Incision *continued*

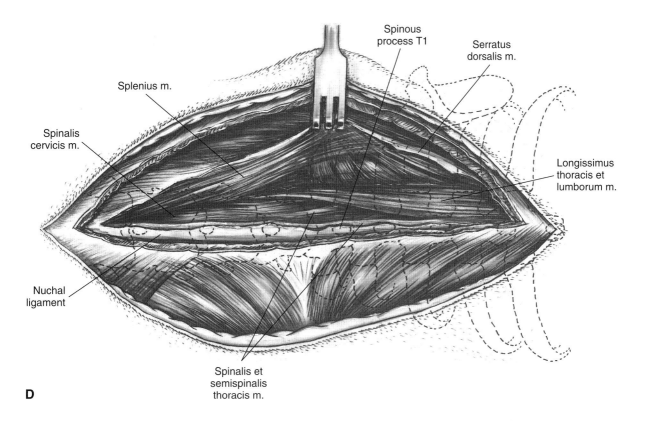

Splenius m.

Spinous
process T1

Serratus
dorsalis m.

Spinalis
cervicis m.

Longissimus
thoracis et
lumborum m.

Nuchal
ligament

Spinalis et
semispinalis
thoracis m.

D

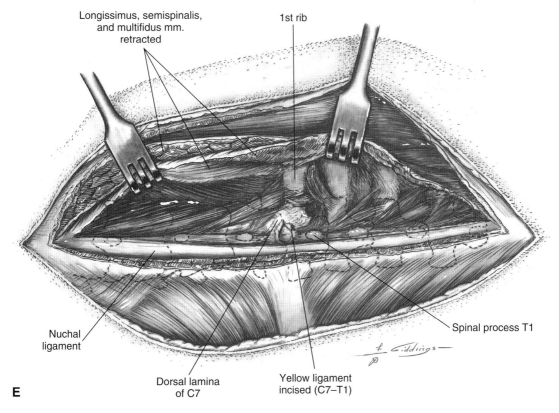

Longissimus, semispinalis,
and multifidus mm.
retracted

1st rib

Nuchal
ligament

Dorsal lamina
of C7

Yellow ligament
incised (C7–T1)

Spinal process T1

E

Approach to the Thoracolumbar Vertebrae Through a Dorsal Incision

Based on a Procedure of Redding[38]

INDICATIONS

1. Open reduction of fractures and luxations of the vertebrae.
2. Dorsal laminectomy and hemilaminectomy.

PATIENT POSITIONING

Dorsal recumbency and supported with a vacuum positioning bag.

EXPLANATORY NOTE

The exposure for left hemilaminectomy is unilateral and is illustrated in Plate 18A-E and described in steps A-E outlined in the description of the procedure that follows. For laminectomy, a bilateral exposure is needed and is achieved by repeating steps B-E on the contralateral side. The final results are illustrated in Plate 18F.

DESCRIPTION OF THE PROCEDURE

A. The length of the dorsal midline incision is determined by the number of vertebrae that are to be exposed. To obtain sufficient muscle retraction, it is necessary to extend the incision the length of two vertebrae cranial and caudal to the vertebra in question. The incision shown here centers on L1, extends from T12 to L3, and is made 5 to 10 mm from the midline.

B. Subcutaneous fat and fascia are incised until the dense lumbodorsal fascia is reached. The fat is undermined to free it from the fascia and to allow its retraction with the skin.

   The fascia and supraspinous ligament are incised around each spinous process and on the midline between each process. The incision is deepened to the laminae to complete the midline muscle separation.

PLATE 18

Approach to the Thoracolumbar Vertebrae Through a Dorsal Incision

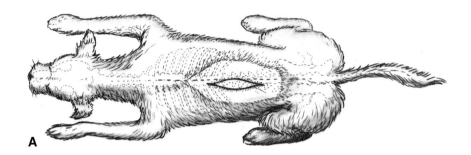

A

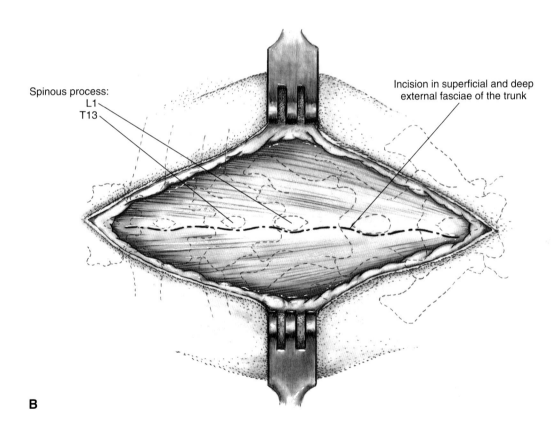

Spinous process:
L1
T13

Incision in superficial and deep
external fasciae of the trunk

B

Approach to the Thoracolumbar Vertebrae Through a Dorsal Incision *continued*

C. The multifidus lumborum muscle is sharply elevated from each spinous process and then bluntly elevated from the laminae laterally to the mammillary processes. This is sufficient exposure for a dorsal laminectomy when done bilaterally. Elevation is most easily done from a caudal-to-cranial direction. See step F.

D. For hemilaminectomy, the multifidus must be incised and freed from the mammillary processes. The incision should be made directly on the bone to limit hemorrhage, and the underlying dorsal nerve root and vessels must be protected.

PLATE 18

Approach to the Thoracolumbar Vertebrae Through a Dorsal Incision *continued*

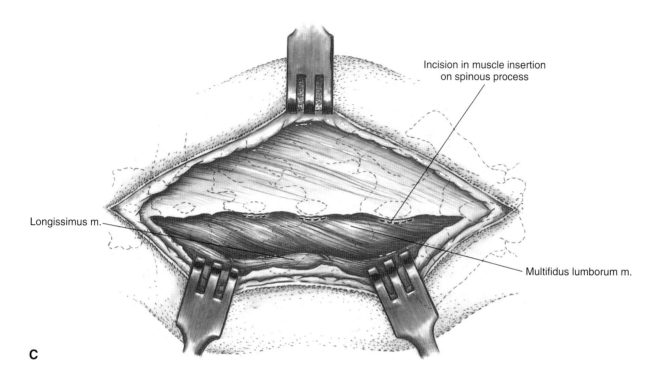

Incision in muscle insertion
on spinous process

Longissimus m.

Multifidus lumborum m.

C

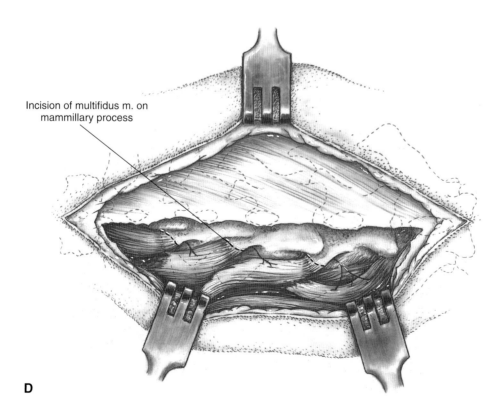

Incision of multifidus m. on
mammillary process

D

Approach to the Thoracolumbar Vertebrae Through a Dorsal Incision *continued*

E. Lateral retraction of the muscles exposes the mammillary processes, nerve roots and vessels, and the rib head or transverse processes.

F. The exposure as done for laminectomy. Compare with steps D and E.

CLOSURE

The lumbodorsal fascia is sutured at the dorsal midline. The subcutaneous fat and fascia are closed with a second layer of sutures, followed by closure of the skin.

PLATE 18

Approach to the Thoracolumbar Vertebrae Through a Dorsal Incision *continued*

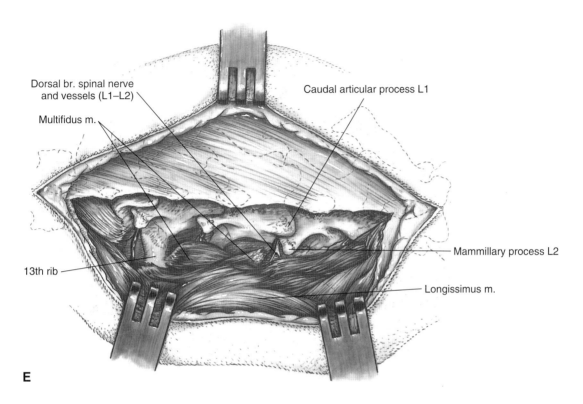

Dorsal br. spinal nerve and vessels (L1–L2)

Multifidus m.

13th rib

Caudal articular process L1

Mammillary process L2

Longissimus m.

E

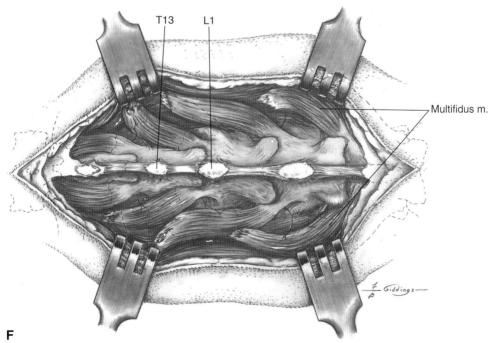

T13   L1

Multifidus m.

F

Approach to the Thoracolumbar Intervertebral Disks Through a Dorsolateral Incision

Based on a Procedure of Yturraspe and Lumb[53]

INDICATIONS

1. Fenestration and curettage of intervertebral disks T10-L5.
2. Hemilaminectomy or pediculectomy for spinal cord decompression from ruptured intervertebral disks or neoplasia.
3. Partial corpectomy for chronic, ventral spinal cord compression caused by a ruptured or protruding intervertebral disk.

ALTERNATIVE APPROACH

Similar exposure of the intervertebral disks is obtained via the lateral approach (see Plate 20).

PATIENT POSITIONING

The dog is positioned in ventral recumbency with the hindlimbs flexed to maintain the normal curvature of the spine (see Plate 19A).

DESCRIPTION OF THE PROCEDURE

A. The skin incision is made slightly to the left side of the midline for a right-handed surgeon. A left-handed surgeon should operate from the dog's right side. The incision extends from the eighth thoracic to the seventh lumbar vertebra.
B. Subcutaneous fat is elevated from the deep fascia of the trunk for a distance of 1.5 cm lateral to the dorsal spinous processes. This exposes the spinalis et semispinalis muscle cranially and the superficial layer of the deep external fascia of the trunk caudally. Both the deep and superficial layers of this fascia originate on the dorsal spinous processes. Both layers of the fascia are incised 5 to 10 mm from the dorsal spines in the midlumbar area, and this incision is continued caudally to the limits of the skin incision. As the fascial incision approaches the spinalis et semispinalis muscle cranially, it is directed medially so that it ends only 1 to 2 mm lateral to the spinous processes. A portion of this muscle must be incised to extend the incision cranially over the ribs.
C. The multifidus and longissimus muscles are separated by blunt dissection of the intermuscular septum. This septum is the first distinct muscle division lateral to the spinous processes and is most obvious in the midlumbar region. This separation is done with sweeping strokes with dissection scissors partially opened and directed in a craniomedial direction. Proceeding from caudal to cranial is advantageous during this dissection.

PLATE 19

Approach to the Thoracolumbar Intervertebral Disks Through a Dorsolateral Incision

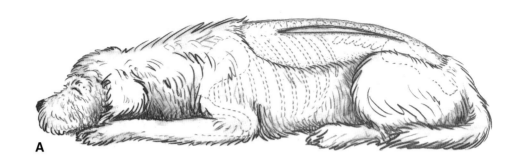

A

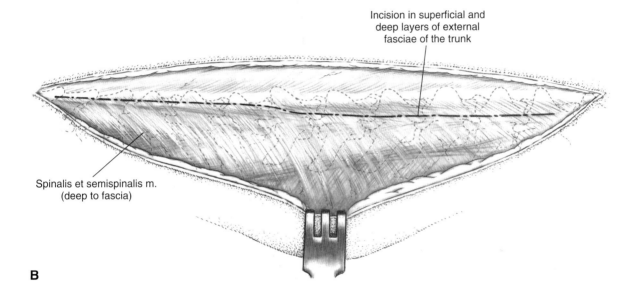

Incision in superficial and deep layers of external fasciae of the trunk

Spinalis et semispinalis m. (deep to fascia)

B

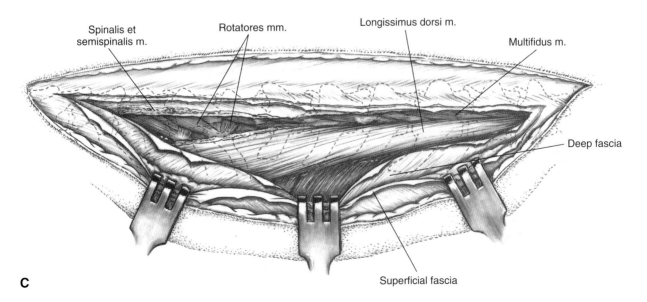

Spinalis et semispinalis m.

Rotatores mm.

Longissimus dorsi m.

Multifidus m.

Deep fascia

Superficial fascia

C

Approach to the Thoracolumbar Intervertebral Disks Through a Dorsolateral Incision *continued*

D. As the dissection deepens, small tendons will be encountered crossing the dissection in a craniomedial direction, and they should be preserved. The tendons are attachments of the longissimus muscle to the accessory processes of the vertebrae. In the thoracic region, the tendon divides and attaches both to the rib and the accessory process. The dorsal branches of the spinal nerves emerge just ventral to these tendinous insertions, and the intervertebral disk space is located caudoventral to the insertions.

E. Exposure of disks is best done with a small curved periosteal elevator. Using the 13th rib as a landmark, the elevator is used to remove muscle and fascia overlying each disk. The insertions of the longissimus tendons are used as landmarks for locating the disk spaces. A nerve root retractor allows the spinal nerves to be retracted cranially and protected from the elevation and fenestrating instruments. T10-T11 is the most cranial disk accessible and L5-L6 the most caudal.

CLOSURE

Both layers of the deep external fascia of the trunk are closed together. Subcutaneous fat and fascia and skin are closed in separate layers.

PLATE 19

Approach to the Thoracolumbar Intervertebral Disks Through a Dorsolateral Incision *continued*

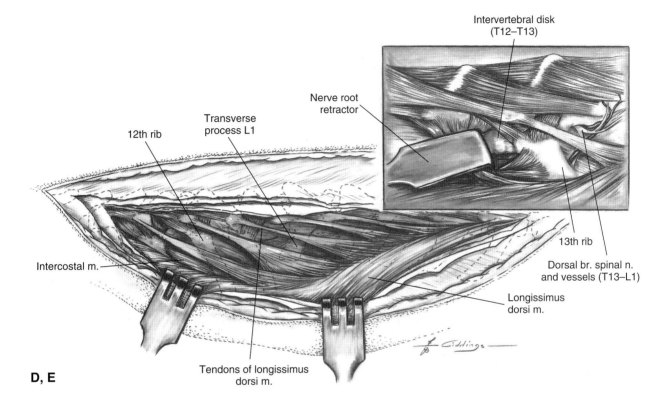

Intervertebral disk
(T12–T13)

Nerve root
retractor

12th rib

Transverse
process L1

Intercostal m.

13th rib

Dorsal br. spinal n.
and vessels (T13–L1)

Longissimus
dorsi m.

Tendons of longissimus
dorsi m.

D, E

Approach to the Thoracolumbar Intervertebral Disks Through a Lateral Incision

Based on Procedures of Flo and Brinker[14] and Seeman[41]

INDICATIONS

1. Fenestration of thoracolumbar disks T10-L5.
2. Hemilaminectomy or pediculectomy for spinal cord decompression from ruptured intervertebral disks or neoplasia.
3. Partial corpectomy for chronic, ventral spinal cord compression caused by ruptured or protruding intervertebral disk.

ALTERNATIVE APPROACH

Similar exposure of the intervertebral disks is obtained via the dorsolateral approach (see Plate 19).

PATIENT POSITIONING

The animal is placed in right lateral recumbency when making the approach to the left side of the intervertebral disks.

DESCRIPTION OF THE PROCEDURE

A. The skin incision is slightly oblique, extending from the base of rib 10 toward the cranioventral iliac spine. The subcutaneous fat is usually quite thick here and is incised on the skin line to reveal the superficial thoracolumbar fascia.
B. The superficial thoracolumbar fascia is incised along the same line.

PLATE 20

Approach to the Thoracolumbar Intervertebral Disks Through a Lateral Incision

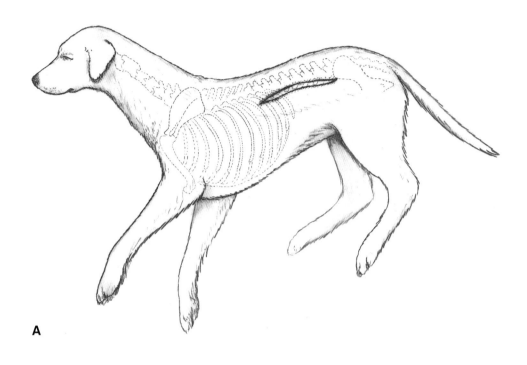

A

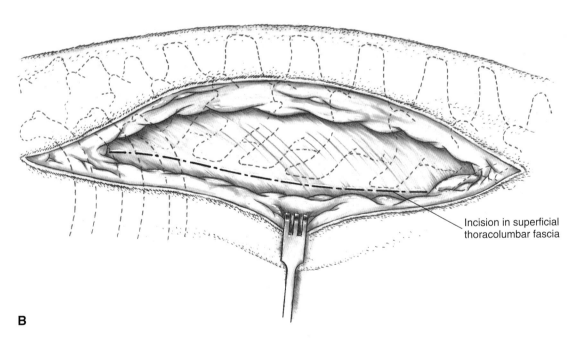

Incision in superficial thoracolumbar fascia

B

Approach to the Thoracolumbar Intervertebral Disks Through a Lateral Incision *continued*

C. The deep thoracolumbar fascia is incised to reveal a second layer of fat and the underlying muscles. The lateral processes can now be palpated quite easily. To approach the thoracic spaces, it is necessary to transect some bundles of the serratus dorsalis muscle.

D. The 13th rib is a good place to start because it allows counting cranially and caudally to identify the other vertebrae. Blunt dissection and separation of the fibers of the iliocostalis lumborum muscle allow the proximal end of the 13th rib to be exposed. A periosteal elevator is used to clear soft tissues from the cranial border of the rib and the lateral surface of the disk. Staying close to the cranial edge of the rib and strong cranial retraction of the muscle will protect the spinal nerve and vessel (see Plate 20D inset drawing). Care must be taken to prevent penetrating the thoracic pleura when clearing the disk surface.

The lumbar disks are exposed by blunt separation of muscle tissue over the end of the appropriate lateral process. Confining the dissection and elevation to the dorsal surface of the process will protect vessels running along the cranial and caudal borders of the tip of the process. The elevation of muscle tissue is continued medially until the disk space is exposed. As the vertebral body and disk are approached, all elevation and retraction should be from a caudal-to-cranial direction to protect the spinal vessel and nerve. A blood vessel will be seen crossing the surface of the disk in the lower lumbar spaces, and it is usually lacerated during the fenestration process.

CLOSURE

The superficial and deep layers of the thoracolumbar fascia are closed with a continuous pattern and absorbable material. They can both be closed in one layer if the intervening fat is not too thick. Subcutaneous and skin layers are closed routinely.

COMMENTS

The choice between this approach and the dorsolateral approach (Plate 19) is a matter of personal preference. The exposure obtained is similar in both.

PLATE 20

Approach to the Thoracolumbar Intervertebral Disks Through a Lateral Incision *continued*

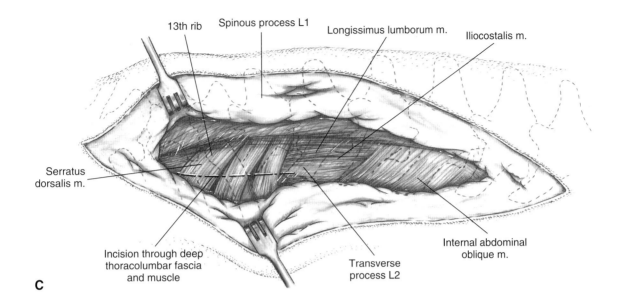

13th rib Spinous process L1 Longissimus lumborum m. Iliocostalis m.

Serratus dorsalis m.

Incision through deep thoracolumbar fascia and muscle

Transverse process L2

Internal abdominal oblique m.

C

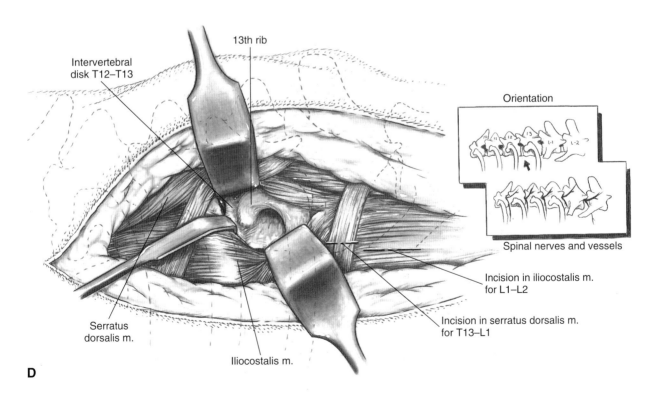

13th rib

Intervertebral disk T12–T13

Orientation

Spinal nerves and vessels

Incision in iliocostalis m. for L1–L2

Incision in serratus dorsalis m. for T13–L1

Serratus dorsalis m.

Iliocostalis m.

D

Approach to Lumbar Vertebra 7 and the Sacrum Through a Dorsal Incision

INDICATIONS

1. Laminectomy of L7-S1.
2. Open reduction of fractures of L7 or S1.

PATIENT POSITIONING

Ventral recumbency and supported under the abdomen and pubis with towels or sandbags.

DESCRIPTION OF THE PROCEDURE

A. A dorsal midline incision is made between the spine of the sixth lumbar vertebra and the caudal median sacral crest. Subcutaneous fat and superficial fascia are incised on the same line to expose the deep gluteal and caudal fasciae, which are also incised on the midline and around each spinous process.

B. The sacrocaudalis dorsal medialis muscles are freed from the spinous processes by incising around each process, then along the midline between processes. Elevation of the muscles is done with a sharp periosteal elevator, working from caudal to cranial.

PLATE 21

Approach to Lumbar Vertebra 7 and the Sacrum Through a Dorsal Incision

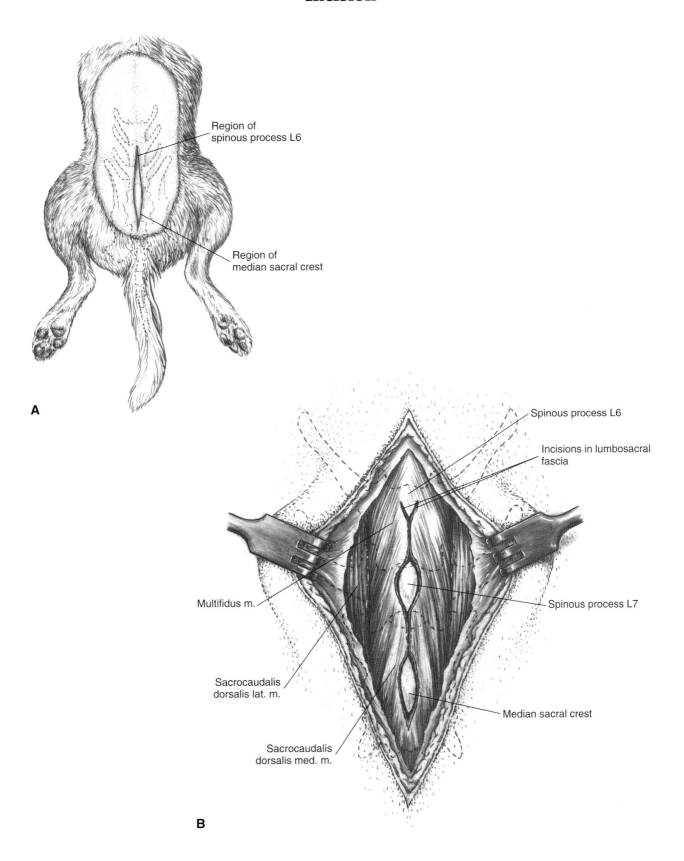

Region of
spinous process L6

Region of
median sacral crest

A

Spinous process L6

Incisions in lumbosacral
fascia

Multifidus m.

Spinous process L7

Sacrocaudalis
dorsalis lat. m.

Median sacral crest

Sacrocaudalis
dorsalis med. m.

B

Approach to Lumbar Vertebra 7 and the Sacrum Through a Dorsal Incision *continued*

C, D. Muscle elevation is continued laterally to the region of L6-L7 and L7-S1 articular processes cranially and to the intermediate sacral crests caudally. Just lateral to the crests are the dorsal sacral foramina, through which pass the dorsal branches of the sacral nerves and vessels. The interarcuate (yellow) ligament between the laminae of L7-S1 is incised to expose the cauda equina nerves.

ADDITIONAL EXPOSURE

This approach can be extended cranially (see Plate 18) or caudally (see Plate 24) if necessary.

CLOSURE

The gluteal and caudal fasciae are closed on the midline. Because of its considerable depth, the subcutaneous fat may need to be closed in two layers.

PLATE 21

Approach to Lumbar Vertebra 7 and the Sacrum Through a Dorsal Incision *continued*

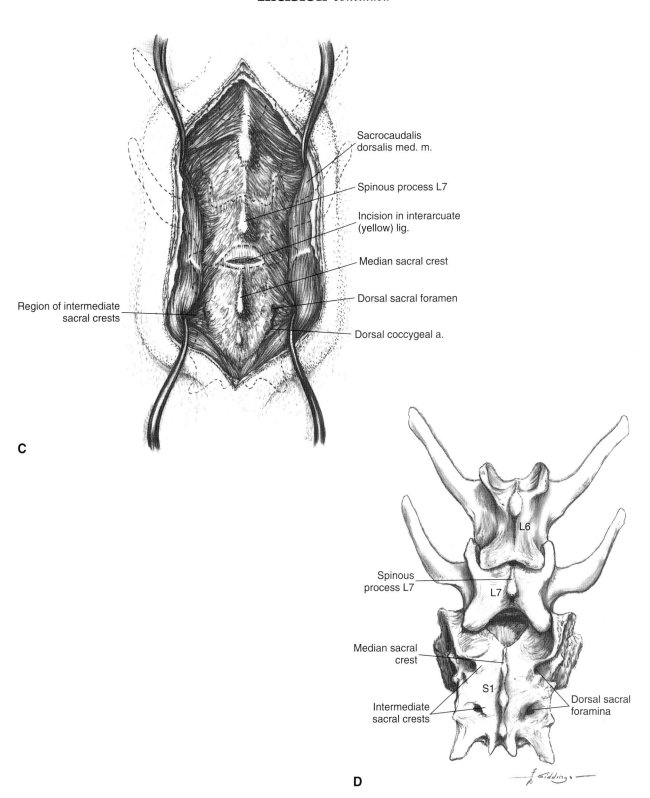

Sacrocaudalis
dorsalis med. m.

Spinous process L7

Incision in interarcuate
(yellow) lig.

Median sacral crest

Dorsal sacral foramen

Dorsal coccygeal a.

Region of intermediate
sacral crests

C

L6

Spinous
process L7

L7

Median sacral
crest

S1

Intermediate
sacral crests

Dorsal sacral
foramina

D

Approach to the Lumbosacral Intervertebral Disk and Foramen Through a Lateral Transilial Osteotomy

Based on a Procedure of Carozzo, Cachon, Genevois, Fau, Remy, Daniaux, Collard, and Viguier[7]

INDICATIONS

1. Fenestration and curettage of the lumbosacral intervertebral disk.
2. Access for endoscopic lumbosacral foraminotomy for foraminal stenosis.

PATIENT POSITIONING

The animal is placed in right lateral recumbency when making the approach to the left side of the lumbosacral intervertebral disk.

DESCRIPTION OF THE PROCEDURE

A. The skin incision is made along the longitudinal axis of the ilium, beginning in the center of the iliac crest, and extending caudoventrally toward the greater trochanter of the femur.
B. Subcutaneous tissue, gluteal fat, and superficial fascia are incised and retracted with the margins of the skin incision. Incision of the deep gluteal fascia in a line overlying the ventral margin of the ilium allows separation of the septum between the middle gluteal muscle and the cranial belly of the sartorius muscle. Some sharp dissection between these two muscles will be required because their muscle fibers blend together.

PLATE 22

Approach to the Lumbosacral Intervertebral Disk and Foramen Through a Lateral Transilial Osteotomy

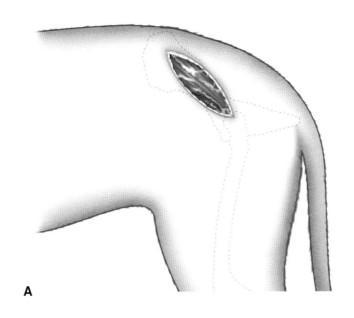

A

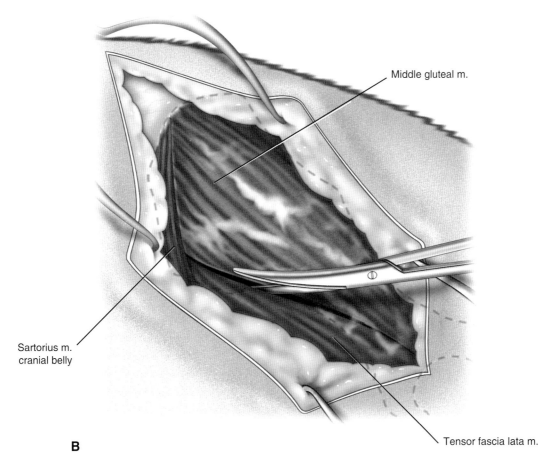

Middle gluteal m.

Sartorius m.
cranial belly

Tensor fascia lata m.

B

Approach to the Lumbosacral Intervertebral Disk and Foramen Through a Lateral Transilial Osteotomy *continued*

C. The middle gluteal muscle is sharply incised along its origin, just inside the edge of the ilial wing. This incision starts at the craniodorsal region of the iliac spine and progresses distally and ventrally toward the ventral iliac spine. The origin of the middle gluteal is elevated from the ilial wing with a periosteal elevator, progressing in a caudal to cranial direction.

PLATE 22

Approach to the Lumbosacral Intervertebral Disk and Foramen Through a Lateral Transilial Osteotomy *continued*

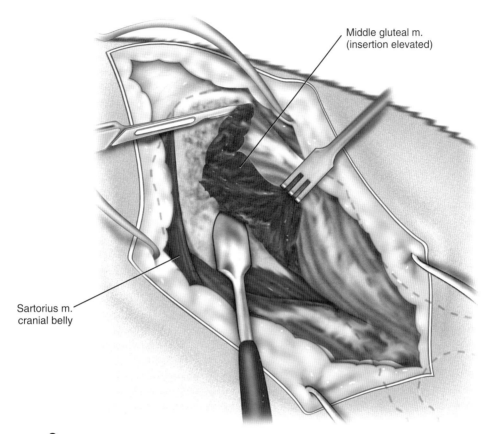

Middle gluteal m.
(insertion elevated)

Sartorius m.
cranial belly

C

Approach to the Lumbosacral Intervertebral Disk and Foramen Through a Lateral Transilial Osteotomy *continued*

D. The reference point for the center of the opening in the ilial wing is the midpoint of a line connecting the cranial dorsal iliac spine and the caudal ventral iliac spine. The location of the lumbosacral disk can be confirmed by digital palpation below the ilium.

E. A round opening about 18 mm in diameter is created in the ilial wing using a bone trephine or high-speed burr.

PLATE 22

Approach to the Lumbosacral Intervertebral Disk and Foramen Through a Lateral Transilial Osteotomy *continued*

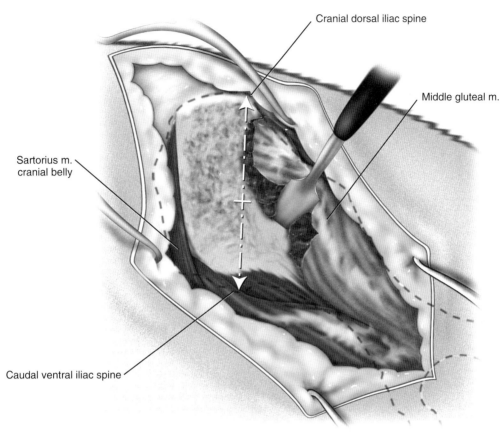

Cranial dorsal iliac spine

Middle gluteal m.

Sartorius m. cranial belly

Caudal ventral iliac spine

D

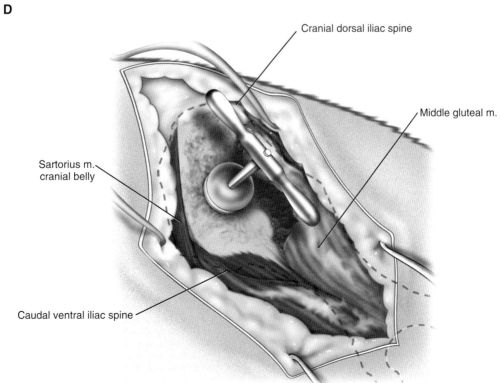

Cranial dorsal iliac spine

Middle gluteal m.

Sartorius m. cranial belly

Caudal ventral iliac spine

E

Approach to the Lumbosacral Intervertebral Disk and Foramen Through a Lateral Transilial Osteotomy *continued*

F. The origins of the quadrates lumborum, iliocostalis, and longissimus lumborum muscles on the medial face of the ilial wing need to incised and displaced cranially. For better exposure of the lumbosacral disk and foramen, the cranial part of the sacral wing can be osteotomized without interfering with the sacroiliac synovial joint.

CLOSURE

The plug of ilial bone is not replaced. Sutures are placed between fasciae of the middle gluteal muscle and the sartorius muscle. Deep gluteal fat and fascia, subcutaneous tissues, and skin are approximated in layers.

PLATE 22

Approach to the Lumbosacral Intervertebral Disk and Foramen Through a Lateral Transilial Osteotomy *continued*

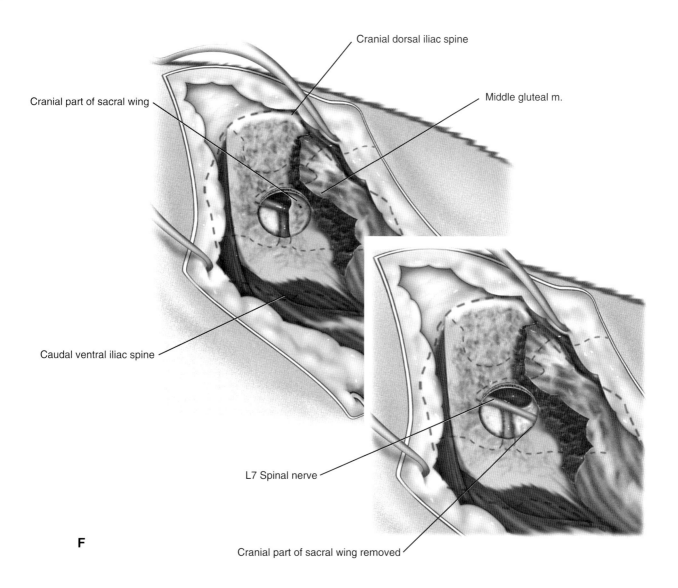

Cranial dorsal iliac spine

Middle gluteal m.

Cranial part of sacral wing

Caudal ventral iliac spine

L7 Spinal nerve

Cranial part of sacral wing removed

F

Approach to Lumbar Vertebrae 6 and 7 and the Sacrum Through a Ventral Abdominal Incision

Based on a Procedure of Montavon and Damur[28]

INDICATIONS

1. Open reduction of fractures and luxations of vertebrae 6 and 7 and the sacrum.
2. Fenestration and curettage of intervertebral disks L6-L7 and L7-S1.
3. Installation of L7-S1 disk prosthesis.

PATIENT POSITIONING

Dorsal recumbency with the hindlimbs abducted.

DESCRIPTION OF THE PROCEDURE

A. The skin incision is made on the midline from the umbilicus to the pelvis in female dogs and cats. In the male dog, the skin incision extends parapreputially to the scrotum.

B. The midline incision continues through the linea alba to open the caudal abdominal cavity. Abdominal organs are retracted cranially and the urinary bladder is retracted laterally toward the surgeon. This exposes the bifurcation of the internal iliac vessels and the median sacral artery.

PLATE 23

Approach to Lumbar Vertebrae 6 and 7 and the Sacrum Through a Ventral Abdominal Incision

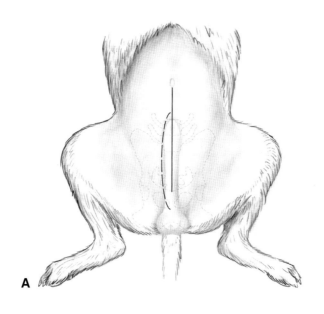

A

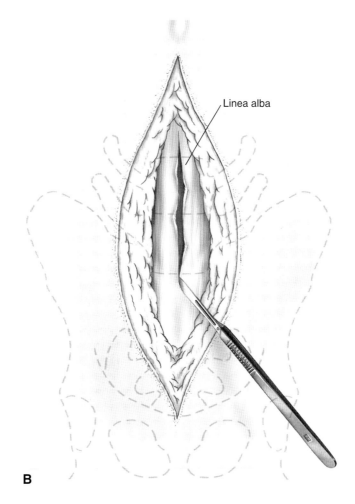

Linea alba

B

Approach to Lumbar Vertebrae 6 and 7 and the Sacrum Through a Ventral Abdominal Incision *continued*

C, D. The median vessels are retracted laterally to allow access to the ventral bodies of L6 and L7 vertebrae, sacrum, and associated intervertebral disks.

PLATE 23

Approach to Lumbar Vertebrae 6 and 7 and the Sacrum Through a Ventral Abdominal Incision *continued*

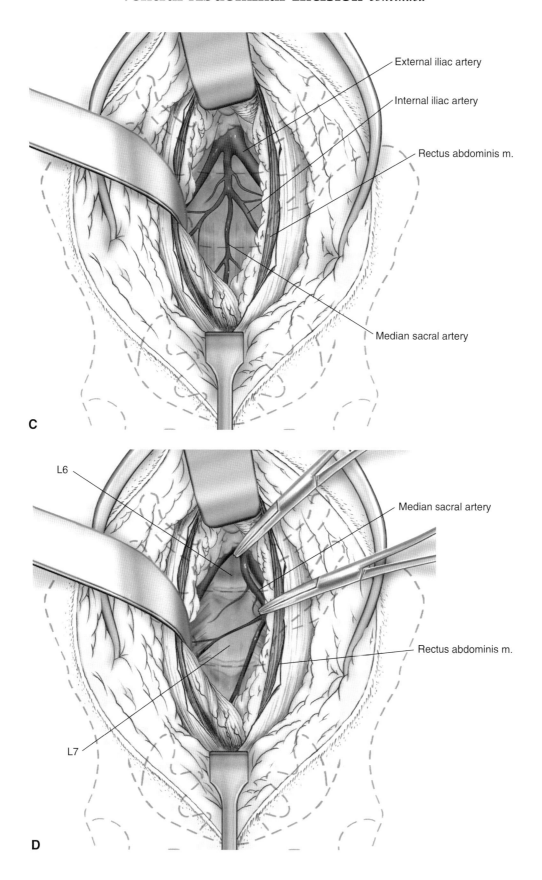

Approach to Lumbar Vertebrae 6 and 7 and the Sacrum Through a Ventral Abdominal Incision *continued*

ADDITIONAL EXPOSURE

E. For complete exposure of the ventral surface of the sacrum, the approach can be extended caudally by osteotomy of the pelvic floor. The gracilis and adductor muscles are sharply divided on midline and then elevated subperiosteally from medial to lateral to expose the obturator nerves and obturator foramina.

PLATE 23

Approach to Lumbar Vertebrae 6 and 7 and the Sacrum Through a Ventral Abdominal Incision *continued*

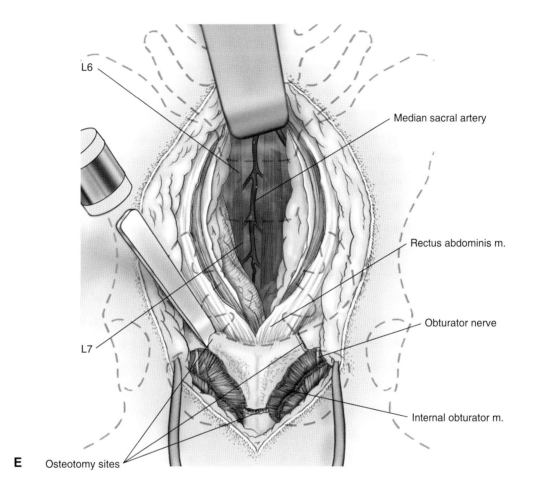

L6

Median sacral artery

Rectus abdominis m.

Obturator nerve

L7

Internal obturator m.

E   Osteotomy sites

Approach to Lumbar Vertebrae 6 and 7 and the Sacrum Through a Ventral Abdominal Incision *continued*

F. The pubic bones are osteotomized transversely at the level of the obturator foramina. The body of each pubic bone is then osteotomized in a parasagittal direction, just medial to the obturator nerve. The internal obturator muscles are subperiosteally elevated from the pubis. The free piece of pelvis is then retracted cranially with insertions of rectus abdominis muscles still attached to the cranial brim of the pelvis.

CLOSURE

The midline celiotomy incision is closed with synthetic absorbable suture in a continuous pattern. Osteotomies of the pelvis are repaired by placement of three hemicerclage wires.

PLATE 23

Approach to Lumbar Vertebrae 6 and 7 and the Sacrum Through a Ventral Abdominal Incision *continued*

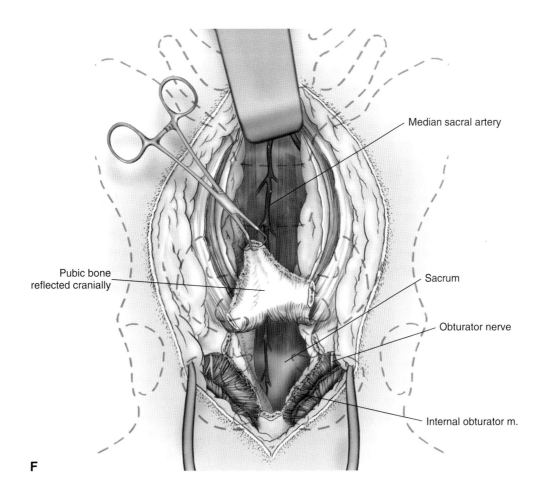

Median sacral artery

Pubic bone reflected cranially

Sacrum

Obturator nerve

Internal obturator m.

F

Approach to the Caudal Vertebrae Through a Dorsal Incision

INDICATIONS

1. Open reduction of fractures and luxations of the caudal vertebrae.
2. Treatment of malunion fractures or congenital malformation of the vertebrae by osteotomy.

PATIENT POSITIONING

Ventral recumbency and supported under the abdomen and pubis with towels or sandbags.

DESCRIPTION OF THE PROCEDURE

A. The skin and subcutaneous fascial incision is made along the dorsal midline of the tail and extends the length of one vertebra proximal and distal to the vertebrae to be exposed.
B. Undermining and retraction of the skin margins reveal the sacrocaudalis muscles under a layer of deep caudal fascia. This fascia is incised on the midline between the paired medial sacrocaudalis dorsalis muscles. The incision is continued into the intermuscular septum until the dorsal surfaces of the vertebrae are reached.
C. A combination of sharp and blunt dissection is used to elevate the muscles from the vertebrae.
D. Only by working close to the bone during the muscular elevation can the dorsal lateral caudal arteries and nerves be avoided.

ADDITIONAL EXPOSURE

This approach can be extended cranially (see Plate 21) to obtain exposure of the sacrum if necessary.

CLOSURE

Deep and subcutaneous fasciae are closed in one layer of sutures, followed by closure of the skin.

COMMENTS

The tail should be bandaged to minimize movement as much as possible for 5 to 7 days postoperatively.

PLATE 24

Approach to the Caudal Vertebrae Through a Dorsal Incision

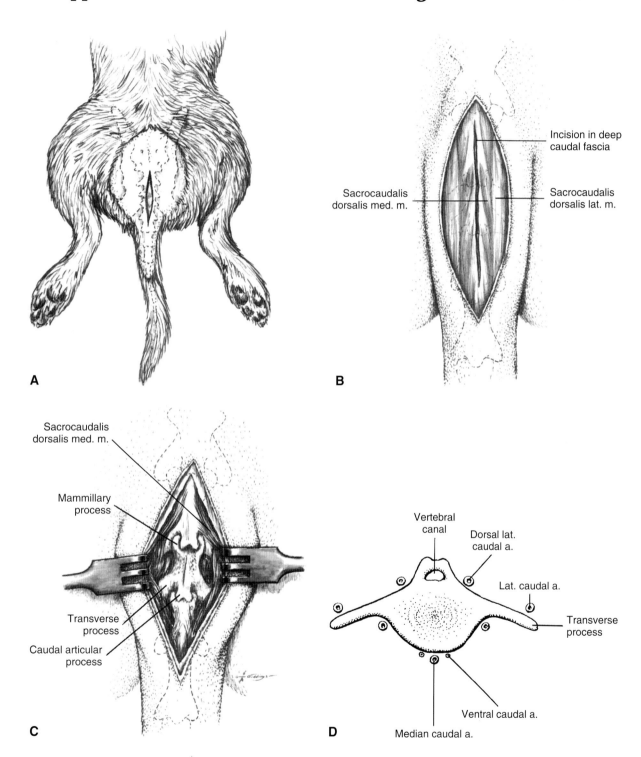

A

B

Incision in deep caudal fascia

Sacrocaudalis dorsalis med. m.

Sacrocaudalis dorsalis lat. m.

Sacrocaudalis dorsalis med. m.

Mammillary process

Transverse process

Caudal articular process

C

Vertebral canal

Dorsal lat. caudal a.

Lat. caudal a.

Transverse process

Ventral caudal a.

Median caudal a.

D

SECTION 4

The Scapula and Shoulder Joint

Approach to the Body, Spine, and Acromion Process of the Scapula

Based on a Procedure of Alexander[1]

INDICATION

Open reduction of fractures of the scapula.

PATIENT POSITIONING

Place the animal in lateral recumbency with the affected limb uppermost.

DESCRIPTION OF THE PROCEDURE

A. Identify the spine of the scapula, acromion process, and greater tubercle of the humerus by palpation. The skin and subcutaneous fascial incision is made directly on the spine of the scapula. The skin and fascia are retracted following the undermining of the edges of the incision. The length of the incision is adjusted to fit the area of interest in the exposure.
B. An incision is now made in the deep fascia along the spine of the scapula and is deepened to free the origin of the scapular part of the deltoideus and the insertions of the omotransversarius and trapezius muscles. These muscles are freed and retracted sufficiently to expose the spine of the scapula and underlying spinatus muscles.
C. The infraspinatus and supraspinatus muscles are elevated from the spine of the scapula. The bellies of the muscles can then be bluntly undermined in a distal to proximal direction using a periosteal elevator (see Figure 19) and then retracted from the body of the scapula. Near the acromion, an incision can be made a short distance into the septum between the acromial and scapular parts of the deltoideus to allow retraction of the scapular part (see Plate 28B, C, D).

ADDITIONAL EXPOSURE

Distal extension to the craniolateral region of the shoulder joint (see Plate 26).
   Distal extension to the craniomedial region of the shoulder joint (see Plates 30 and 32).

CLOSURE

A single row of sutures will suffice to close all the incised deep structures. The suture line runs directly along the spine and includes the deep fascia and the omotransversarius, trapezius, and deltoideus muscles. Subcutaneous tissues and skin are closed in separate layers.

COMMENTS

Elevation of the infraspinatus muscle from the scapular spine is complicated by the presence of the metacromion in the cat. This caudally projecting protuberance, located on the spine 1 to 2 cm proximal to the acromion, overhangs the infraspinatus slightly, but it does not actually alter the procedure.

PRECAUTIONS

Distally the exposure of the neck of the scapula is complicated by the suprascapular nerve and artery. The suprascapular nerve emerges around the scapular notch, supplying a branch to the overlying supraspinatus muscle. The nerve then crosses the neck of the scapula distal to the scapular spine to supply the infraspinatus muscle.

PLATE 25

Approach to the Body, Spine, and Acromion Process of the Scapula

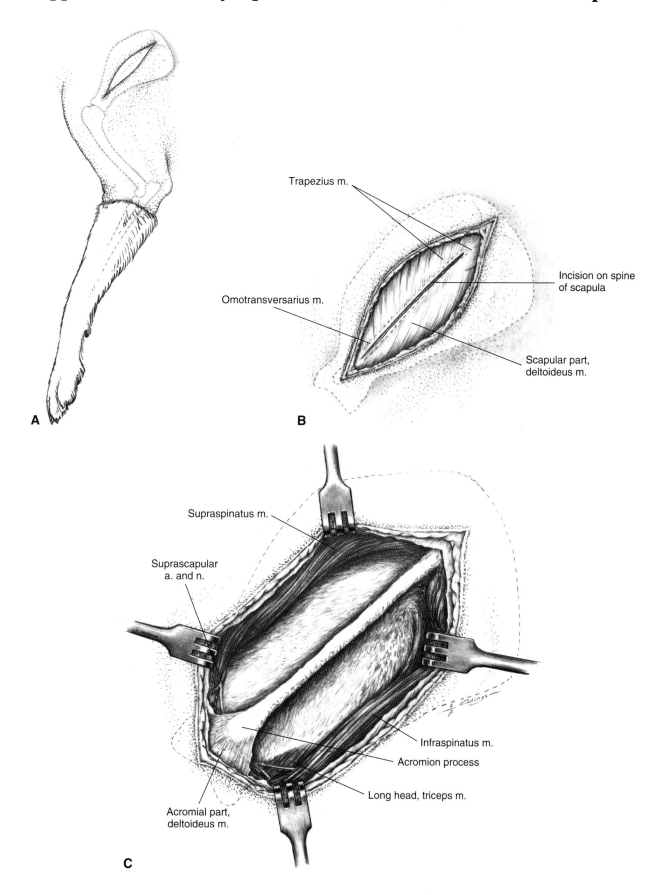

Trapezius m.

Incision on spine of scapula

Omotransversarius m.

Scapular part, deltoideus m.

A

B

Supraspinatus m.

Suprascapular a. and n.

Infraspinatus m.

Acromion process

Long head, triceps m.

Acromial part, deltoideus m.

C

Approach to the Craniolateral Region of the Shoulder Joint

INDICATIONS

1. Open reduction of fractures of the neck and glenoid cavity of the scapula.
2. Open reduction of luxations of the shoulder joint.
3. Osteochondroplasty for osteochondritis dissecans of the humeral head.
4. Open reduction of fractures of the humeral head.

ALTERNATIVE APPROACHES

The exposure provided by this craniolateral approach (see Plate 26) is generally much greater than is needed for osteochondritis dissecans surgery. It is only recommended when the surgeon has no assistant to retract and position the limb, as is needed for the other recommended approaches (see Plates 27, 28, and 29).

PATIENT POSITIONING

Place the animal in lateral recumbency with the affected limb uppermost.

DESCRIPTION OF THE PROCEDURE

A. Identify the spine of the scapula, acromion process, and greater tubercle by palpation. The curved incision begins at the middle of the scapula and follows the spine distally, crossing the joint and continuing over the lateral surface of the humerus to the midpoint of the shaft. The skin margins are undermined and retracted after the subcutaneous fascia and fat are incised in the same line as the skin incision.

B. An incision is made in the deep fascia, starting distally at the omobrachial vein and centered over the belly of the acromial part of the deltoideus. It continues proximally toward the acromial process, passing through the craniodistal insertion of the omotransversarius muscle, and onto the spine of the scapula. The scapular incision encompasses the distal one third of the spine and is deepened both cranial and caudal to the spine to include the insertions. Protect the branches of the axillary nerve entering the deep surface of the deltoideus muscle as it is retracted distally of the omotransversarius and trapezius and the origin of the scapular part of the deltoideus muscle. Take care not to incise the underlying spinatus muscles.

PLATE 26

Approach to the Craniolateral Region of the Shoulder Joint

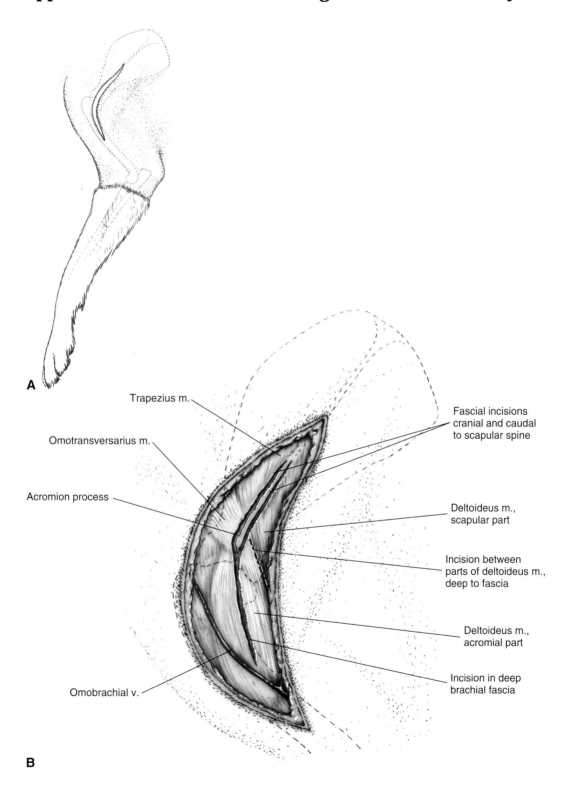

Trapezius m.

Omotransversarius m.

Acromion process

Omobrachial v.

Fascial incisions
cranial and caudal
to scapular spine

Deltoideus m.,
scapular part

Incision between
parts of deltoideus m.,
deep to fascia

Deltoideus m.,
acromial part

Incision in deep
brachial fascia

A

B

Approach to the Craniolateral Region of the Shoulder Joint *continued*

C. The omotransversarius and trapezius muscles are retracted craniodorsally. An incision is made between the two parts of the deltoideus muscle (shown in Plate 26B) and is developed bluntly to allow freeing of the scapular part of the deltoideus and its caudoventral retraction. Use care during this dissection to preserve as many as possible of the muscular branches of the axillary nerve that will be found in this area. The area of the acromion is cleared of adherent tissue to allow an osteotomy (see Plate 26C1 for detail). Using a small curved hemostat, separate between the acromial part of the deltoideus muscle and the underlying infraspinatus and supraspinatus muscles, while staying close to the acromion.

D. The acromion is osteotomized to include all of the origin of the acromial part of the deltoideus (see Plate 26C1 for detail). Either an osteotome or a bone-cutting forceps can be used for the osteotomy; in either case, care must be used to protect the underlying suprascapular nerve. Protect the branches of the axillary nerve entering the deep surface of the deltoideus muscle as it is retracted distally. Some surgeons prefer tenotomy of the origin of the deltoideus near the acromion. In young animals the acromion may not be ossified. In these cases, a tenotomy of the acromial part of the

PLATE 26

Approach to the Craniolateral Region of the Shoulder Joint *continued*

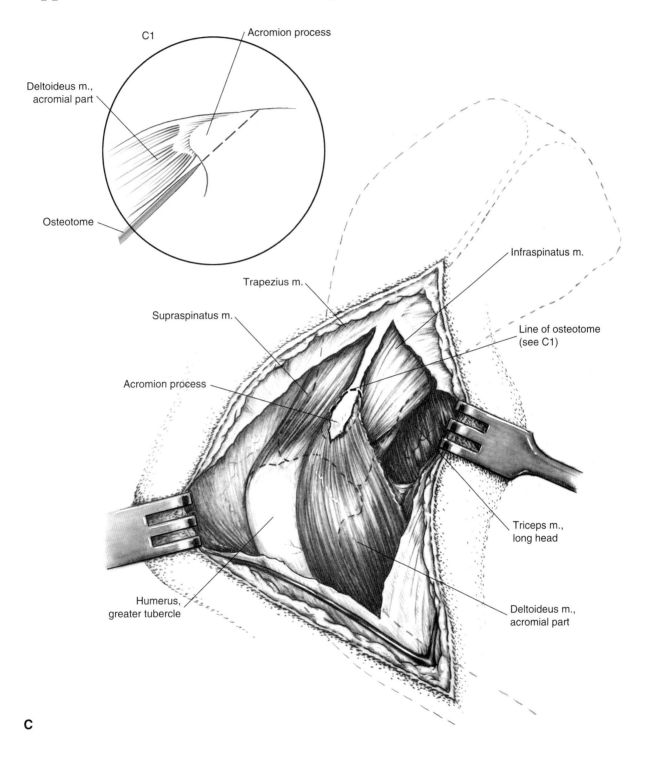

C1
Acromion process
Deltoideus m., acromial part
Osteotome

Trapezius m.
Supraspinatus m.
Acromion process
Humerus, greater tubercle

Infraspinatus m.
Line of osteotome (see C1)
Triceps m., long head
Deltoideus m., acromial part

C

Approach to the Craniolateral Region of the Shoulder Joint *continued*

deltoideus is performed close to the acromion. Tenotomy is also more satisfactory in small dogs and cats. Holes drilled in the acromion allow for reattachment of the tendon (see Figure 22).

F. The supraspinatus and infraspinatus muscles are bluntly elevated from the spine and body of the scapula sufficiently to allow their retraction as shown. Note the position of the suprascapular nerve and avoid this structure during the elevation and retraction of the infraspinatus.

Exposure of the joint requires tenotomy of the infraspinatus muscle. This cut is made near the muscle's insertion on the humerus, with enough stump being left to receive one or two sutures. In some cases it may be necessary to treat the teres minor muscle in a like manner, thus allowing greater exposure of the ventrolateral aspect of the joint capsule.

ADDITIONAL EXPOSURE

Proximal extension to the body and spine of the scapula (see Plate 25).

Extension of the approach to the cranial region of the shoulder joint with osteotomy of the greater tubercle of the humerus provides total exposure of the scapular neck and most of the glenoid cavity (see Plate 32).

CLOSURE

A modified Bunnell-Mayer or locking-loop suture (Figure 21A, C), reinforced with one or two mattress sutures, is used to join the transected infraspinatus muscle. The acromion is attached to the spine by two 20- to 22-gauge monofilament stainless steel sutures placed through holes drilled in the bones (Figure 24B). Several sutures are placed between the two parts of the deltoideus muscle. A single tier of sutures may be used to close the remaining muscles and deep fascia. Starting at the proximal end of the incision the suture engages the deep fascia, the trapezius, the scapular part of the deltoideus, and the deep fascia. This pattern is continued distally, with the omotransversarius replacing the trapezius as the acromion is approached. Distal to the acromion, the deep fascia alone is closed.

COMMENTS

Elevation of the infraspinatus muscle from the scapular spine is complicated by the presence of the metacromion in the cat. This caudally projecting protuberance, located 1 to 2 cm proximal to the acromion, overhangs the infraspinatus slightly, but it does not actually alter the procedure.

PRECAUTIONS

The suprascapular nerve emerges around the scapular notch, supplying a branch to the overlying supraspinatus muscle. The nerve then crosses the neck of the scapula, distal to the scapular spine, to supply the infraspinatus muscle. The axillary nerve curves around the caudal border of the subscapularis muscle and neck of the scapula, and then it crosses the caudal aspect of the shoulder joint between the joint capsule and long head of the triceps muscle.

PLATE 26

Approach to the Craniolateral Region of the Shoulder Joint *continued*

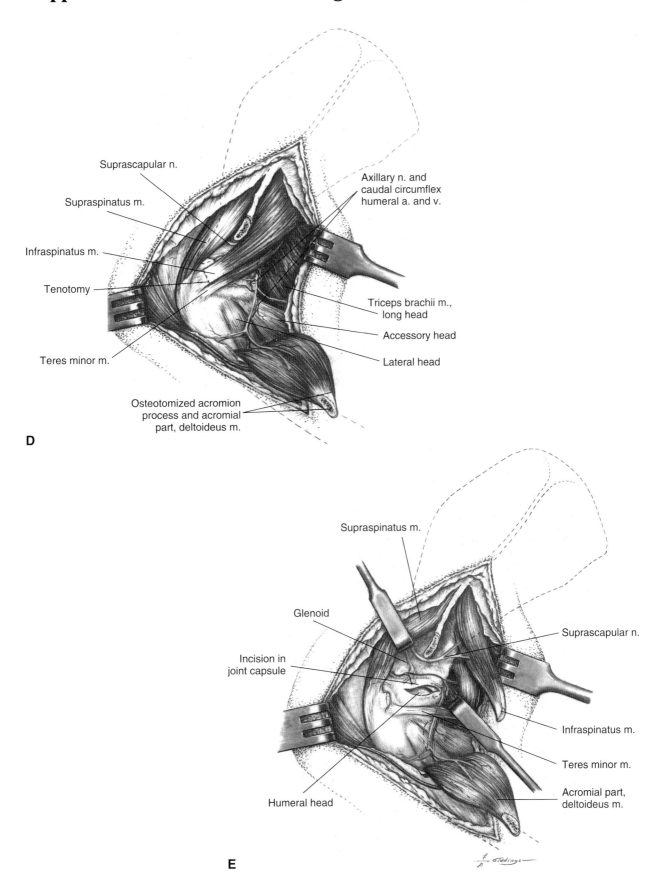

D

Suprascapular n.

Supraspinatus m.

Infraspinatus m.

Tenotomy

Teres minor m.

Osteotomized acromion process and acromial part, deltoideus m.

Axillary n. and caudal circumflex humeral a. and v.

Triceps brachii m., long head

Accessory head

Lateral head

Suprascapular m.

Glenoid

Incision in joint capsule

Humeral head

Suprascapular n.

Infraspinatus m.

Teres minor m.

Acromial part, deltoideus m.

E

Approach to the Craniolateral Region of the Shoulder Joint by Tenotomy of the Infraspinatus Muscle

Based on a Procedure of Hohn[20]

INDICATIONS

1. Osteochondroplasty of the humeral head for osteochondritis dissecans.
2. Tenotomy for contracture of the infraspinatus muscle.

ALTERNATIVE APPROACHES

An alternative is the approach to the craniolateral region of the shoulder with osteotomy of the acromion process (see Plate 26), but it provides more exposure than generally needed for surgical correction of osteochondritis dissecans or infraspinatus contracture and may unnecessarily produce greater surgical trauma.

This craniolateral approach (see Plate 27) gives good exposure to the articular surface of the humeral head, but poorer access to the caudal compartment of the joint for removal of joint mice, compared to the caudolateral (see Plate 28) and caudal (see Plate 29) approaches.

PATIENT POSITIONING

Place the animal in lateral recumbency with the affected limb uppermost.

DESCRIPTION OF THE PROCEDURE

A. Identify the spine of the scapula, acromion process, and greater tubercle of the humerus by palpation. A curved incision begins at the distal one third of the scapular spine and follows the spine distally, crossing the joint and continuing over the craniolateral surface of the humerus to the midshaft region. Skin margins are undermined and retracted after the subcutaneous fat and fascia are incised in the same line as the skin.
B. Deep fascia is incised, beginning at the acromion and continuing distally over the cranial border of the acromial part of the deltoideus. This incision is continued to the insertion of the acromial part of the deltoideus on the humerus.
C. The belly of the acromial part of the deltoideus is retracted to allow tenotomy of the infraspinatus tendon 5 mm from its humeral insertion. Elevation of a portion of the insertion of the deltoideus may be necessary to permit adequate retraction of this muscle.

PLATE 27

Approach to the Craniolateral Region of the Shoulder Joint by Tenotomy of the Infraspinatus Muscle

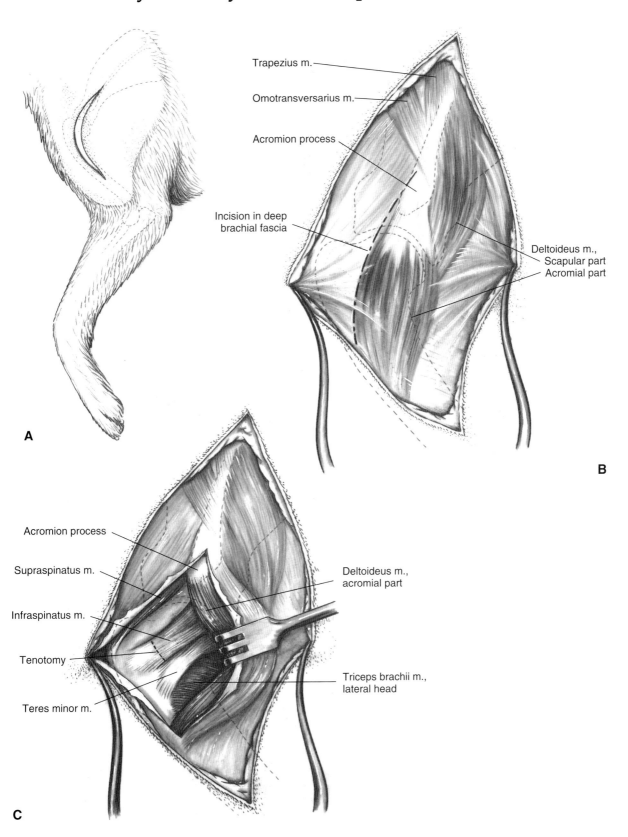

A

B

Trapezius m.

Omotransversarius m.

Acromion process

Incision in deep brachial fascia

Deltoideus m., Scapular part Acromial part

C

Acromion process

Supraspinatus m.

Infraspinatus m.

Tenotomy

Teres minor m.

Deltoideus m., acromial part

Triceps brachii m., lateral head

Approach to the Craniolateral Region of the Shoulder Joint by Tenotomy of the Infraspinatus Muscle *continued*

    D. Retraction of the infraspinatus tendon and acromial part of the deltoideus will allow incision of the joint capsule midway between the glenoid rim and the humeral head. Additional exposure can be obtained by tenotomy of the teres minor muscle.

    E. After retraction of the joint capsule, the humerus is strongly rotated internally to increase exposure of the caudal portion of the head. The humeral head can be partially luxated in the lateral direction for better exposure of a large lesion.

CLOSURE

The joint capsule is closed with interrupted absorbable sutures of 3-0 size. The tendon of the infraspinatus is reattached with a modified Bunnell-Mayer or locking-loop suture (Figure 21A, C) and reinforced with one or two mattress sutures, nonabsorbable material of 0 or 2-0 size being used. The deep fascial incision, subcutaneous fat and fascia, and skin are closed in separate layers.

PLATE 27

Approach to the Craniolateral Region of the Shoulder Joint by Tenotomy of the Infraspinatus Muscle *continued*

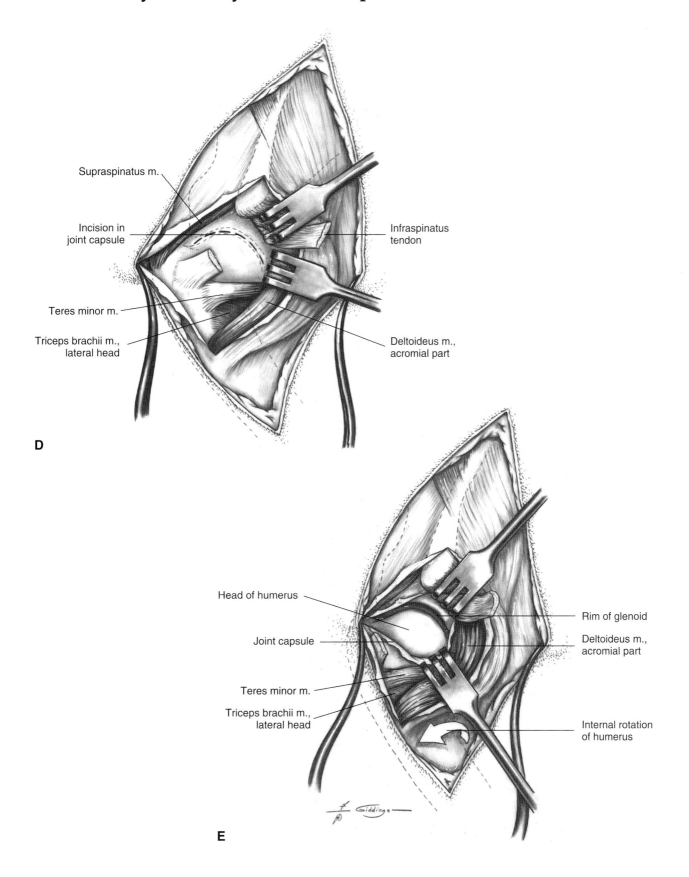

Supraspinatus m.

Incision in joint capsule

Infraspinatus tendon

Teres minor m.

Triceps brachii m., lateral head

Deltoideus m., acromial part

D

Head of humerus

Rim of glenoid

Joint capsule

Deltoideus m., acromial part

Teres minor m.

Triceps brachii m., lateral head

Internal rotation of humerus

E

Approach to the Caudolateral Region of the Shoulder Joint

INDICATIONS

1. Osteochondroplasty of the humeral head for osteochondritis dissecans.
2. Open reduction of caudoventral luxations of the shoulder.
3. Open reduction of fractures of the ventral portion of the glenoid cavity.

ALTERNATIVE APPROACHES

The approach to the craniolateral region of the shoulder joint with osteotomy of the acromion process (see Plate 26) provides improved access for reduction of shoulder luxations and glenoid fractures but more surgical exposure than generally needed for osteochondritis dissecans lesions.

The approach to the craniolateral region of the shoulder joint by tenotomy of the infraspinatus muscle (see Plate 27) provides better exposure to osteochondritis dissecans lesions of the humeral head. However, access to the caudal compartment of the shoulder joint for removal of joint mice is better with this caudolateral approach (see Plate 28) or the caudal approach (see Plate 29).

PATIENT POSITIONING

Place the animal in lateral recumbency with the affected limb uppermost.

DESCRIPTION OF THE PROCEDURE

A. Identify the spine of the scapula, acromion process, and greater tubercle of the humerus by palpation. A curved incision begins at the middle of the scapula and follows the spine distally, crossing the joint and continuing over the lateral surface of the humerus to the midpoint of the shaft. Skin margins are undermined and retracted after subcutaneous fascia and fat are incised in the same line as the skin incision.

B. Deep fascia is incised over the ventral border of the distal scapular spine to free the origin of the scapular part of the deltoideus muscle. This fascial incision is continued distally over the acromial part of the deltoideus to the omobrachial vein. The incised fascia is elevated and retracted cranially and caudally from the underlying deltoideus muscle.

C. An incision is made on the ventral border of the spine of the scapula and continued distally between the scapular and acromial parts of the deltoideus muscle.

PLATE 28

Approach to the Caudolateral Region of the Shoulder Joint

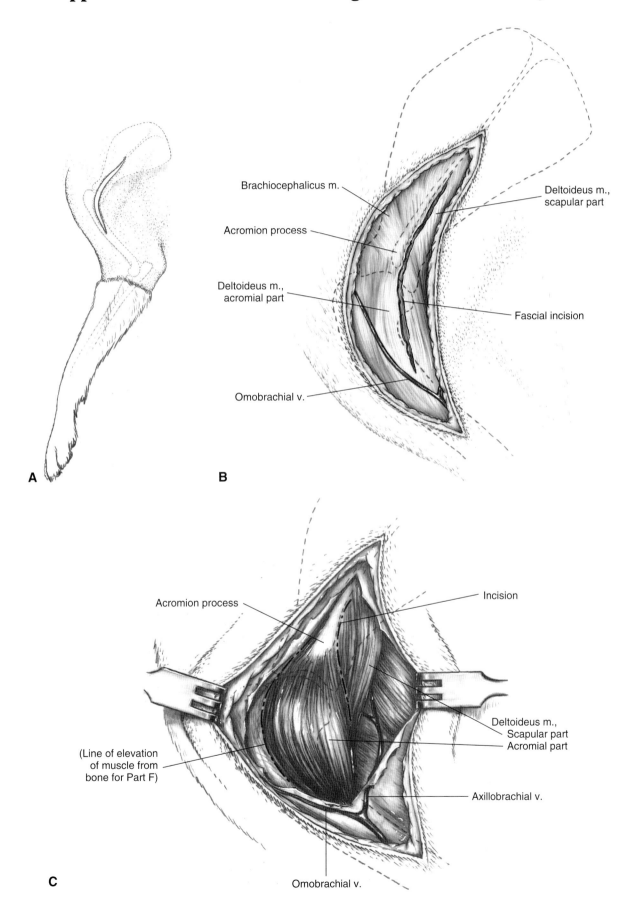

B

Brachiocephalicus m.

Deltoideus m.,
scapular part

Acromion process

Deltoideus m.,
acromial part

Fascial incision

Omobrachial v.

A

C

Acromion process

Incision

Deltoideus m.,
Scapular part

Acromial part

(Line of elevation
of muscle from
bone for Part F)

Axillobrachial v.

Omobrachial v.

Approach to the Caudolateral Region of the Shoulder Joint *continued*

D. The division between the two parts of deltoideus muscle is developed by blunt dissection to allow freeing of the scapular part of the muscle and its caudal retraction with the deep fascia. A muscular branch of the axillary nerve is found between the two parts of the deltoideus. It is usually possible to preserve this structure.

There are two possible ways to proceed from this point. Plate 28E illustrates the simpler method, but it may not provide sufficient exposure in some animals. Continuing as shown in Plate 28F and G will give additional exposure.

E. Working along the ventral border of the teres minor muscle, bluntly dissect between this muscle and the underlying joint capsule. Strong dorsocranial retraction of the teres minor muscle with a Senn retractor will expose the joint capsule. An incision is made parallel and close to the rim of the glenoid cavity. Care is taken to protect the subscapular vessels and axillary nerve lying between the joint capsule and the long head of the triceps muscle. Internal rotation and adduction of the humerus provides maximal exposure of the humeral head.

As an alternative, the junction between the infraspinatus and teres minor muscles is separated. The teres minor muscle is elevated from the underlying joint capsule and retracted caudoventrally, whereas the infraspinatus and acromial part of the deltoideus muscles are retracted craniodorsally. Although there is less risk of damage to the branches of the axillary nerve and caudal circumflex humeral vessels, less of the articular cartilage on the humeral head can be seen as compared to the standard caudolateral approach described previously.

PLATE 28

Approach to the Caudolateral Region of the Shoulder Joint *continued*

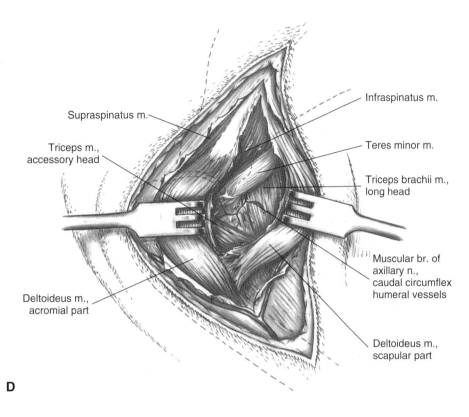

Supraspinatus m.

Triceps m.,
accessory head

Deltoideus m.,
acromial part

Infraspinatus m.

Teres minor m.

Triceps brachii m.,
long head

Muscular br. of
axillary n.,
caudal circumflex
humeral vessels

Deltoideus m.,
scapular part

D

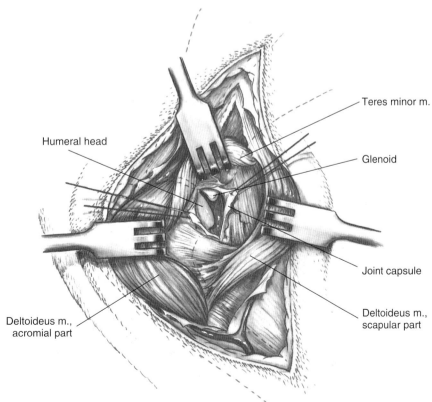

Humeral head

Deltoideus m.,
acromial part

Teres minor m.

Glenoid

Joint capsule

Deltoideus m.,
scapular part

E

Approach to the Caudolateral Region of the Shoulder Joint *continued*

F. The belly of the acromial part of the deltoideus is undermined along its cranial border and elevated from the underlying humerus (see incision in Plate 28C). The deltoideus is then retracted caudally to expose the tendons of insertion of the infraspinatus and teres minor muscles on the greater tubercle of the humerus. Fascia overlying the tendon of the teres minor is incised to allow tenotomy about 5 mm from its insertion. Place a modified mattress or locking-loop suture in the tendon before its transection, leaving the needle attached to the suture (see Figure 21).

G. The tendon suture is passed caudally under the acromial part of the deltoideus, and the two bellies of the deltoideus are separated with Gelpi self-retaining retractors. The tendon suture in the teres minor is used to apply gentle traction as the muscle is dissected free from the underlying joint capsule. The infraspinatus is retracted dorsally and the joint capsule is incised parallel to the rim of the glenoid. As this incision is carried caudally to the flexor surface of the joint, care must be taken to preserve the subscapular artery and axillary nerve that lie very close to the joint. Internal rotation of the humerus will provide maximum exposure of the caudal surface of the humeral head.

CLOSURE

The joint capsule is closed with interrupted sutures of 3-0 absorbable material. If the teres minor tendon was cut, the preplaced tendon suture is placed through the tendon insertion and tied. External rotation of the humerus will facilitate tying this suture. Additional small mattress sutures are used in the tendon if necessary to gain adequate closure. The intermuscular septum between the two parts of the deltoideus is next sutured with the suture material of choice, and the cranial border of the acromial part of the deltoideus is reattached to the fascia on the proximal portion of the humeral shaft. The next step is to suture the fascial origin of the scapular part of the deltoideus to the spine of the scapula. This suture line is continued distally to close the fascia overlying the acromial part of the deltoideus. Subcutaneous closure is made with care because of the tendency for subcutaneous seroma to form.

PRECAUTIONS

The axillary nerve curves around the caudal border of the neck of the scapula, branching to innervate teres minor and deltoideus muscles. These nerves, together with the subscapular and cranial circumflex humeral arteries, cross the caudal aspect of the shoulder joint between the joint capsule and long head of the triceps muscle.

PLATE 28

Approach to the Caudolateral Region of the Shoulder Joint *continued*

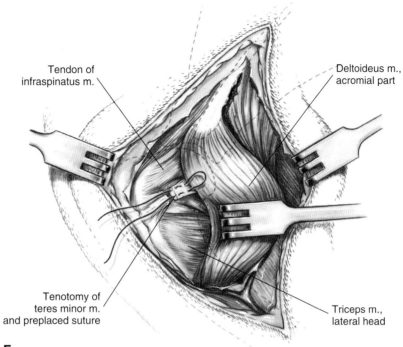

Tendon of
infraspinatus m.

Deltoideus m.,
acromial part

Tenotomy of
teres minor m.
and preplaced suture

Triceps m.,
lateral head

F

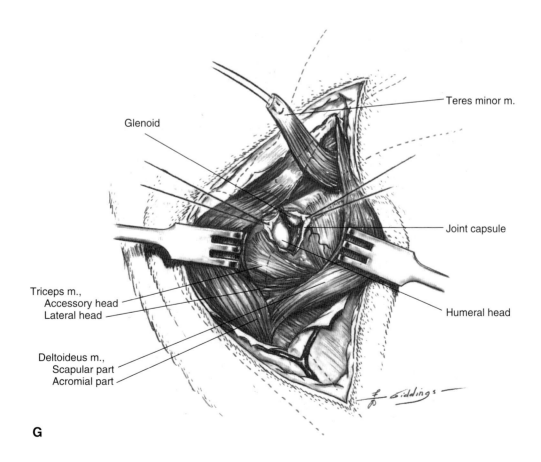

Glenoid

Teres minor m.

Joint capsule

Triceps m.,
Accessory head
Lateral head

Humeral head

Deltoideus m.,
Scapular part
Acromial part

G

Approach to the Caudal Region of the Shoulder Joint

Based on a Procedure of Gahring[16]

INDICATION

Osteochondroplasty for osteochondritis dissecans of the humeral head.

ALTERNATIVE APPROACHES

The caudolateral approach (see Plate 28) and this caudal approach (see Plate 29) both provide good exposure to osteochondritis dissecans lesions of the humeral head and the caudal compartment of the shoulder joint for removal of joint mice. The caudal approach has the advantage of not requiring any tenotomies.

The approach to the craniolateral region of the shoulder joint by tenotomy of the infraspinatus muscle (see Plate 27) provides better exposure to osteochondritis dissecans lesions of the humeral head but poor access to the caudal compartment of the shoulder joint for removal of joint mice.

The approach to the craniolateral region of the shoulder joint with osteotomy of the acromion process (see Plate 26) provides improved access for reduction of shoulder luxations and glenoid fractures but more surgical exposure than generally needed for osteochondritis dissecans lesions.

PATIENT POSITIONING

Place the animal in lateral recumbency with the affected limb uppermost.

DESCRIPTION OF THE PROCEDURE

A. Identify the spine of the scapula, acromion process, and greater tubercle of the humerus by palpation. The skin incision extends from the middle of the scapular spine to the midshaft of the humerus.

B. Subcutaneous fat and deep fascia of the shoulder are incised and elevated to reveal the scapular part of the deltoideus muscle and the lateral and long heads of the triceps brachii muscle. An incision is made in the intermuscular septum between the caudal border of the deltoideus and the long head of the triceps and is continued distally over the lateral head of the triceps.

C. Blunt dissection under the deltoideus and strong elevation of that muscle will reveal the caudal circumflex artery and vein and a muscular branch of the axillary nerve. The teres minor muscle and the joint capsule lie directly under these structures.

PLATE 29
Approach to the Caudal Region of the Shoulder Joint

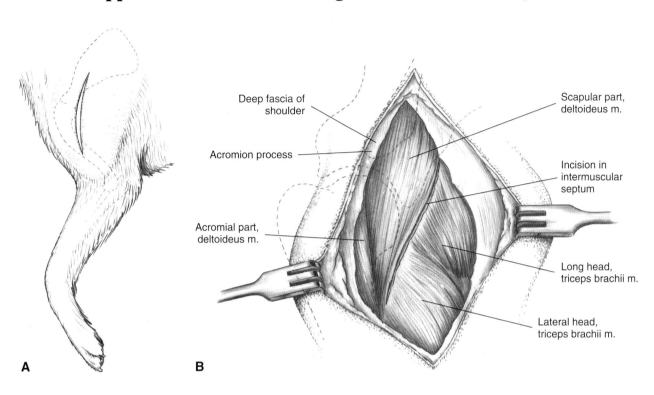

A

B

Deep fascia of shoulder

Acromion process

Acromial part, deltoideus m.

Scapular part, deltoideus m.

Incision in intermuscular septum

Long head, triceps brachii m.

Lateral head, triceps brachii m.

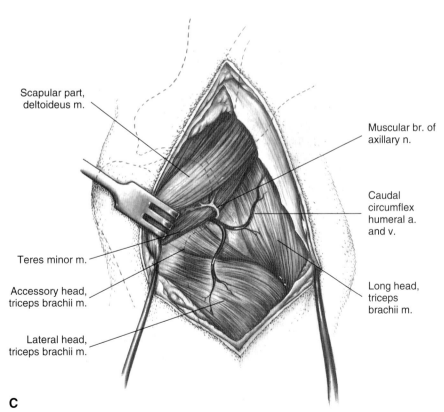

C

Scapular part, deltoideus m.

Teres minor m.

Accessory head, triceps brachii m.

Lateral head, triceps brachii m.

Muscular br. of axillary n.

Caudal circumflex humeral a. and v.

Long head, triceps brachii m.

Approach to the Caudal Region of the Shoulder Joint *continued*

D. Craniodorsal retraction of the teres minor will expose the axillary nerve.

PLATE 29

Approach to the Caudal Region of the Shoulder Joint *continued*

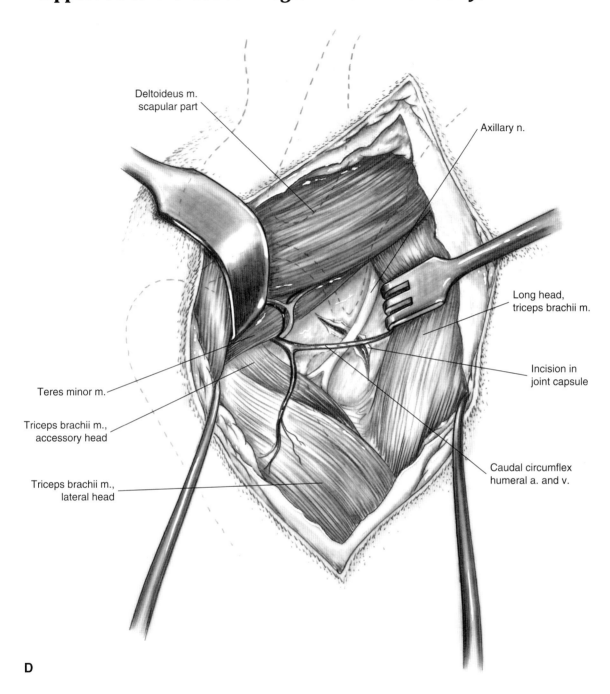

Deltoideus m.
scapular part

Axillary n.

Long head,
triceps brachii m.

Incision in
joint capsule

Teres minor m.

Triceps brachii m.,
accessory head

Triceps brachii m.,
lateral head

Caudal circumflex
humeral a. and v.

D

Approach to the Caudal Region of the Shoulder Joint *continued*

    E. The axillary nerve and accompanying vessels are elevated and gently retracted with a rubber Penrose drain or umbilical tape. Palpation will identify the inferior rim of the glenoid cavity and the caudal aspect of the humeral head. The joint capsule is incised 5 mm from and parallel to the rim of the glenoid cavity.

    F. Retraction of the joint capsule gives good exposure of the caudal cul-de-sac of the joint. Strong internal rotation of the limb, combined with varying degrees of flexion and extension of the shoulder, will provide exposure of the osteochondritis dissecans lesion.

CLOSURE

The joint capsule is closed with interrupted sutures of 3-0 absorbable material. The intermuscular septum between the deltoideus and triceps muscles is closed, followed by closure of the deep fascial layer, subcutaneous tissues, and skin.

PRECAUTIONS

This approach is more complicated than the caudolateral approach (see Plate 28) because of the axillary nerve and caudal circumflex humeral vessels. The axillary nerve curves around the caudoventral border of the scapula, at which point it divides into two portions. One portion innervates the subscapularis and teres major muscles. The other portion crosses the shoulder joint caudally between the joint capsule and long head of the triceps muscle. Accompanied by the caudal circumflex humeral vessels, it runs laterally to innervate the laterally overlying teres minor and deltoideus muscles.

PLATE 29

Approach to the Caudal Region of the Shoulder Joint *continued*

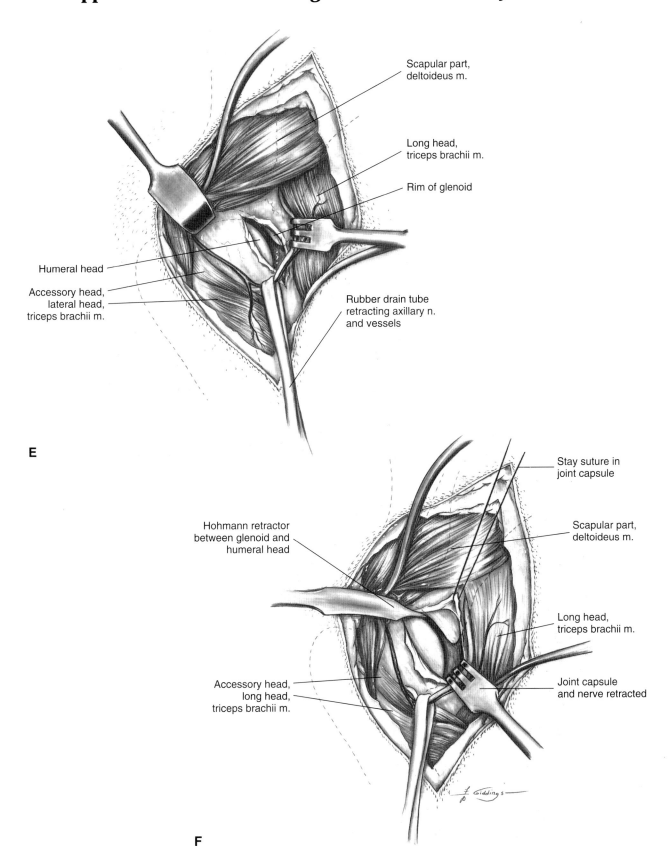

Scapular part,
deltoideus m.

Long head,
triceps brachii m.

Rim of glenoid

Humeral head

Accessory head,
lateral head,
triceps brachii m.

Rubber drain tube
retracting axillary n.
and vessels

E

Stay suture in
joint capsule

Scapular part,
deltoideus m.

Hohmann retractor
between glenoid and
humeral head

Long head,
triceps brachii m.

Accessory head,
long head,
triceps brachii m.

Joint capsule
and nerve retracted

F

Approach to the Craniomedial Region of the Shoulder Joint

Based on a Procedure of Hohn et al[23]

INDICATIONS

1. Exposure of the biceps brachii tendon and intertubercular groove.
2. Open reduction of medial shoulder luxations.
3. Open reduction of fractures of the neck and glenoid cavity of the scapula.
4. Open reduction of fractures of the lesser tubercle of the humerus.

ALTERNATIVE APPROACH

The craniolateral approach to the shoulder with acromial osteotomy (see Plate 26) may provide better exposure for open reduction of lateral shoulder luxations and fractures of the neck and glenoid cavity of the scapula. However, if transposition of the biceps brachii tendon is needed for stabilization of a luxating shoulder, then a combined craniomedial approach (see Plate 30) and cranial approach (see Plate 32) with osteotomy of the greater tubercle is recommended.

PATIENT POSITIONING

The animal is in dorsal recumbency (see Plate 30A) with the forelimb suspended for draping (see Figure 2).

DESCRIPTION OF THE PROCEDURE

A. Palpate the cranial border and acromion of the scapula and the greater tubercle and diaphysis of the humerus. The skin incision starts medial and slightly cranial to the acromion of the scapula. It continues distally, medial to the midline of the humerus, and ends at the midshaft of this bone.
B. After incision and retraction of the subcutaneous tissues with the skin, the brachiocephalicus muscle is identified. This muscle is retracted medially, following a fascial incision along its lateral border for the entire length of the exposure. The omobrachial vein is ligated to allow this incision.
C. The limb is externally rotated and the insertion of the superficial pectoral muscle is freed from the humerus from its proximal border distally to the cephalic vein, which crosses the muscle. This muscle will not be reattached at its insertion; therefore it can be cut very close to the bone.

PLATE 30

Approach to the Craniomedial Region of the Shoulder Joint

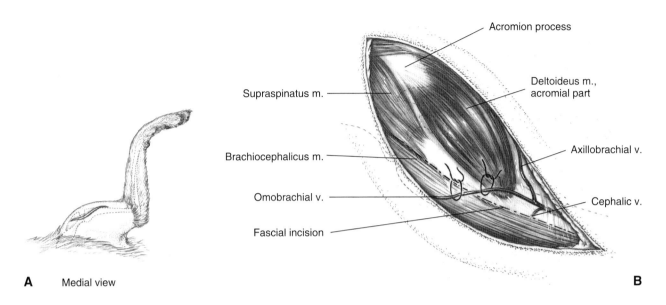

Supraspinatus m.

Brachiocephalicus m.

Omobrachial v.

Fascial incision

Acromion process

Deltoideus m., acromial part

Axillobrachial v.

Cephalic v.

A   Medial view

B

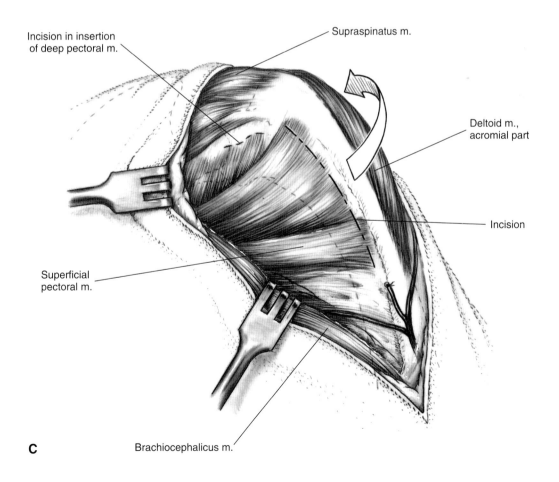

Incision in insertion of deep pectoral m.

Supraspinatus m.

Deltoid m., acromial part

Incision

Superficial pectoral m.

Brachiocephalicus m.

C

Approach to the Craniomedial Region of the Shoulder Joint *continued*

D. The deep pectoral is similarly incised to free its entire insertion. After separating the fascial attachments between the supraspinatus and the deep pectoral, both pectoral muscles are retracted medially. When separating the deep pectoral from the supraspinatus muscle, be aware of the position of the suprascapular nerve (see Plate 32A). The tendon of the coracobrachialis muscle is transected near its origin. This exposes the tendon of insertion of the subscapularis muscle on the lesser tubercle of the humerus.

PLATE 30

Approach to the Craniomedial Region of the Shoulder Joint *continued*

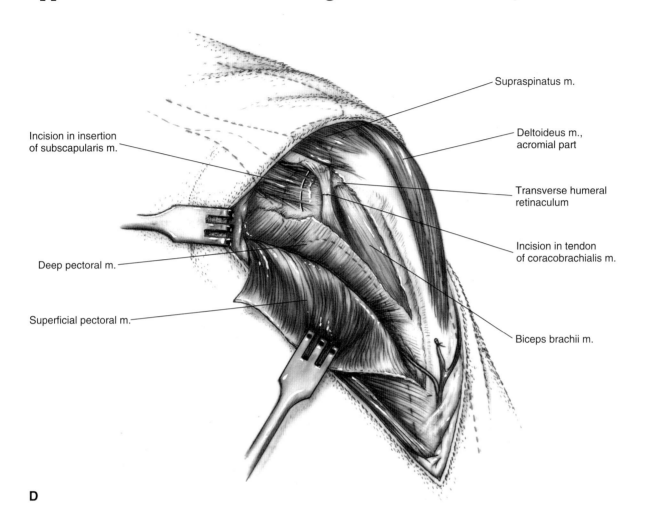

Supraspinatus m.

Incision in insertion
of subscapularis m.

Deltoideus m.,
acromial part

Transverse humeral
retinaculum

Deep pectoral m.

Incision in tendon
of coracobrachialis m.

Superficial pectoral m.

Biceps brachii m.

D

Approach to the Craniomedial Region of the Shoulder Joint *continued*

E. The tendinous insertion of the subscapularis muscle on the lesser tubercle of the humerus is transected close to the bone, but enough tendon is left on the bone to allow suturing. The joint capsule is incised parallel to the medial rim of the glenoid cavity. Retraction of the belly of the subscapularis muscle exposes the medial joint capsule, which is incised as needed to gain access to the interior of the joint.

ADDITIONAL EXPOSURE

Further exposure of the neck and glenoid cavity of the scapula and the humeral head is obtained by combining this craniomedial approach with the cranial (see Plate 32) and craniolateral (see Plate 26) approaches.

The entire proximal two thirds of the humerus is exposed for fracture reduction and application of a cranial plate by combining this craniomedial approach with the craniolateral approach to the humerus (see Plate 34).

CLOSURE

The joint capsule is sutured with 2-0 or 3-0 interrupted absorbable sutures. Mattress sutures of 0 or 2-0 nonabsorbable material are used to reattach the tendon of the subscapularis muscle. Both pectoral muscles are advanced cranially to attach to deltoideus and deep brachial fascia. The brachiocephalicus muscle is sutured to brachial fascia, and subcutaneous tissues are closed in layers.

PLATE 30

Approach to the Craniomedial Region of the Shoulder Joint *continued*

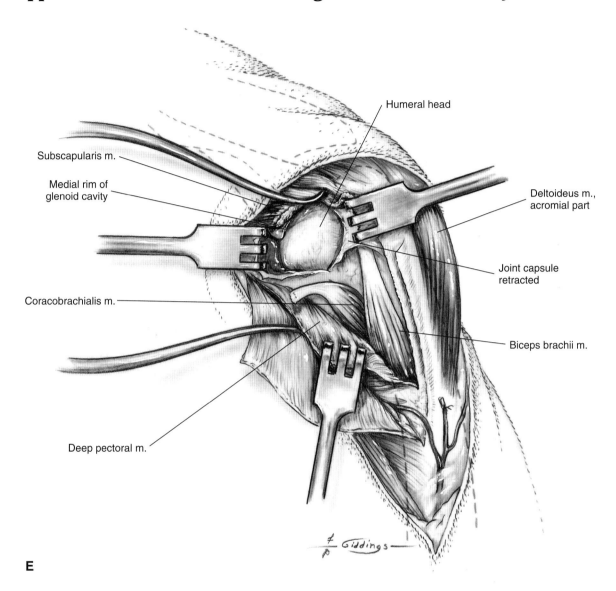

Subscapularis m.

Medial rim of
glenoid cavity

Coracobrachialis m.

Deep pectoral m.

Humeral head

Deltoideus m.,
acromial part

Joint capsule
retracted

Biceps brachii m.

E

Approach to the Medial Region of the Shoulder Joint

INDICATIONS

1. Open reduction of medial shoulder luxation.
2. Open reduction of fractures of the neck and glenoid cavity of the scapula.
3. Open reduction of fractures of the lesser tubercle of the humerus.

PATIENT POSITIONING

The animal is in dorsal recumbency (see Plate 31A) with the forelimb suspended for draping (see Figure 2).

DESCRIPTION OF THE PROCEDURE

A. Palpate the cranial border of the scapula and the greater tubercle and diaphysis of the humerus. The skin incision starts on the cranial border of the scapula and extends slightly caudomedial to the greater tubercle of the humerus. It continues distally, medial to the midline of the humerus, and ends at the midshaft of this bone.

B. After incision and retraction of the subcutaneous tissues with the skin, the brachiocephalicus muscle is identified. This muscle is retracted laterally, following a fascial incision along its craniomedial border for the entire length of the exposure.

PLATE 31
Approach to the Medial Region of the Shoulder Joint

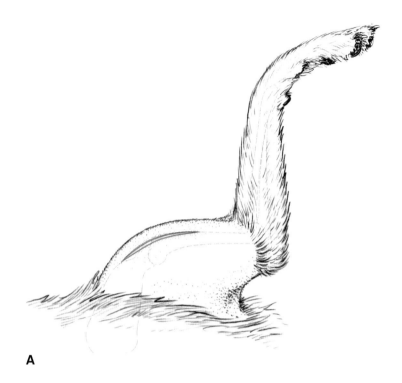

A

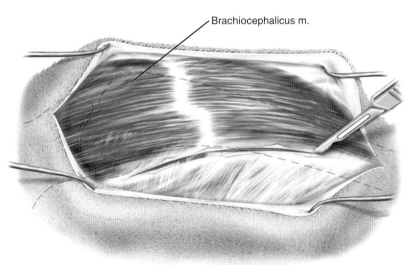

Brachiocephalicus m.

B

Approach to the Medial Region of the Shoulder Joint *continued*

C. The limb is externally rotated, and the insertion of the superficial pectoral muscle is freed from the humerus from its proximal border distally to the cephalic vein, which crosses the muscle. This muscle will not be reattached at its insertion; therefore it can be cut very close to the bone.

D. The deep pectoral is similarly incised to free its entire insertion. After separating the fascial attachments between the supraspinatus and the deep pectoral, both pectoral muscles are retracted medially. When separating the deep pectoral from the supraspinatus muscle, be aware of the position of the suprascapular nerve (see Plate 32A). The biceps brachii and coracobrachialis muscles are identified and retracted cranially. This exposes the tendon of insertion of the subscapularis muscle on the lesser tubercle of the humerus.

PLATE 31

Approach to the Medial Region of the Shoulder Joint *continued*

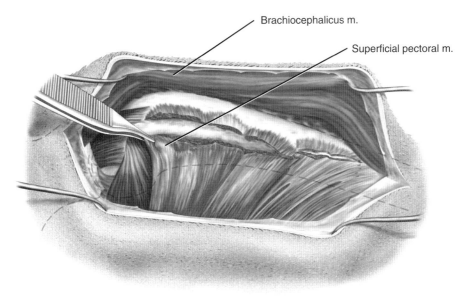

Brachiocephalicus m.

Superficial pectoral m.

C

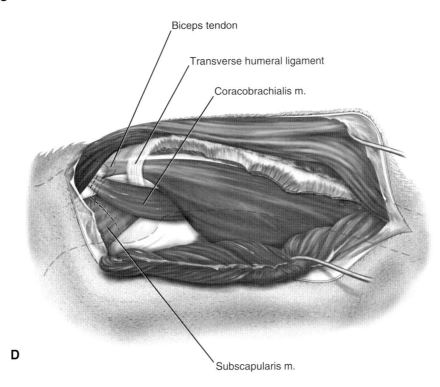

Biceps tendon

Transverse humeral ligament

Coracobrachialis m.

Subscapularis m.

D

Approach to the Medial Region of the Shoulder Joint *continued*

E. The tendinous insertion of the subscapularis muscle on the lesser tubercle of the humerus is transected close to the bone, but enough tendon is left on the bone to allow suturing. Proximally, retraction of the belly of the subscapularis muscle exposes the medial joint capsule, which is incised as needed to gain access to the interior of the joint. Great care should be taken to preserve the two components of the medial glenohumeral ligament. Transection of this ligament destabilizes the shoulder joint and can result in subluxation of the shoulder.

CLOSURE

The joint capsule is sutured with 2-0 or 3-0 interrupted absorbable sutures. Mattress sutures of 0 or 2-0 nonabsorbable material are used to reattach the tendon of the subscapularis muscle. Both pectoral muscles are advanced cranially to attach to deltoideus and deep brachial fascia. The brachiocephalicus muscle is sutured to brachial fascia, and subcutaneous tissues are closed in layers.

PLATE 31

Approach to the Medial Region of the Shoulder Joint *continued*

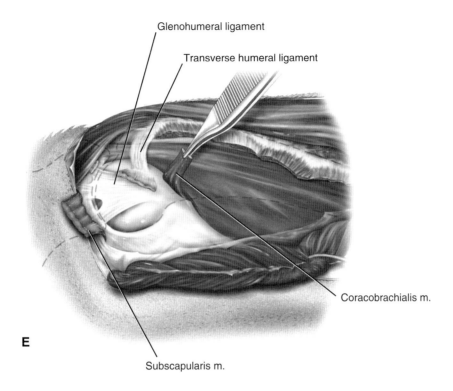

Glenohumeral ligament

Transverse humeral ligament

Coracobrachialis m.

E

Subscapularis m.

Approach to the Cranial Region of the Shoulder Joint

Based on a Procedure of De Angelis and Schwartz[10]

INDICATIONS

1. Open reduction of cranial luxations of the shoulder.
2. Open reduction of fractures of the neck and glenoid of the scapula.
3. Open reduction of fractures of the head of the humerus.
4. Arthrodesis of the shoulder.

EXPLANATORY NOTE

The procedure is initiated as shown in Plate 30A-D.

DESCRIPTION OF THE PROCEDURE

A, B. Following elevation and retraction of the superficial and deep pectoral muscles, the fascial attachments between the deep pectoral and supraspinatus muscles are divided sufficiently to allow retraction of the supraspinatus. An osteotome is used to osteotomize the greater tubercle containing the tendinous insertion of the supraspinatus muscle. Note that the cut is made at two different angles to better resist the shearing forces of muscle pull after reattachment. Care must be taken to not cut the tendinous insertion of the infraspinatus muscle and to protect the tendon of the biceps muscle during the osteotomy.

PLATE 32
Approach to the Cranial Region of the Shoulder Joint

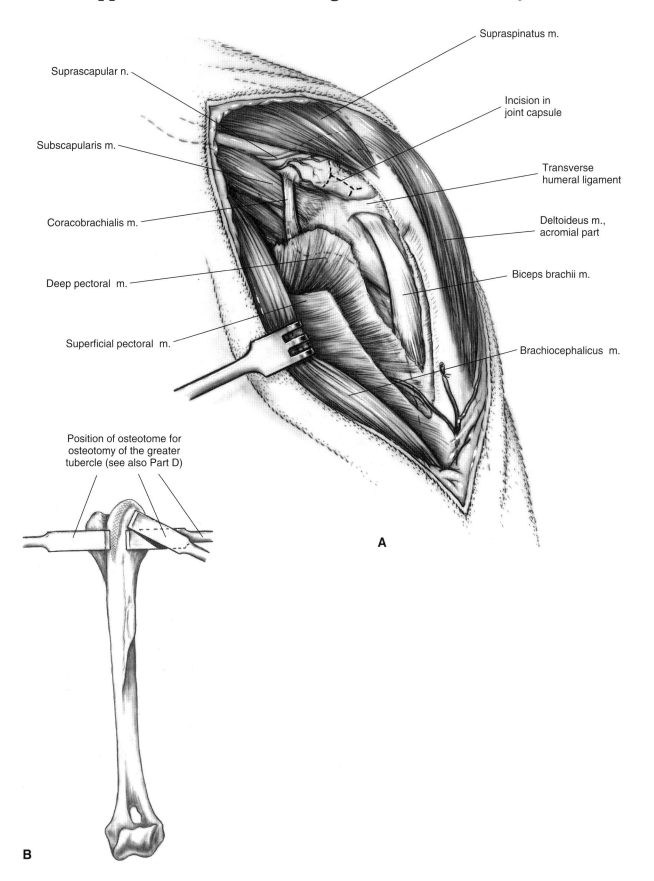

Suprascapular n.

Subscapularis m.

Coracobrachialis m.

Deep pectoral m.

Superficial pectoral m.

Supraspinatus m.

Incision in
joint capsule

Transverse
humeral ligament

Deltoideus m.,
acromial part

Biceps brachii m.

Brachiocephalicus m.

Position of osteotome for
osteotomy of the greater
tubercle (see also Part D)

A

B

Approach to the Cranial Region of the Shoulder Joint *continued*

C.   The supraspinatus muscle can now be reflected proximally and dorsally after dissecting it free of the joint capsule. Continued elevation of the muscle from the scapula will expose the scapular neck and glenoid. Identify and protect the suprascapular nerve (also see Plate 26E).

ADDITIONAL EXPOSURE

For total exposure of the scapular neck and most of the glenoid cavity, the cranial approach is combined with the approach to the craniolateral region of the shoulder (see Plate 26).

For arthrodesis of the shoulder joint and stabilization with a cranial plate, this cranial approach is combined with the craniodorsal exposure of the scapular spine (see Plate 25), craniolateral approach to the shoulder (see Plate 26), and craniolateral approach to the shaft of the humerus (see Plate 34).

CLOSURE

The greater tubercle is reattached with two lag screws or two Kirschner wires of 0.045- to 0.062-inch diameter as shown in Plate 32D. The superficial and deep pectoral muscles are sutured to the fascia of the deltoideus muscle. The remaining fascial layers, subcutaneous tissues, and skin are closed separately.

PLATE 32

Approach to the Cranial Region of the Shoulder Joint *continued*

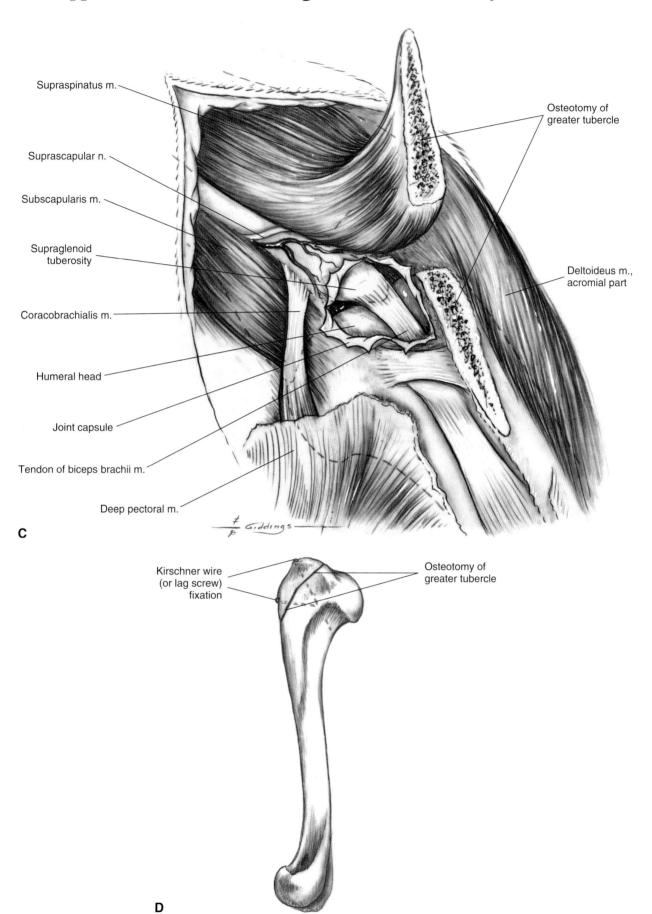

Supraspinatus m.

Suprascapular n.

Subscapularis m.

Supraglenoid tuberosity

Coracobrachialis m.

Humeral head

Joint capsule

Tendon of biceps brachii m.

Deep pectoral m.

Osteotomy of greater tubercle

Deltoideus m., acromial part

C

Kirschner wire (or lag screw) fixation

Osteotomy of greater tubercle

D

SECTION 5

The Forelimb

■ **Approach to the Proximal Shaft and Trochlear Notch of the Ulna**

■ **Approach to the Tuber Olecrani**

■ **Approach to the Distal Shaft and Styloid Process of the Ulna**

■ **Approach to the Head and Proximal Metaphysis of the Radius**

■ **Approach to the Shaft of the Radius Through a Medial Incision**

■ **Approach to the Shaft of the Radius Through a Lateral Incision**

■ **Approach to the Distal Radius and Carpus Through a Dorsal Incision**

■ **Approach to the Distal Radius and Carpus Through a Palmaromedial Incision**

■ **Approach to the Accessory Carpal Bone and Palmarolateral Carpal Joints**

■ **Approaches to the Metacarpal Bones**

■ **Approach to the Proximal Sesamoid Bones**

■ **Approaches to the Phalanges and Interphalangeal Joints**

Approach to the Proximal Shaft of the Humerus

INDICATIONS

Open reduction of fractures of the proximal half of the shaft of the humerus.

ALTERNATIVE APPROACH

Medial exposure of the proximal shaft of the humerus is obtained with the approach to the craniomedial region of the shoulder (see Plate 30). For greater exposure distally, the cephalic vein is ligated where it disappears under the caudal edge of the brachiocephalicus muscle. The insertions of superficial pectoral and deep pectoral muscles are incised along their entire lengths on the humerus.

PATIENT POSITIONING

Lateral recumbency with the affected limb uppermost.

DESCRIPTION OF THE PROCEDURE

A. Identify the acromion process, greater tubercle of the humerus, and deltoid tuberosity by palpation. The skin incision is made slightly lateral to the cranial midline of the bone and extends from the greater tubercle of the humerus distally to a point near the midshaft of the bone, just beyond the deltoid tuberosity.
B. Following undermining and retraction of the skin, an incision is made through the deep fascia along the lateral border of the brachiocephalicus muscle. The insertion of the acromial part of the deltoideus muscle is also incised.

PLATE 33

Approach to the Proximal Shaft of the Humerus

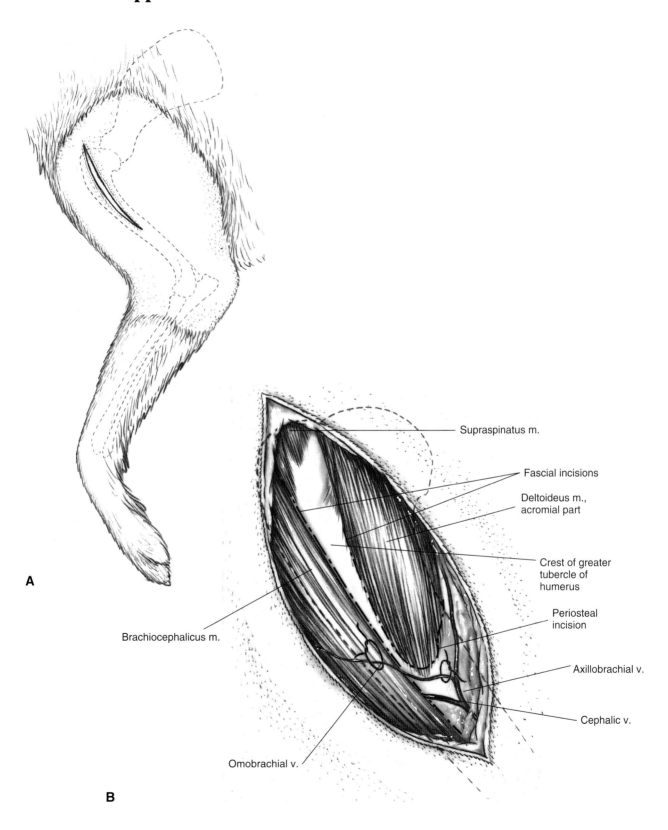

A

B

Supraspinatus m.

Fascial incisions

Deltoideus m.,
acromial part

Crest of greater
tubercle of
humerus

Periosteal
incision

Axillobrachial v.

Cephalic v.

Brachiocephalicus m.

Omobrachial v.

Approach to the Proximal Shaft of the Humerus *continued*

C. The brachiocephalicus can be retracted cranially following blunt dissection between the muscle and the bone. The deltoideus muscle is retracted caudally to reveal the tendons of insertion of the teres minor and infraspinatus muscles. If more exposure of bone is needed, the insertions of the superficial pectoral muscle and the lateral head of the triceps muscle can be incised.

D. Periosteal elevation of the lateral head of the triceps exposes the lateral and caudal aspects of the shaft. If the craniomedial shaft must be exposed, a portion of the insertion of the deep pectoral muscle can be elevated. This muscle insertion is just medial to that of the superficial pectoral muscle.

ADDITIONAL EXPOSURE

Proximal extension of this approach to the cranial region of the shoulder, with osteotomy of the greater tubercle of the humerus, provides total exposure of the scapular neck and most of the glenoid cavity (see Plate 32).

Medial extension of this approach to the craniomedial region of the shoulder (see Plate 30) provides exposure of the tendon of origin of the biceps brachii muscle, supraglenoid tuberosity, and medial aspect of the humeral head.

Distal extension of this approach to the shaft of the humerus, through a craniolateral incision (see Plate 34), provides good exposure of the proximal two thirds of the humerus.

The entire length of the humerus is exposed from the craniolateral aspect by the combination of the craniolateral approaches to the proximal (see Plate 33), middle (see Plate 34), and distal (see Plate 37) portions of the humerus. The brachialis muscle and radial nerve cover the humeral shaft distally and need to be protected and retracted.

CLOSURE

The deep pectoral and triceps muscles are not reattached because they are only partially elevated and will reattach to the periosteum by fibrosis. The external fasciae of the superficial pectoral and deltoideus muscles are sutured to each other over the cranial border of the bone. The deep fascia is reattached to the edge of the brachiocephalicus muscle, followed by closure of the subcutaneous tissues and skin.

PLATE 33

Approach to the Proximal Shaft of the Humerus *continued*

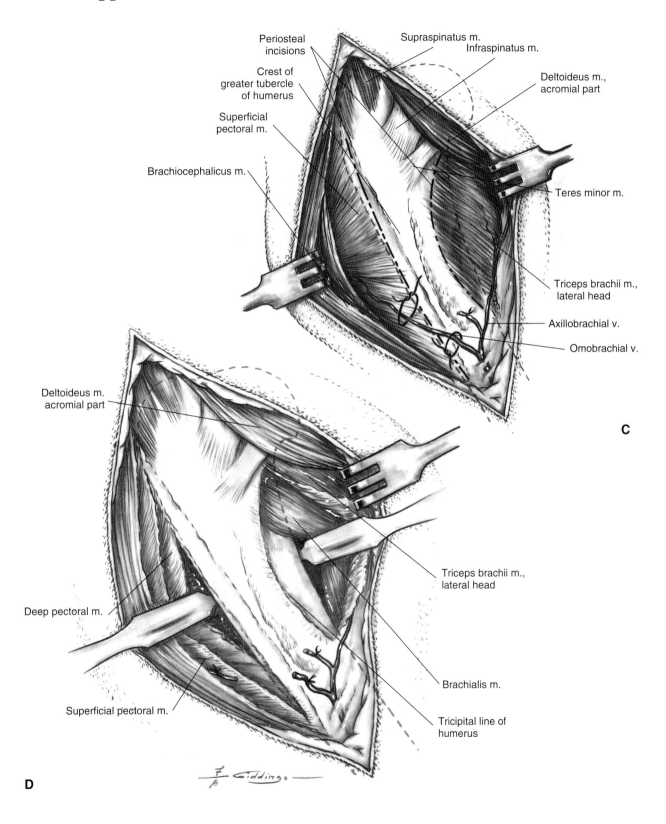

Periosteal
incisions

Crest of
greater tubercle
of humerus

Superficial
pectoral m.

Brachiocephalicus m.

Supraspinatus m.

Infraspinatus m.

Deltoideus m.,
acromial part

Teres minor m.

Triceps brachii m.,
lateral head

Axillobrachial v.

Omobrachial v.

C

Deltoideus m.
acromial part

Deep pectoral m.

Superficial pectoral m.

Triceps brachii m.,
lateral head

Brachialis m.

Tricipital line of
humerus

D

Approach to the Midshaft of the Humerus Through a Craniolateral Incision

INDICATION

Internal fixation of midshaft fractures of the humerus.

ALTERNATIVE APPROACH

The approach to the shaft of the humerus through a medial incision is an alternative (see Plate 35). It provides exposure of the entire diaphysis of the humerus that may be valuable for bone plate application.

PATIENT POSITIONING

Lateral recumbency with the affected limb uppermost.

DESCRIPTION OF THE PROCEDURE

A. Palpate the greater tubercle, deltoid tuberosity, and lateral epicondyle of the humerus. The skin incision extends from the greater tubercle of the humerus proximally to the lateral epicondyle distally, following the craniolateral border of the humerus.
B. Subcutaneous fat and fascia are incised on the same line and mobilized and retracted with the skin. Fat and brachial fascia are incised and dissected away to allow visualization of the cephalic vein. Brachial fascia is incised along the lateral border of the brachiocephalicus muscle and distally over the cephalic vein. The cephalic vein is ligated at the distal end of the field and again proximally, where it disappears under the edge of the brachiocephalicus muscle. The axillobrachial and omobrachial veins are similarly ligated and the isolated venous segment is removed. An incision is made in the craniomedial fascia of the brachialis muscle and in the insertion of the lateral head of the triceps brachii on the humerus.

PLATE 34

Approach to the Midshaft of the Humerus Through a Craniolateral Incision

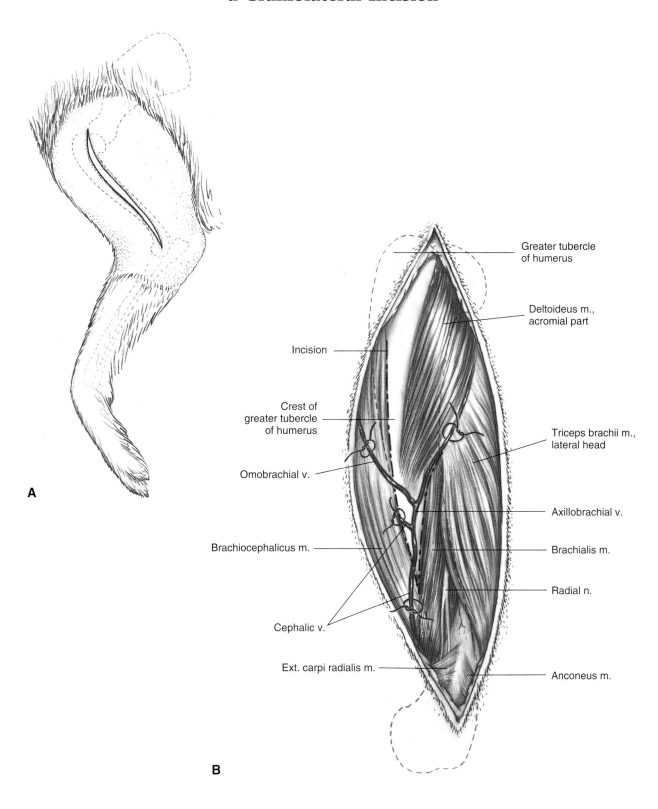

A

B

Greater tubercle
of humerus

Deltoideus m.,
acromial part

Incision

Crest of
greater tubercle
of humerus

Triceps brachii m.,
lateral head

Omobrachial v.

Axillobrachial v.

Brachiocephalicus m.

Brachialis m.

Radial n.

Cephalic v.

Ext. carpi radialis m.

Anconeus m.

Approach to the Midshaft of the Humerus Through a Craniolateral Incision *continued*

C. An incision is next made in the periosteal insertion of the superficial pectoral and brachiocephalicus muscles on the humeral shaft. The radial nerve overlying the brachialis muscle should be identified and protected when making these incisions.

D. Hohmann retractors are used to retract the brachialis and triceps muscles caudally and expose the musculospiral groove of the humerus. Cranial retraction will elevate the biceps brachii, superficial pectoral, and brachiocephalicus muscles from the shaft. Again, the radial nerve must be protected during retraction. Avoid continuation of dissection farther distally between the brachialis and brachiocephalicus muscles because the superficial branch of the radial nerve may be inadvertently damaged. For additional exposure of the humerus distally, retract the brachialis muscle and radial nerve cranially (see Plate 37E).

ADDITIONAL EXPOSURE

Based on a procedure of Wallace and Berg,[51] and a procedure of Newton.[31] Greater visualization of the distal shaft of the humerus can be obtained by transection of the brachialis muscle, with the transected muscle being used as a physiologic retractor of the radial nerve, its preservation being paramount.

Extension of this approach more proximally with subperiosteal elevation of the acromial head of the deltoideus muscle (see Plate 33) provides good exposure of the proximal two thirds of the humerus.

More distal exposure of the humeral shaft can be obtained by cranial retraction of the brachialis muscle and radial nerve (see Plate 37E).

The entire length of the humerus is exposed by the combination of the craniolateral approaches to the proximal (see Plate 33), middle (see Plate 34), and distal (see Plate 37) portions of the humerus. The brachialis muscle and radial nerve cover the humeral shaft distally and need to be protected and retracted.

CLOSURE

The insertions of the superficial pectoral and brachiocephalicus muscles are sutured to the superficial fascia of the brachialis muscle distally and to the deltoideus muscle proximally. The insertion of the lateral head of the triceps is attached to the brachiocephalicus. Brachial fascia, subcutaneous fat and fascia, and skin are closed in separate layers.

PRECAUTIONS

The brachialis muscle and overlying radial nerve cover the distal one third of the humeral shaft and need to be protected and gently retracted.

PLATE 34

Approach to the Midshaft of the Humerus Through a Craniolateral Incision *continued*

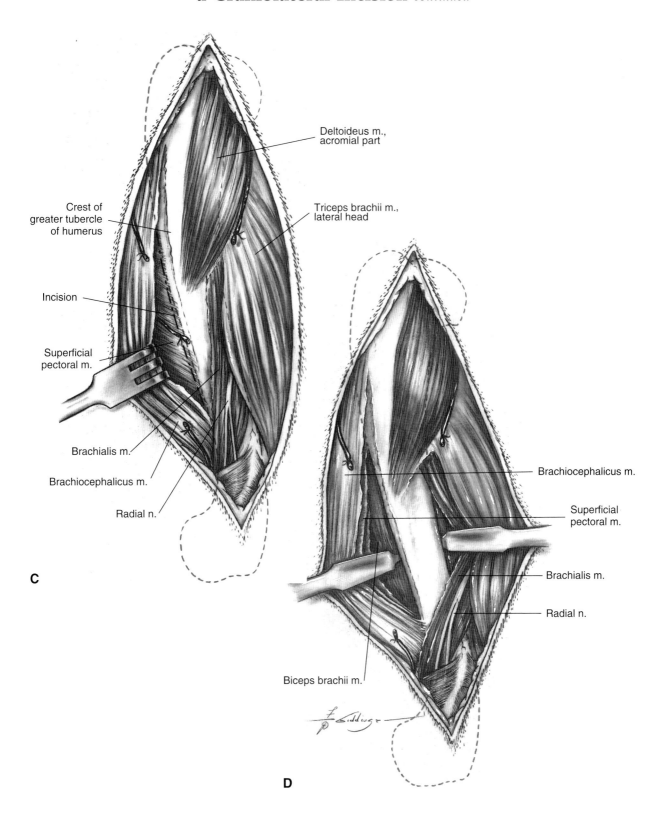

Deltoideus m., acromial part

Crest of greater tubercle of humerus

Triceps brachii m., lateral head

Incision

Superficial pectoral m.

Brachialis m.

Brachiocephalicus m.

Radial n.

C

Brachiocephalicus m.

Superficial pectoral m.

Brachialis m.

Radial n.

Biceps brachii m.

D

Approach to the Shaft of the Humerus Through a Medial Incision

Based on a Procedure of Montgomery, Milton, and Mann[29]

INDICATION

Open reduction and internal fixation of midshaft fractures of the humerus.

ALTERNATIVE APPROACH

This approach through a medial incision allows visualization of the entire shaft of the humerus, which is valuable when applying a bone plate to a highly comminuted fracture. As an alternative, more limited exposure is obtained with the craniolateral approach to the midshaft (see Plate 34), the distal shaft (see Plate 37), or a combination of both. Lateral exposure of the distal one third of the shaft is impaired by the overlying brachialis muscle and radial nerve.

PATIENT POSITIONING

Dorsal recumbency with the affected limb abducted and suspended for draping.

DESCRIPTION OF THE PROCEDURE

A. Identify by palpation the greater tubercle and medial epicondyle of the humerus. The medial skin incision begins proximally at the level of the greater tubercle and extends distally to the medial epicondyle. Subcutaneous fat and fascia are incised on the same line and retracted with the skin.
B. Deep brachial fascia is incised along the cranial border of the brachiocephalicus muscle and along the distal border of the superficial pectoral muscle. The distal part of this incision is made carefully to preserve the underlying neurovascular structures.
C. Fascia distal to the superficial pectoral muscle is carefully dissected from the vessels and nerves. The brachiocephalicus muscle is retracted cranially to expose the insertion of the superficial pectoral muscle on the shaft of the humerus. This insertion is incised close to the bone, beginning at the distal border of the muscle and extending proximally to the level of the cephalic vein.

PLATE 35

Approach to the Shaft of the Humerus Through a Medial Incision

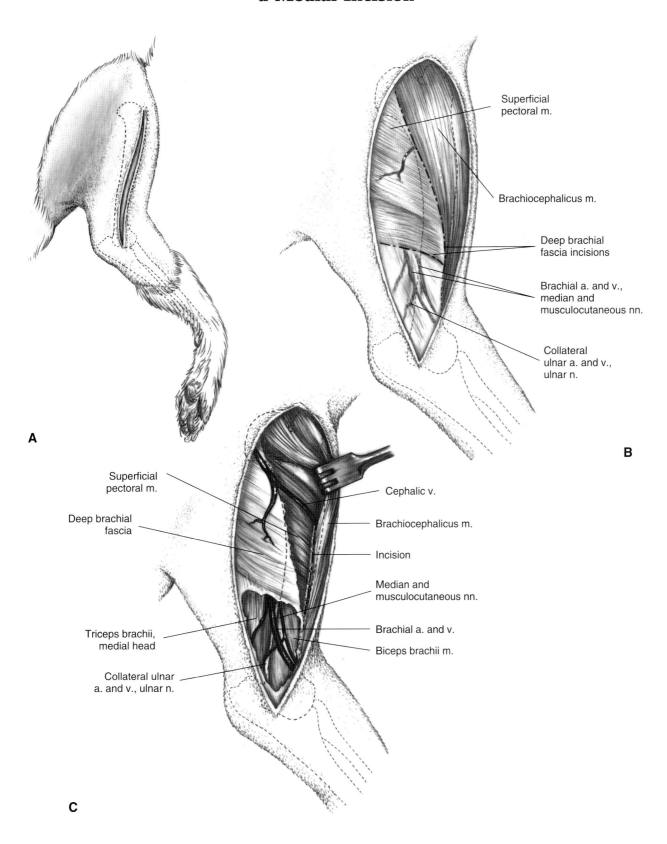

Superficial
pectoral m.

Brachiocephalicus m.

Deep brachial
fascia incisions

Brachial a. and v.,
median and
musculocutaneous nn.

Collateral
ulnar a. and v.,
ulnar n.

A

B

Superficial
pectoral m.

Deep brachial
fascia

Triceps brachii,
medial head

Collateral ulnar
a. and v., ulnar n.

Cephalic v.

Brachiocephalicus m.

Incision

Median and
musculocutaneous nn.

Brachial a. and v.

Biceps brachii m.

C

Approach to the Shaft of the Humerus Through a Medial Incision *continued*

D. The superficial pectoral incision is extended into the muscle, parallel to the cephalic vein, by blunt dissection between muscle fibers. The aponeurosis from the superficial part of the deep pectoral muscle is incised along the shaft of the humerus and retracted, exposing the underlying biceps brachii muscle.

PLATE 35

Approach to the Shaft of the Humerus Through a Medial Incision *continued*

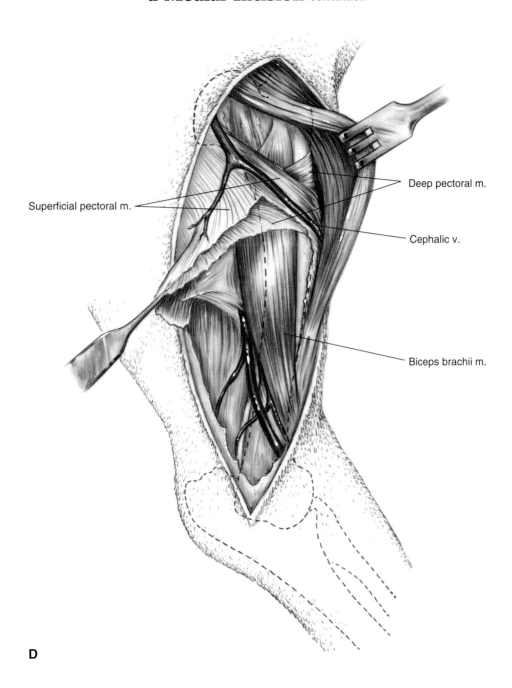

Superficial pectoral m.

Deep pectoral m.

Cephalic v.

Biceps brachii m.

D

Approach to the Shaft of the Humerus Through a Medial Incision *continued*

E. Exposure of the proximal portion and midportion of the bone is optimal if the brachiocephalicus muscle is retracted cranially and the biceps brachii muscle is retracted caudally. Flexion of the elbow joint will facilitate caudal retraction of the biceps brachii muscle. The remaining attached portion of the superficial pectoral muscle is retracted as necessary, and bone plates are placed under it. If essential, the cephalic vein can be ligated and the entire insertion of the muscle incised.

PLATE 35

Approach to the Shaft of the Humerus Through a Medial Incision *continued*

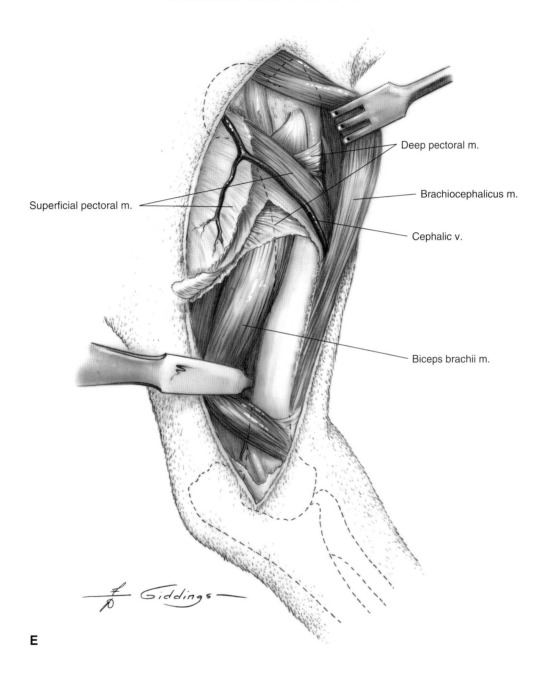

Superficial pectoral m.

Deep pectoral m.

Brachiocephalicus m.

Cephalic v.

Biceps brachii m.

E

Approach to the Shaft of the Humerus Through a Medial Incision *continued*

F. The middle and distal regions of the humerus are best exposed by cranial retraction of the biceps brachii muscle, which requires careful dissection along the caudal border of the muscle to separate it from the neurovascular structures. The proximal and distal branches of the musculocutaneous nerve must be protected where they penetrate the muscle.

ADDITIONAL EXPOSURE

More proximal exposure of the intertubercular groove, lesser tubercle, and medial side of the head of the humerus can be obtained by transecting the insertion of the deep pectoral muscle on the greater tubercle (see Plate 32A). The transverse humeral ligament is transected and retraction of the tendon of the biceps brachii muscle from the intertubercular groove is facilitated by flexion of the elbow.

Additional distal exposure is obtained in combination with the approach to the distal shaft and supracondylar region of the humerus through a medial incision (see Plate 38). These two approaches are not completely continuous but are interrupted by the brachial artery and vein and musculocutaneous and median nerves (see Plate 35F). These must be protected and retracted caudally for the midshaft approach (see Plate 35F) and cranially for the more distal exposure (see Plate 38C and D).

CLOSURE

The superficial pectoral muscle is sutured to its insertion or to the fascia of the brachialis muscle. The deep fascial incisions are closed, followed by subcutaneous fat and fascia and skin.

PRECAUTIONS

The brachial artery and vein and musculocutaneous and median nerves cross the medial surface of the distal humerus caudal to the biceps brachii muscle.

PLATE 35

Approach to the Shaft of the Humerus Through a Medial Incision *continued*

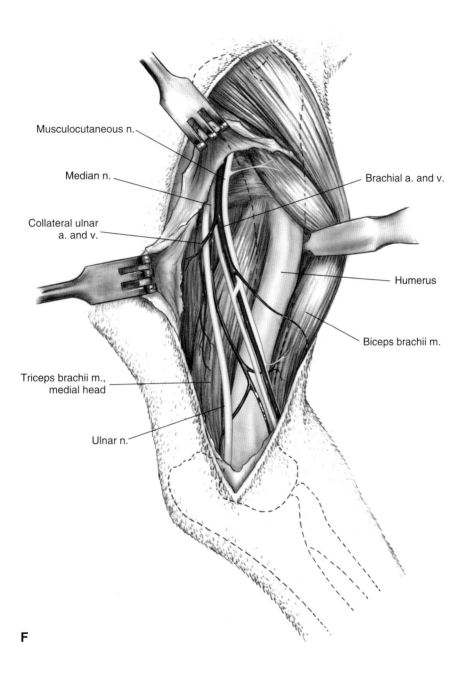

Musculocutaneous n.

Median n.

Collateral ulnar
a. and v.

Brachial a. and v.

Humerus

Biceps brachii m.

Triceps brachii m.,
medial head

Ulnar n.

F

Minimally Invasive Approach to the Shaft of the Humerus

Based on a Procedure of Déjardin and Guiot[11]

INDICATION

Minimally invasive plate osteosynthesis of fractures involving the midshaft and supracondylar regions of the humerus.

ALTERNATIVE APPROACH

The alternative minimally invasive approach is a combination of exposure of the craniolateral part of the proximal humerus (Plate 33) with the lateral approach to the humeral condyle and epicondyle (Plate 39). This lateral approach is valuable when applying an interlocking nail, but the contouring of a bone plate to the lateral epicondyle of the humerus is more difficult than it is for the medial epicondyle.

PATIENT POSITIONING

Dorsal recumbency with the affected limb suspended for draping (see Plate 36A).

DESCRIPTION OF THE PROCEDURE

The magnitude of exposure has been intentionally enlarged in the following descriptive illustrations, to highlight the relevant features of the surgical anatomy. Once familiar with the anatomy, the field of dissection and exposure can be reduced by at least 50% to obtain a true minimally invasive approach to the humerus.

A. The patient is positioned in dorsal recumbency with the affected limb suspended for draping. This position permits two orthogonal fluoroscopic images to be obtained before making the surgical approach, as well as during the surgical procedure.

PLATE 36
Minimally Invasive Approach to the Shaft of the Humerus

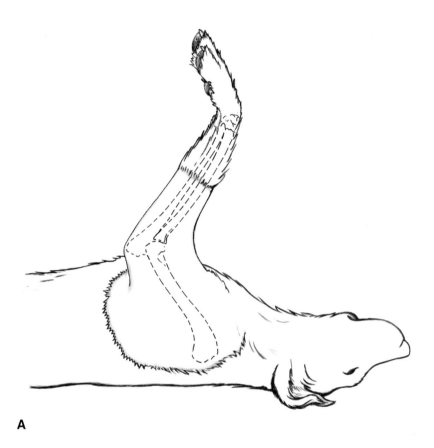

A

Minimally Invasive Approach to the Shaft of the Humerus *continued*

B. The limb is abducted, and the distal approach is commenced with a skin incision that is centered over the caudal aspect of the medial epicondyle of the humerus.

C. The skin margins are mobilized and retracted. The antebrachial fascia is incised to expose the caudal and distal aspect of the medial epicondyle.

PLATE 36

Minimally Invasive Approach to the Shaft of the Humerus *continued*

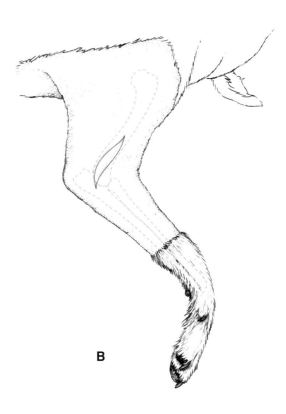

B

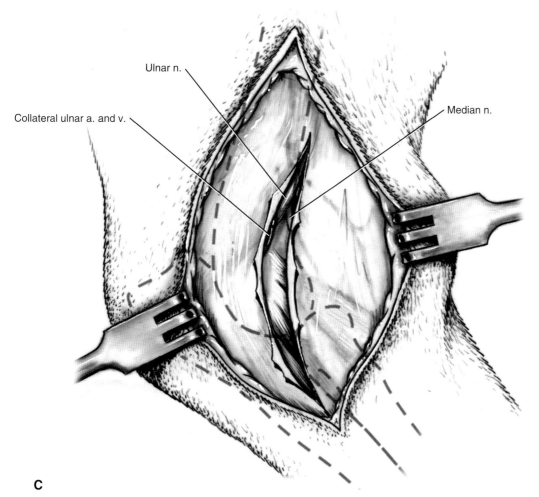

Ulnar n.

Collateral ulnar a. and v.

Median n.

C

Minimally Invasive Approach to the Shaft of the Humerus *continued*

D. The medial head of the triceps muscle and the ulnar nerve are mobilized and retracted caudally. The median nerve is not exposed, but care is taken to preserve it. If required, the origin of the superficial digital flexor muscle on the medial epicondylar ridge is partially transected by a few millimeters to expose the distal edge of the bone for intramedullary pin insertion.

E. A blunt instrument, such as the soft-tissue retractor illustrated here, is passed along the medial side of the humeral shaft to create an epiperiosteal tunnel. The tunnel is directed toward the craniomedial surface of the proximal part of the humerus.

PLATE 36

Minimally Invasive Approach to the Shaft of the Humerus *continued*

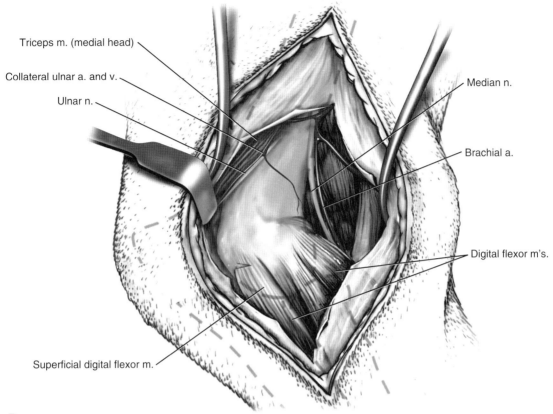

Triceps m. (medial head)

Collateral ulnar a. and v.

Ulnar n.

Median n.

Brachial a.

Digital flexor m's.

Superficial digital flexor m.

D

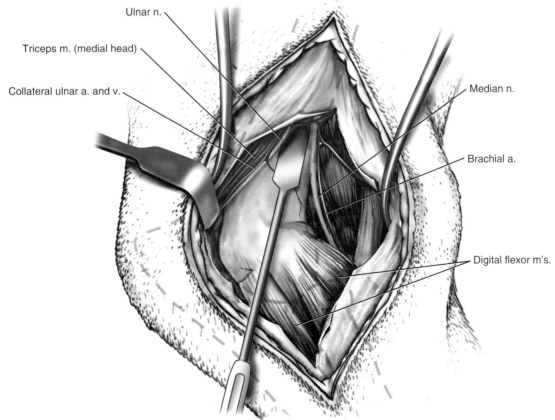

Ulnar n.

Triceps m. (medial head)

Collateral ulnar a. and v.

Median n.

Brachial a.

Digital flexor m's.

E

Minimally Invasive Approach to the Shaft of the Humerus *continued*

F. The second skin incision is made over the craniomedial aspect of the humerus in the region of the insertion of the supraspinatus muscle on the greater tubercle.

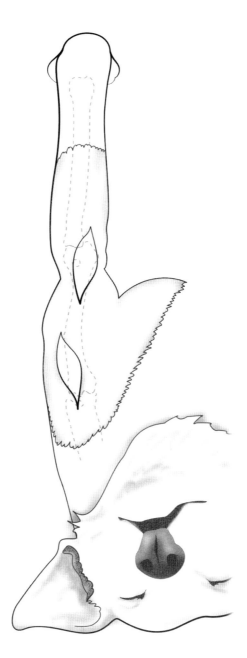

PLATE 36

Minimally Invasive Approach to the Shaft of the Humerus *continued*

F

Minimally Invasive Approach to the Shaft of the Humerus *continued*

G. The incision continues through the subcutaneous fat and the fascia along the caudal edge of the brachiocephalicus muscle.

PLATE 36

Minimally Invasive Approach to the Shaft of the Humerus *continued*

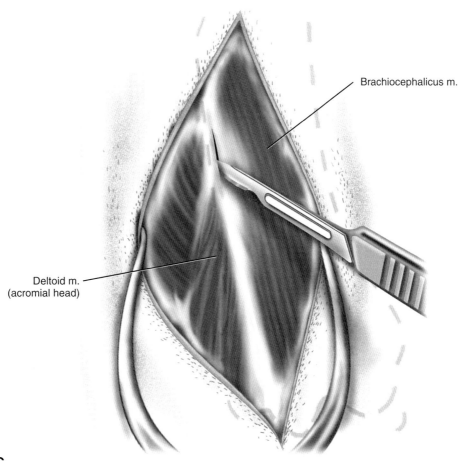

Brachiocephalicus m.

Deltoid m.
(acromial head)

G

Minimally Invasive Approach to the Shaft of the Humerus *continued*

H. The brachiocephalicus muscle is retracted medially, and the origin of the superficial pectoral muscle is incised in the proximal region to allow passage of the soft tissue retractor and completion of the epiperiosteal tunnel.

PLATE 36

Minimally Invasive Approach to the Shaft of the Humerus *continued*

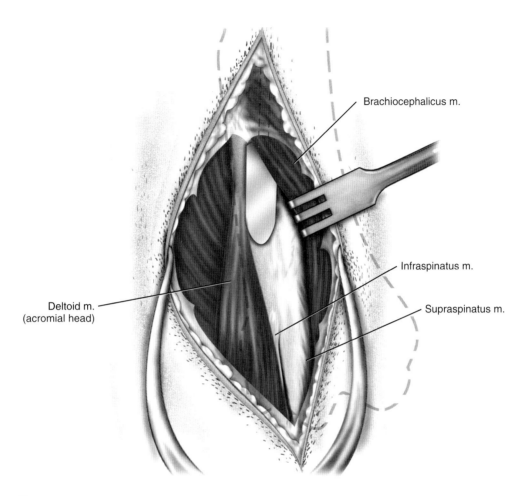

Brachiocephalicus m.

Infraspinatus m.

Supraspinatus m.

Deltoid m.
(acromial head)

H

Minimally Invasive Approach to the Shaft of the Humerus *continued*

I. Overview showing passage of soft tissue retractor from the medial epicondyle to the greater tubercle of the humerus.

ADDITIONAL EXPOSURE

If necessary, the minimally invasive approach to the humerus can be extended to provide complete exposure of the medial aspect of the humerus (Plate 35).

CLOSURE

The distal incision is closed with sutures placed in the brachial fascia and subcutaneous fat, taking care to avoid injury of the ulnar nerve. The proximal incision is closed by suturing the superficial pectoral muscle to the deltoideus muscle. The external fascia of the brachiocephalicus muscle is sutured to brachial fascia. The subcutaneous tissue and skin are closed in layers.

PLATE 36

Minimally Invasive Approach to the Shaft of the Humerus *continued*

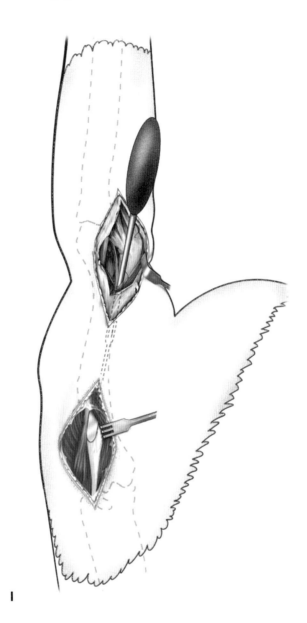

I

Approach to the Distal Shaft of the Humerus Through a Craniolateral Incision

Based on a Procedure of Brinker[4]

INDICATION

Open reduction of fractures between the midshaft and the supracondylar area of the humerus.

ALTERNATIVE APPROACH

The alternative approach through a medial incision to the midshaft (see Plate 35) and distal shaft (see Plate 38) provides exposure to the entire shaft of the humerus, which is valuable when applying a bone plate.

PATIENT POSITIONING

Lateral recumbency with the affected limb uppermost.

DESCRIPTION OF THE PROCEDURE

A. The craniolateral border of the humerus is the guide for this incision, which commences at the midshaft and ends at the lateral epicondyle.
B. The skin margins are mobilized and retracted. Subcutaneous fascia and fat are incised in the same line as the skin, avoiding the cephalic and axillobrachial veins. The deep fascia of the brachium is incised along the cranial border of the triceps. The incision parallels the cephalic and axillobrachial veins to allow their mobilization. The radial nerve must be protected when the distal end of this incision is opened.

PLATE 37
Approach to the Distal Shaft of the Humerus Through a Craniolateral Incision

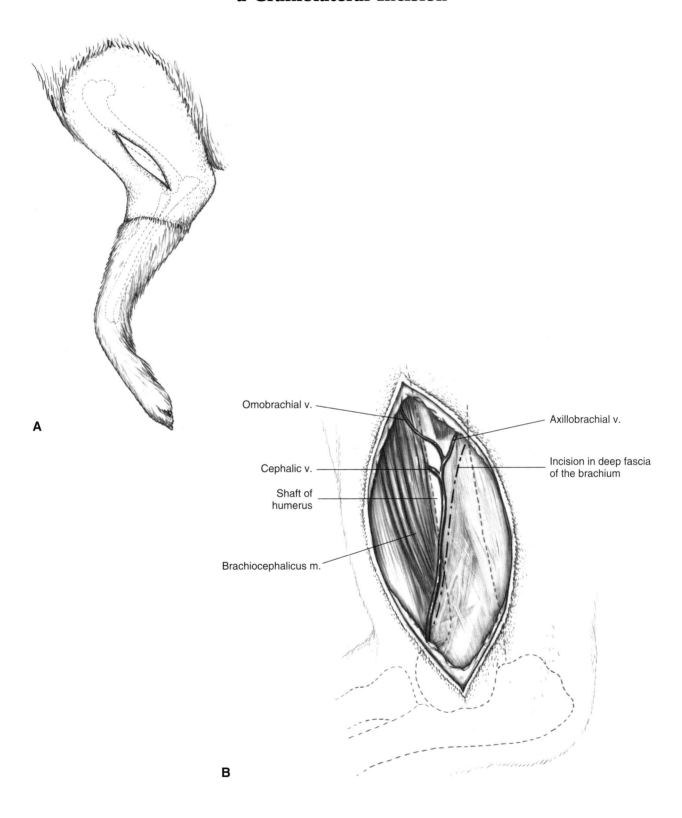

A

Omobrachial v.

Axillobrachial v.

Cephalic v.

Incision in deep fascia
of the brachium

Shaft of
humerus

Brachiocephalicus m.

B

Approach to the Distal Shaft of the Humerus Through a Craniolateral Incision *continued*

C. The deep fascia is undermined to allow cranial retraction of the brachiocephalicus muscle and the cephalic vein and exposure of the radial nerve. An incision is made in the periosteal insertion of the superficial pectoral muscle.

PLATE 37

Approach to the Distal Shaft of the Humerus Through a Craniolateral Incision *continued*

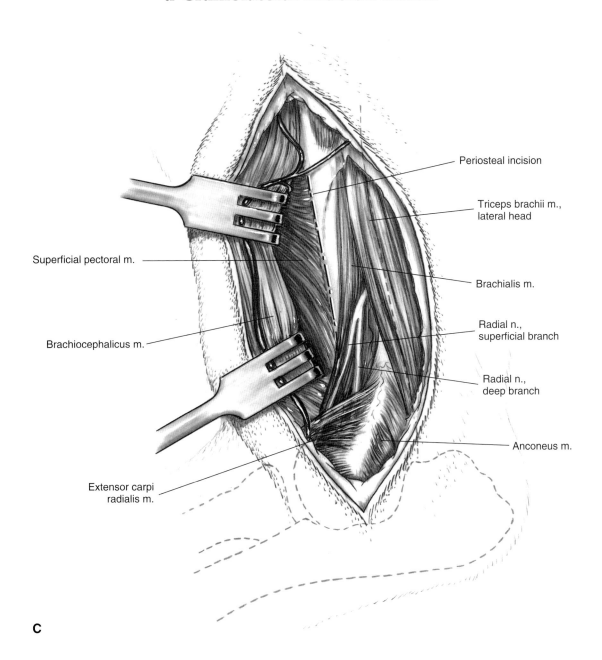

Periosteal incision

Triceps brachii m., lateral head

Superficial pectoral m.

Brachialis m.

Radial n., superficial branch

Brachiocephalicus m.

Radial n., deep branch

Anconeus m.

Extensor carpi radialis m.

C

Approach to the Distal Shaft of the Humerus Through a Craniolateral Incision *continued*

     D. The superficial pectoral muscle is elevated at its insertion on the humerus as necessary to allow cranial retraction. The brachialis muscle is freed from the bone by blunt dissection and is retracted caudally with the triceps and the radial nerve.

PLATE 37

Approach to the Distal Shaft of the Humerus Through a Craniolateral Incision *continued*

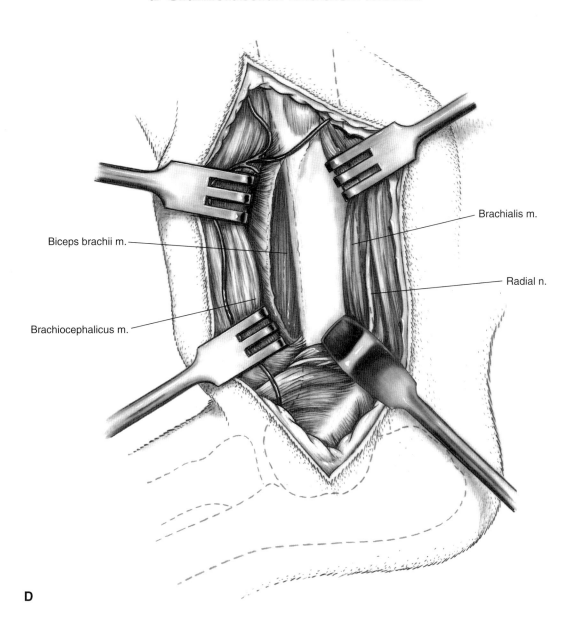

Brachialis m.

Biceps brachii m.

Radial n.

Brachiocephalicus m.

D

Approach to the Distal Shaft of the Humerus Through a Craniolateral Incision *continued*

E. To obtain better exposure of the distal portion of the bone, the lateral head of the triceps brachii muscle can be retracted caudally and the brachialis muscle and radial nerve retracted cranially.

ADDITIONAL EXPOSURE

Proximal extension of this approach through a craniolateral incision provides exposure to the midshaft (see Plate 34) and proximal shaft (see Plate 33) of the humerus.

Distally this approach can be extended to provide exposure of the lateral aspect of the humeral condyle and epicondyle (see Plate 39) or the lateral humeroulnar part of the elbow joint (see Plate 41).

CLOSURE

Interrupted sutures are placed between the external fasciae of the brachialis and brachiocephalicus/superficial pectoral muscles. Deep brachial fascia is attached to the triceps, and subcutaneous tissue and skin are closed in layers.

PRECAUTIONS

As the radial nerve emerges from under the lateral and accessory heads of the triceps muscle, it provides branches innervating the lateral, medial, and accessory heads of this muscle before coursing laterally over the brachialis muscle. Shortly thereafter it bifurcates into the deep branch that innervates the supinator muscle and all the extensor muscles of the carpus and digits, as well as the superficial branch that provides sensory innervation to the dorsum of the paw.

PLATE 37

Approach to the Distal Shaft of the Humerus Through a Craniolateral Incision *continued*

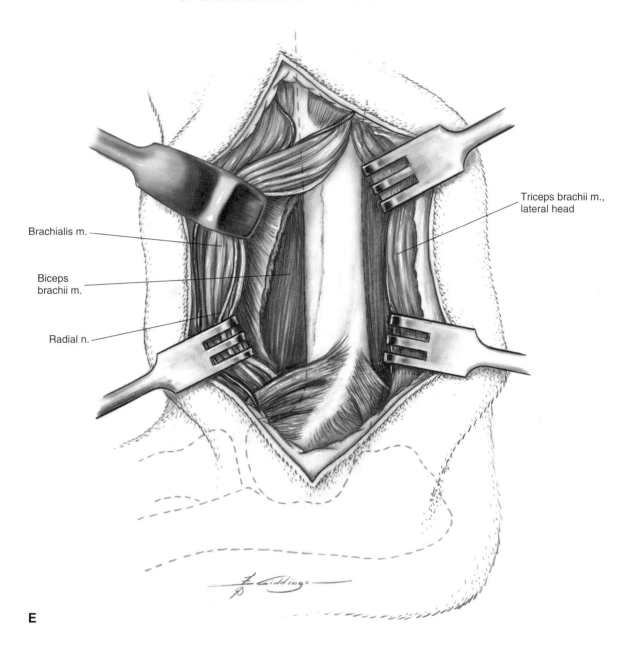

Brachialis m.

Biceps brachii m.

Radial n.

Triceps brachii m., lateral head

E

Approach to the Distal Shaft and Supracondylar Region of the Humerus Through a Medial Incision

Based on a Procedure of Brinker[4]

INDICATION

Open reduction of fractures of the humerus at midshaft or distally.

ALTERNATIVE APPROACHES

The approach to the shaft of the humerus through a medial incision (see Plate 35) is preferred when complete exposure of the midshaft is required.

The approach to the distal shaft of the humerus through a craniolateral incision (see Plate 37) is an alternative, but exposure of the bone is hindered laterally by the overlying radial nerve and brachialis muscle.

PATIENT POSITIONING

Dorsal recumbency with the affected limb abducted and suspended for draping.

DESCRIPTION OF THE PROCEDURE

A. Palpate the greater tubercle and medial epicondyle of the humerus. The skin incision extends from the medial epicondyle proximally along the cranial border of the humerus to the midshaft of the bone.
B. The skin is retracted and the subcutaneous fat is elevated sufficiently to allow visualization of the brachial and collateral ulnar vessels. The ulnar and median nerves that accompany these vessels are not yet visible; they lie slightly deeper. An incision is made in the deep fascia directly over the distal shaft of the humerus and between the blood vessels. It will be necessary to continue the incision proximally over the vessels.
C. Beginning at the medial epicondyle, bluntly dissect the subfascial fat and fascia overlying the humerus to allow initial identification of the ulnar nerve caudally and median nerve cranially.

PLATE 38

Approach to the Distal Shaft and Supracondylar Region of the Humerus Through a Medial Incision

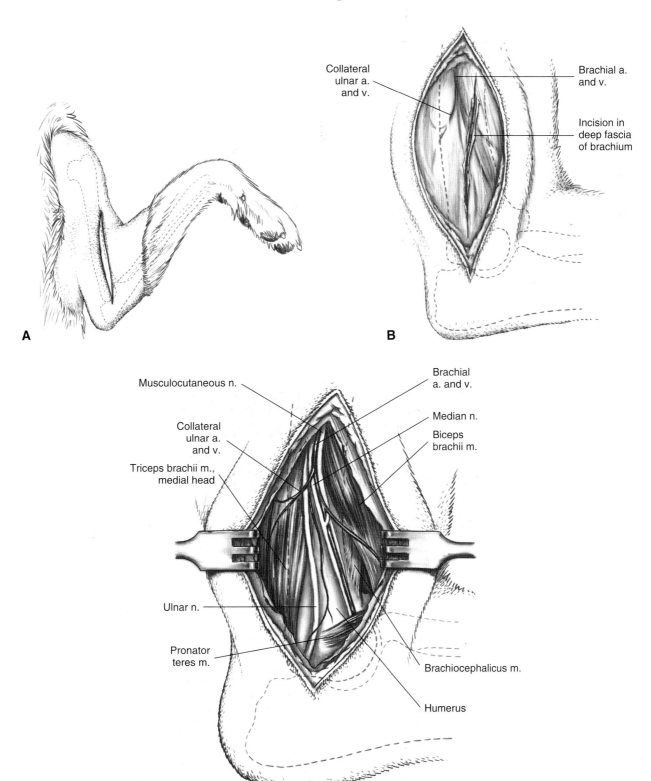

A

B

Collateral ulnar a. and v.

Brachial a. and v.

Incision in deep fascia of brachium

C

Musculocutaneous n.

Collateral ulnar a. and v.

Triceps brachii m., medial head

Ulnar n.

Pronator teres m.

Brachial a. and v.

Median n.

Biceps brachii m.

Brachiocephalicus m.

Humerus

Approach to the Distal Shaft and Supracondylar Region of the Humerus Through a Medial Incision *continued*

D. The manner in which the vessels and the nerves are mobilized depends on the area of the bone that is to be exposed. The method illustrated is used when the distal and supracondylar portions of the humerus are involved. If great care is taken to protect the vessels and nerves, sufficient exposure of the midshaft can be obtained for insertion of the proximal screws in a bone plate. For further exposure of the midshaft of the humerus, the median and musculocutaneous nerves and brachial artery and vein are freed and retracted caudally with the triceps and the collateral ulnar vessels (see Plate 35F).

The biceps brachii and triceps brachii muscles are elevated from the shaft of the bone. The periosteal branches of blood vessels are ligated or coagulated as required. Subperiosteal elevation of a portion of the insertion of the superficial pectoral and brachiocephalicus muscles is necessary to fully expose the cranial surface of the bone.

E. In the cat, retraction of the neurovascular components is complicated by the passage of the brachial artery and median nerve through the supracondylar foramen of the humerus. Note also the short part of the medial head of the triceps brachii muscle running caudal to the medial aspect of the humeral condyle and inserting on the medial side of the olecranon process. If this muscle is elevated to expose a fracture line, care must be taken to protect the ulnar nerve deep to it.

ADDITIONAL EXPOSURE

Proximally, exposure of the medial side of the humerus is limited by the median nerve, which bifurcates from the ulnar nerve about the midshaft of the humerus and then courses craniodistally. Additional proximal exposure can be obtained by combining with the medial approach (see Plate 35), but these two approaches are not continuous. The brachial artery and vein and median and musculocutaneous nerves must be protected and carefully retracted (see Plate 35F).

Distally, exposure can be readily extended by combining with the approach to the medial humeral epicondyle (see Plate 48).

A separate approach to the lateral aspect of the humeral condyle and epicondyle (see Plate 39), in combination with this medial approach (see Plate 38), can be used for open reduction of supracondylar T-Y fractures of the distal humerus.

CLOSURE

The deep fascia, subcutaneous tissues, and skin are closed in separate layers.

PRECAUTIONS

Although this approach provides good exposure of the supracondylar region, a good knowledge of the neurovascular anatomy of the region is imperative.

PLATE 38

Approach to the Distal Shaft and Supracondylar Region of the Humerus Through a Medial Incision *continued*

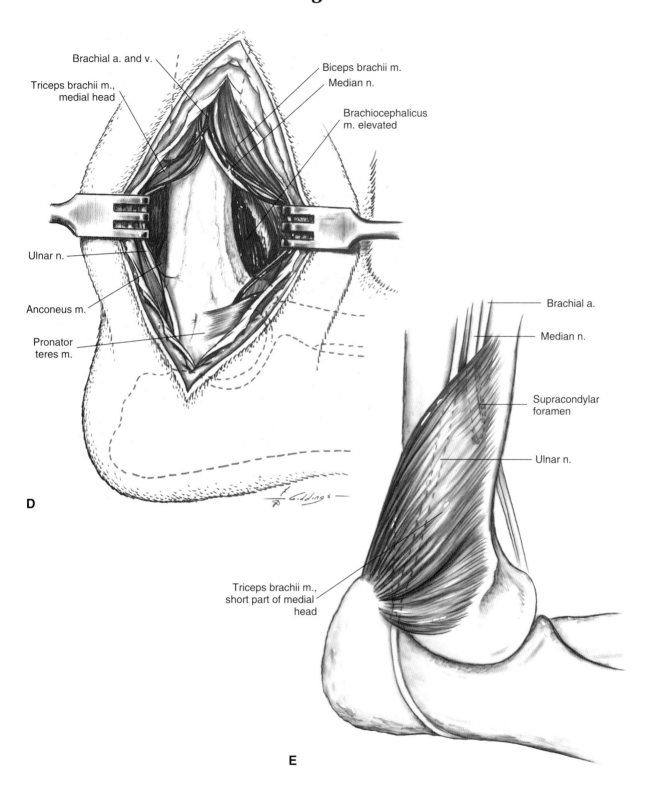

Brachial a. and v.

Triceps brachii m., medial head

Biceps brachii m.

Median n.

Brachiocephalicus m. elevated

Ulnar n.

Anconeus m.

Pronator teres m.

D

Brachial a.

Median n.

Supracondylar foramen

Ulnar n.

Triceps brachii m., short part of medial head

E

Approach to the Lateral Aspect of the Humeral Condyle and Epicondyle in the Dog

Based on a Procedure of Turner and Hohn[49]

INDICATIONS

1. Open reduction of fractures of the humeral condyle.
2. Open reduction of lateral elbow luxation.

ALTERNATIVE APPROACHES

The approaches to the lateral (see Plate 40) and caudal (see Plate 42) humeroulnar parts of the elbow joint are alternatives, but exposure of the humeral articular surface for evaluation of intra-articular fracture reduction is very limited.

PATIENT POSITIONING

Lateral recumbency with the affected limb uppermost.

DESCRIPTION OF THE PROCEDURE

A. Identify the lateral head of triceps muscle, lateral epicondyle, and olecranon by palpation. The skin incision extends along the lower fourth of the humerus and crosses the joint to end distally on the ulna. The incision passes over or slightly caudal to the lateral epicondyle. The subcutaneous fascia is incised on the same line.
B. As the skin and subcutaneous fascia are retracted, the deep brachial and antebrachial fascia and the lateral head of the triceps muscle are exposed. An incision is made through the deep fascia along the cranial border of the triceps and is continued distally over the extensor muscles.

PLATE 39

Approach to the Lateral Aspect of the Humeral Condyle and Epicondyle in the Dog

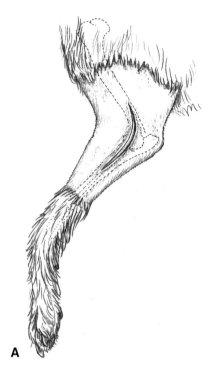

A

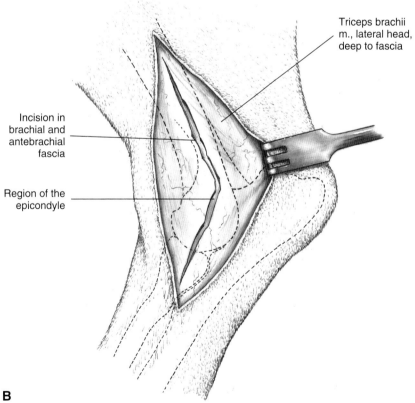

Triceps brachii m., lateral head, deep to fascia

Incision in brachial and antebrachial fascia

Region of the epicondyle

B

Approach to the Lateral Aspect of the Humeral Condyle and Epicondyle in the Dog *continued*

C. Retraction of the fascia exposes the condylar region of the humerus. Although it is proximal to the main area of exposure, it is well to note the location of the radial nerve. An incision is started distally in the intermuscular septum between the extensor carpi radialis and the common digital extensor muscles. This incision continues proximally into the periosteal origin of the lateral half of the extensor carpi radialis muscle on the lateral epicondylar crest of the humerus.

PLATE 39

Approach to the Lateral Aspect of the Humeral Condyle and Epicondyle in the Dog *continued*

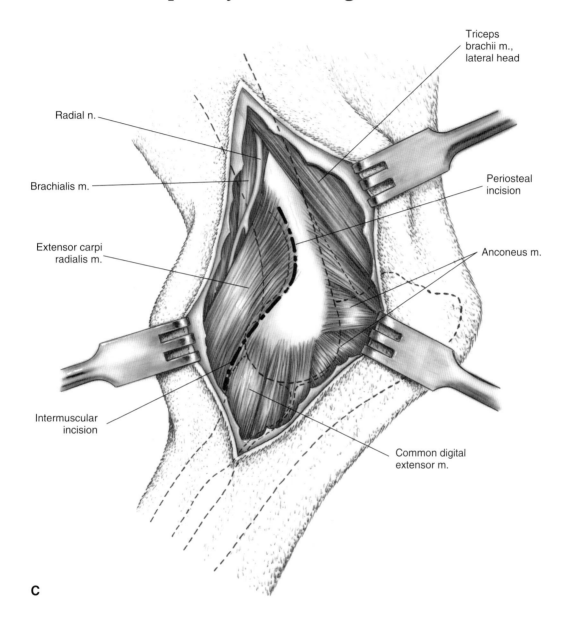

Triceps brachii m., lateral head

Radial n.

Brachialis m.

Extensor carpi radialis m.

Periosteal incision

Anconeus m.

Intermuscular incision

Common digital extensor m.

C

Approach to the Lateral Aspect of the Humeral Condyle and Epicondyle in the Dog *continued*

D. The extensor carpi radialis muscle is elevated from the bone and underlying joint capsule, and the capsule is opened with an L-shaped incision. Care must be taken to protect the articular cartilage of the condyle.
E. Retraction of the joint capsule reveals the humeral condyle.

ADDITIONAL EXPOSURE

Additional proximal exposure is obtained in combination with the approach to the distal shaft of the humerus through a craniolateral incision (see Plate 37).

Additional distal exposure is obtained in combination with the approach to the head of the radius (see Plate 46) or the proximal metaphysis of the radius (see Plate 54).

This lateral approach (see Plate 39) can be used in combination with the medial approach to the distal shaft and supracondylar region of the humerus (see Plate 38) for open reduction of T-Y fractures of the distal humerus to avoid the need for olecranon osteotomy (see Plate 43) or triceps tenotomy (see Plate 44).

CLOSURE

The joint capsule is closed with interrupted sutures. A continuous pattern can be used in the intermuscular incision. If there is no tissue available to reattach the extensor carpi radialis to the humerus, the muscle can be sutured to the external fascia of the anconeus muscle. The brachial and antebrachial fascia is closed with a continuous pattern.

PRECAUTIONS

Although not directly in the field, the radial nerve emerges from under the lateral head of the triceps muscle and runs obliquely craniodistal on the brachialis muscle. It bifurcates into superficial and deep branches that cross the flexor surface of the elbow medial to the origin of the extensor carpi radialis muscle.

PLATE 39

Approach to the Lateral Aspect of the Humeral Condyle and Epicondyle in the Dog *continued*

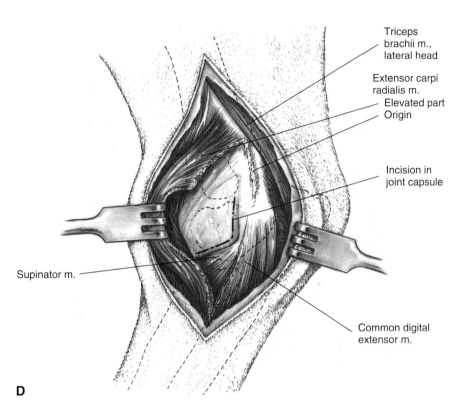

Triceps brachii m., lateral head

Extensor carpi radialis m.
Elevated part
Origin

Incision in joint capsule

Supinator m.

Common digital extensor m.

D

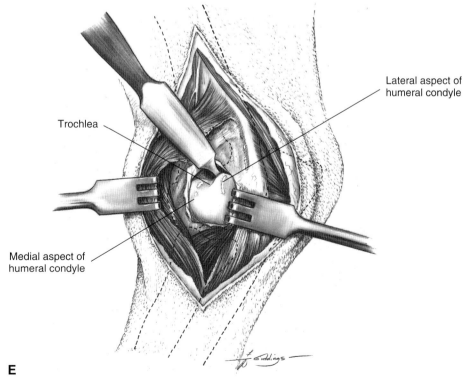

Lateral aspect of humeral condyle

Trochlea

Medial aspect of humeral condyle

E

Approach to the Lateral Aspect of the Humeral Condyle and Epicondyle in the Cat

INDICATIONS

1. Open reduction of fractures of the humeral condyle.
2. Open reduction of lateral elbow luxation.

PATIENT POSITIONING

Lateral recumbency with the affected limb uppermost.

DESCRIPTION OF THE PROCEDURE

Although the steps in this approach for the cat are similar to those followed in the dog (Plate 39), the lateral head of the triceps muscle is relatively larger and overlies the lateral epicondyle of the humerus in the cat.

A. Identify the lateral head of triceps muscle, lateral epicondyle, and olecranon by palpation. The skin incision extends along the lower fourth of the humerus and crosses the joint to end distally on the ulna. The incision passes over the lateral epicondyle. The subcutaneous fascia is incised on the same line.

B. As the skin and subcutaneous fascia are retracted, the deep brachial and antebrachial fascia and the lateral head of the triceps muscle are exposed. An incision is made through the deep fascia along the cranial border of the triceps and is continued distally over the extensor muscles. It may be necessary to partially transect some of the insertion of the lateral head of the triceps muscle on the lateral surface of the olecranon.

PLATE 40

Approach to the Lateral Aspect of the Humeral Condyle and Epicondyle in the Cat

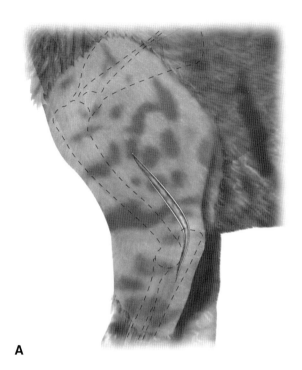

A

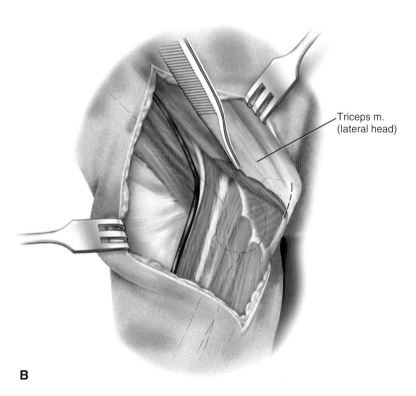

Triceps m.
(lateral head)

B

Approach to the Lateral Aspect of the Humeral Condyle and Epicondyle in the Cat *continued*

C. Retraction of the lateral head of the triceps muscle exposes the condylar region of the humerus. Although it is proximal to the main area of exposure, it is well to note the location of the radial nerve. An incision is started distally in the intermuscular septum between the extensor carpi radialis and the common digital extensor muscles. This incision continues proximally into the periosteal origin of the extensor carpi radialis muscle on the lateral epicondylar crest of the humerus.

D. The extensor carpi radialis muscle is elevated from the bone and underlying joint capsule, and the capsule is opened with an L-shaped incision. Care must be taken to protect the articular cartilage of the condyle. Retraction of the joint capsule reveals the humeral condyle.

CLOSURE

The joint capsule is closed with interrupted sutures. A continuous pattern can be used in the intermuscular incision. If there is no tissue available to reattach the extensor carpi radialis to the humerus, the muscle can be sutured to the external fascia of the anconeus muscle. The brachial and antebrachial fascia is closed with a continuous pattern.

PRECAUTIONS

Although not directly in the field, the radial nerve emerges from under the lateral head of the triceps muscle and runs obliquely craniodistal on the brachialis muscle. It bifurcates into superficial and deep branches that cross the flexor surface of the elbow medial to the origin of the extensor carpi radialis muscle.

PLATE 40

Approach to the Lateral Aspect of the Humeral Condyle and Epicondyle in the Cat *continued*

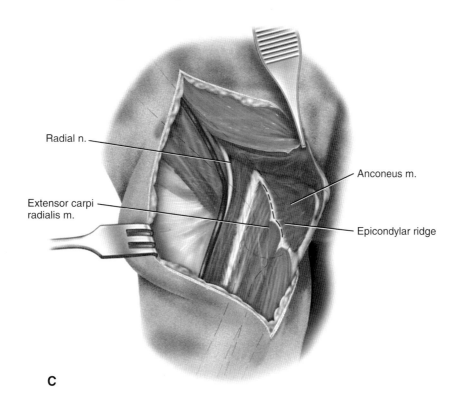

Radial n.

Anconeus m.

Extensor carpi radialis m.

Epicondylar ridge

C

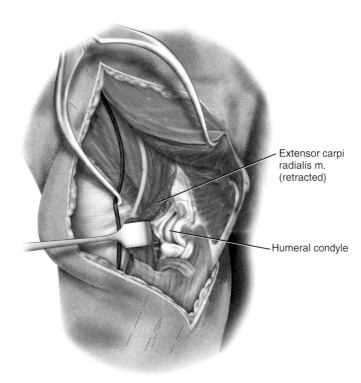

Extensor carpi radialis m. (retracted)

Humeral condyle

D

Approach to the Lateral Humeroulnar Part of the Elbow Joint

Based on a Procedure of Snavely and Hohn[46]

INDICATIONS

1. Excision or fixation of an ununited anconeal process.
2. Open reduction of lateral elbow luxation.

ALTERNATIVE APPROACHES

Alternative approaches through a lateral incision provide exposure of the lateral aspect of the condyle and epicondyle (see Plate 39) and the caudal humeroulnar joint compartment (see Plate 42).

PATIENT POSITIONING

Lateral recumbency with the affected limb uppermost.

DESCRIPTION OF THE PROCEDURE

A. The skin incision is centered on the lateral humeral epicondyle, which is easily palpated. The incision curves to follow the lateral epicondylar crest and the proximal radius.
B. Subcutaneous fascia is incised on the same line as the skin. The fascia of the brachium is incised along the cranial border of the lateral head of the triceps brachii to its insertion on the olecranon.

PLATE 41

Approach to the Lateral Humeroulnar Part
of the Elbow Joint

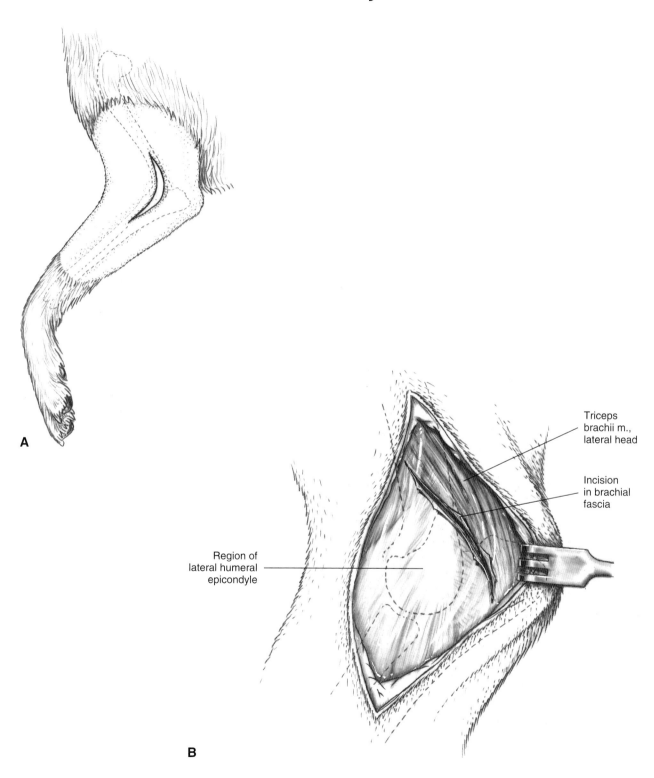

A

Triceps
brachii m.,
lateral head

Incision
in brachial
fascia

Region of
lateral humeral
epicondyle

B

Approach to the Lateral Humeroulnar Part of the Elbow Joint *continued*

    C. Elevation of the triceps brachii exposes the anconeus muscle, which is incised at its periosteal origin on the lateral epicondylar crest.

    D. Subperiosteal elevation of the origin of the anconeus muscle exposes the caudolateral compartment of the elbow and the anconeal process of the ulna.

ADDITIONAL EXPOSURE

Additional proximal exposure is obtained in combination with the approach to the distal shaft of the humerus through a craniolateral incision (see Plate 37).

    Additional distal exposure is obtained in combination with the approach to the head of the radius (see Plate 46).

    This lateral approach (see Plate 41) can be used in combination with the medial approach to the distal shaft and supracondylar region of the humerus (see Plate 38) for open reduction of T-Y fractures of the distal humerus to avoid the need for olecranon osteotomy (see Plate 43) or triceps tenotomy (see Plate 44).

CLOSURE

The origin of the anconeus muscle is sutured to the origins of the extensor muscles of the antebrachium. The fascia of the triceps brachii, subcutaneous fascia, and skin are closed in separate layers.

PRECAUTIONS

Although not directly in the field, the radial nerve emerges from under the lateral head of the triceps muscle and runs obliquely craniodistal on the brachialis muscle. It bifurcates into superficial and deep branches that cross the flexor surface of the elbow medial to the origin of the extensor carpi radialis muscle.

PLATE 41

Approach to the Lateral Humeroulnar Part
of the Elbow Joint *continued*

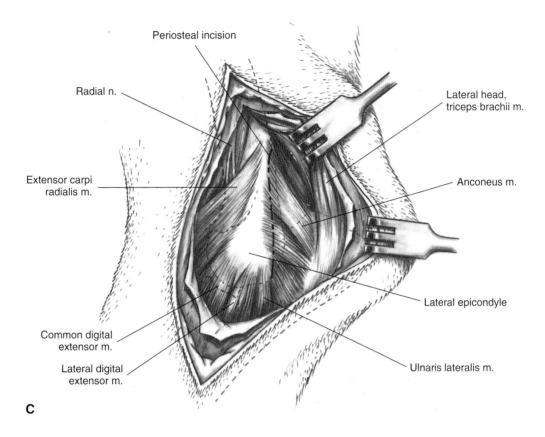

Periosteal incision

Radial n.

Extensor carpi
radialis m.

Common digital
extensor m.

Lateral digital
extensor m.

Lateral head,
triceps brachii m.

Anconeus m.

Lateral epicondyle

Ulnaris lateralis m.

C

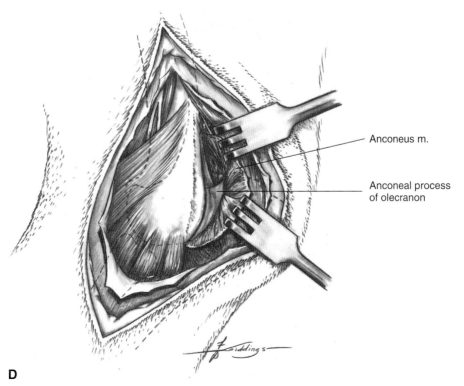

Anconeus m.

Anconeal process
of olecranon

D

Approach to the Supracondylar Region of the Humerus and the Caudal Humeroulnar Part of the Elbow Joint

Based on a Procedure of Chalman and Slocum[8]

INDICATIONS

1. Reduction of supracondylar or lateral condylar fractures of the humerus (see Comment).
2. Reduction of lateral luxation of the elbow joint.
3. Excision or fixation of an ununited anconeal process.

ALTERNATIVE APPROACHES

Other approaches through a lateral incision provide exposure of the lateral aspect of the condyle and epicondyle (see Plate 39) or lateral compartment of the humeroulnar joint (see Plate 41). Exposure of the anconeal process is inferior to that obtained with the caudal approach (see Plate 42).

Approaches to the humeroulnar compartment by olecranon osteotomy (see Plate 43), triceps tenotomy (see Plate 44), and proximal ulnar osteotomy (see Plate 45) provide much greater exposure of the caudal aspect of the humeral condyle, which may be useful in the reduction of chronic elbow luxation.

PATIENT POSITIONING

Lateral recumbency with the affected limb uppermost.

DESCRIPTION OF THE PROCEDURE

A. The skin incision starts just distal to the midshaft of the humerus and follows the caudal edge of the bone distally. At the level of the lateral humeral epicondyle, the incision curves between the epicondylar crest and the tuber olecrani and continues distally along the ulna.
B. Subcutaneous fat and fascia are incised on the same line as the skin and then elevated from the deep brachial fascia to allow wide retraction of the skin margins. An incision is made in the deep brachial fascia over the division between the long and lateral heads of the triceps brachii muscle. This incision is slightly caudal and roughly parallel to the shaft of the humerus. Distally, it extends into the tendon of insertion of the lateral head of the triceps brachii muscle on the tuber olecrani, where a few millimeters of tendon are left on the olecranon to facilitate closure.

PLATE 42

Approach to the Supracondylar Region of the Humerus and the Caudal Humeroulnar Part of the Elbow Joint

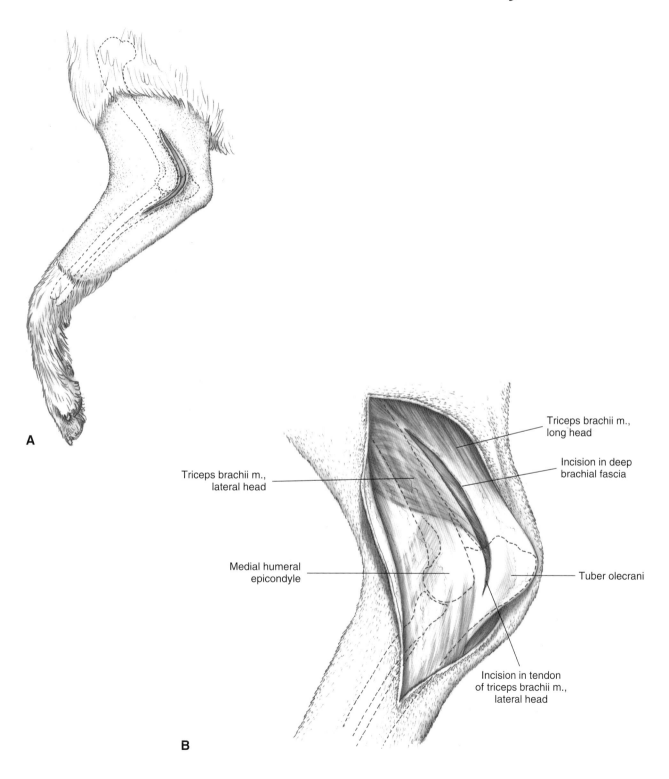

A

Triceps brachii m., long head

Incision in deep brachial fascia

Triceps brachii m., lateral head

Medial humeral epicondyle

Tuber olecrani

Incision in tendon of triceps brachii m., lateral head

B

Approach to the Supracondylar Region of the Humerus and the Caudal Humeroulnar Part of the Elbow Joint *continued*

C. The separation between the heads of the triceps is developed by blunt dissection; it is limited by the collateral radial vessels and a muscular branch of the radial nerve proximally and by the tuber olecrani distally. Blunt dissection is also used to separate the long head of the triceps brachii muscle from the underlying anconeus muscle. The periosteal insertions of the anconeus muscle on the tuber olecrani and medial epicondylar crest are incised.

D. Retraction of the elevated anconeus muscle and the long head of the triceps brachii muscle exposes the anconeal process, the lateral aspect of the humeral condyle, and the supracondylar region of the humerus. A variation is elevation of the anconeus muscle from the lateral epicondylar crest, similar to that shown in Plate 41C and D.

ADDITIONAL EXPOSURE

Proximal extension of this approach is not possible because the muscular branches of the radial nerve supply the lateral head of the triceps muscle (see Plate 42C).

Additional distal exposure to the proximal shaft of the ulna is obtained in combination with the approach to the tuber olecrani (see Plate 52).

CLOSURE

The anconeus muscle is sutured to fascia and remnants of periosteum on the medial epicondylar crest and ulna. The deep antebrachial fascia and tendon of insertion of the triceps brachii muscle are closed in the next layer. Subcutaneous tissues and skin are closed in two layers.

PRECAUTIONS

As the radial nerve emerges from under the lateral and accessory heads of the triceps muscle, it provides branches innervating the lateral, medial, and accessory heads of this muscle before coursing laterally over the brachialis muscle.

COMMENT

This approach is particularly useful for supracondylar fractures, where it may eliminate the need for a combined medial and lateral approach.

PLATE 42

Approach to the Supracondylar Region of the Humerus and the Caudal Humeroulnar Part of the Elbow Joint *continued*

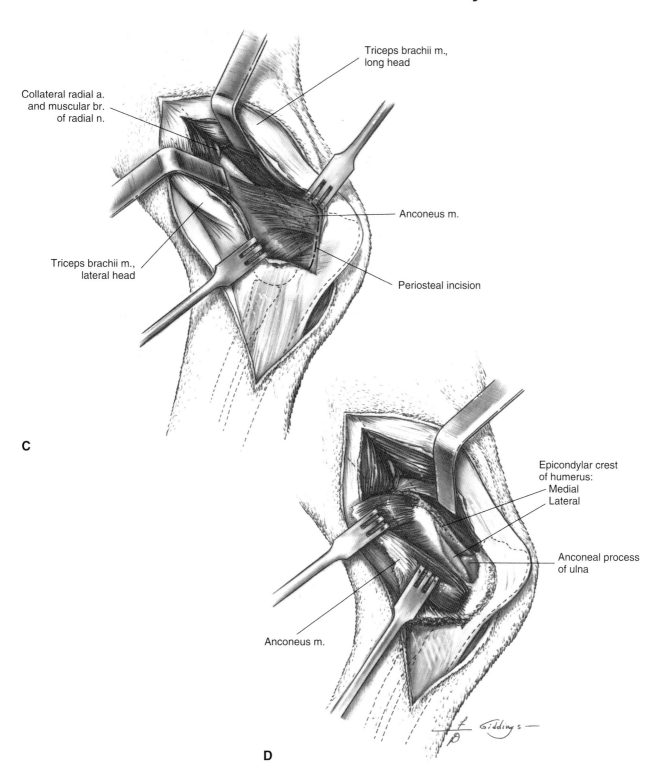

Triceps brachii m., long head

Collateral radial a. and muscular br. of radial n.

Anconeus m.

Triceps brachii m., lateral head

Periosteal incision

C

Epicondylar crest of humerus:
Medial
Lateral

Anconeal process of ulna

Anconeus m.

D

Approach to the Humeroulnar Part of the Elbow Joint by Osteotomy of the Tuber Olecrani

Based on a Procedure of Mostosky, Cholvin, and Brinker[30]

INDICATIONS

1. Open reduction of fractures of the condylar and supracondylar regions of the humerus.
2. Open reduction of chronic luxations of the elbow joint.
3. Exploration of the caudal compartment of the elbow joint.

ALTERNATIVE APPROACHES

The approach to the humeroulnar part of the elbow joint by triceps tenotomy (see Plate 44) provides similar exposure and avoids the need for repair of the olecranon osteotomy. The choice between these two approaches is largely a matter of the surgeon's preference. The tension band wire repair (see Figure 23C) is more secure than a sutured tenorrhaphy; this difference is more critical in larger dogs.

More limited exposure of fractures of the condylar and supracondylar regions of the humerus can be obtained with the medial approach (see Plate 38) in combination with one of the lateral approaches (see Plate 39, 41, or 42). Although this avoids ulnar osteotomy or triceps tenotomy, fracture reduction is generally more difficult.

The approach to the elbow by osteotomy of the proximal ulnar diaphysis (see Plate 45) provides total exposure of the humeral condyle and is more than needed for reduction of most condylar fractures.

PATIENT POSITIONING

Lateral recumbency with the affected limb uppermost (see Plate 43A) or dorsal recumbency with the affected limb abducted and suspended for draping (see Plate 44A).

DESCRIPTION OF THE PROCEDURE

A. A skin incision is made slightly lateral to the caudal midline of the limb. The incision extends from the distal third of the humerus to the proximal third of the ulna and crosses the elbow joint between the olecranon process and the lateral epicondyle.
B. Subcutaneous fat and fascia are incised and then widely undermined to allow retraction of the cranial skin margin beyond the lateral epicondyle and the caudal margin medial to the olecranon process. An incision is made in the fascia of the triceps brachii along the cranial border of the lateral head to allow elevation of its tendon from the olecranon.
C. The limb is elevated and the elbow flexed to allow dissection of the medial side of the joint.

PLATE 43

Approach to the Humeroulnar Part of the Elbow Joint by Osteotomy of the Tuber Olecrani

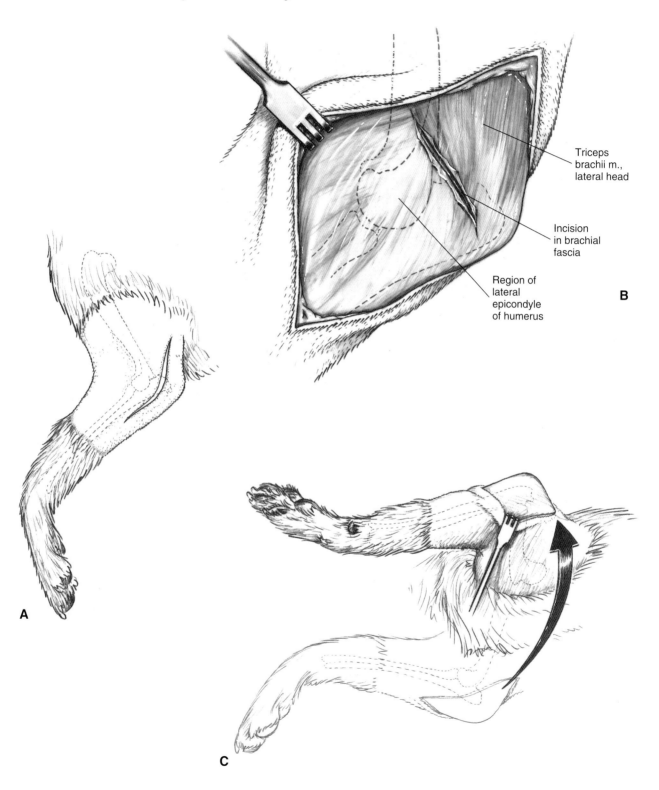

Triceps brachii m., lateral head

Incision in brachial fascia

Region of lateral epicondyle of humerus

A

B

C

Approach to the Humeroulnar Part of the Elbow Joint by Osteotomy of the Tuber Olecrani *continued*

    D. Undermining of the subcutaneous fat and fascia continues around the joint to the medial side until the caudal skin margin can be retracted beyond the medial epicondyle. After incising the triceps fascia, the cranial border of the medial head of the triceps is undermined from the proximal to the medial condyle to the olecranon. The ulnar nerve and collateral ulnar vessels lie parallel to the cranial border of the medial head and deep to it, under the antebrachial fascia (see Plate 38C). The nerve and vessels should be identified and protected throughout the procedure by retracting them distally.

    When operating on the cat, refer at this point to Plate 38E.

    E. A Gigli wire saw is pulled between the two fascial incisions cranial to the tendon of the triceps brachii on the olecranon, resting on the bone in the notch between the olecranon and anconeal process. Transection of the caudal cutaneous antebrachial nerve and vessels is unavoidable. However, care must be exercised at this point to be certain the ulnar nerve and collateral ulnar vessels are free from the wire. The olecranon process is then osteotomized with the wire saw at approximately a 45-degree angle to the shaft of the ulna. A power saw also can be used, but osteotomes should be avoided. The bone is so hard that it shatters easily.

PLATE 43

Approach to the Humeroulnar Part of the Elbow Joint by Osteotomy of the Tuber Olecrani *continued*

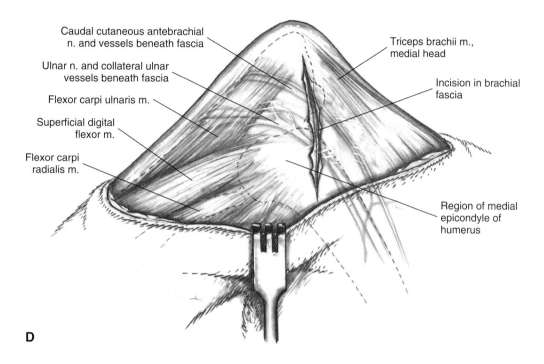

Caudal cutaneous antebrachial n. and vessels beneath fascia

Ulnar n. and collateral ulnar vessels beneath fascia

Flexor carpi ulnaris m.

Superficial digital flexor m.

Flexor carpi radialis m.

Triceps brachii m., medial head

Incision in brachial fascia

Region of medial epicondyle of humerus

D

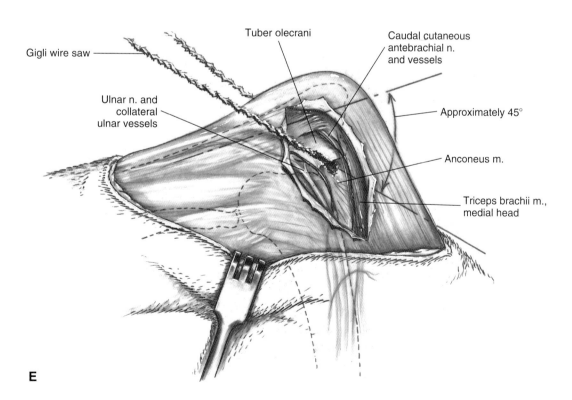

Gigli wire saw

Ulnar n. and collateral ulnar vessels

Tuber olecrani

Caudal cutaneous antebrachial n. and vessels

Approximately 45°

Anconeus m.

Triceps brachii m., medial head

E

Approach to the Humeroulnar Part of the Elbow Joint by Osteotomy of the Tuber Olecrani *continued*

F. The olecranon process with the attached triceps brachii muscle can now be reflected proximally to reveal the entire caudal surface of the joint. If the anconeus muscle is intact, an incision is made through the muscle and the underlying joint capsule near their attachments from just proximal to the medial aspect of the humeral condyle, continuing distally onto the olecranon. If possible, the branch of the collateral ulnar vessel that penetrates the muscle is preserved.

G. Maximum exposure of the intra-articular area is gained by complete flexion of the joint and retraction of the anconeus muscle.

ADDITIONAL EXPOSURE

Proximal extension of the approach medially is achieved in combination with the approaches to the distal shaft (see Plate 38) and midshaft (see Plate 35) of the humerus. However, these approaches are not continuous and the ulnar nerve (see Plate 38C) and median and musculocutaneous nerves (see Plate 35F) must be identified and protected.

Proximal extension of the approach laterally is limited by the muscular branches of the radial nerve innervating the lateral and accessory heads of the triceps muscle (see Plate 44I).

Distal extension of the approach provides exposure of the proximal shaft and trochlear notch of the ulna (see Plates 51 and 52).

CLOSURE

No attempt is made to close the incision in the anconeus. The olecranon process is reattached by the tension band wire technique (see Figure 23C). Predrilling of the olecranon before making the osteotomy can facilitate subsequent insertion of Kirschner wires used in the repair. The cranial borders of the triceps are sutured to the surrounding deep fascia, and subcutaneous sutures are used to pull the fat and fascia together and to take some of the tension off the skin sutures.

PRECAUTIONS

At the middle of the brachium, the ulnar nerve diverges from the median nerve and runs distally along the cranial border of the medial head of the triceps muscle. Medial to the elbow it is covered by heavy fascia. After crossing the medial epicondyle, it runs under the head of the flexor carpi ulnaris muscle.

Proximal retraction of the triceps muscles is limited by the radial nerve, which emerges from the interval between the medial and long heads. It branches to innervate the medial, accessory, and long heads and passes distally across the lateral surface of the brachialis muscle (see Plate 44I).

PLATE 43

Approach to the Humeroulnar Part of the Elbow Joint by Osteotomy of the Tuber Olecrani *continued*

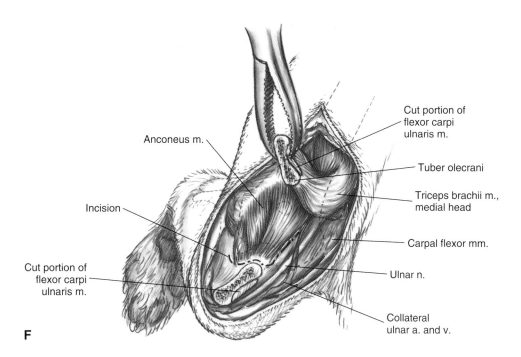

Anconeus m.

Incision

Cut portion of flexor carpi ulnaris m.

Cut portion of flexor carpi ulnaris m.

Tuber olecrani

Triceps brachii m., medial head

Carpal flexor mm.

Ulnar n.

Collateral ulnar a. and v.

F

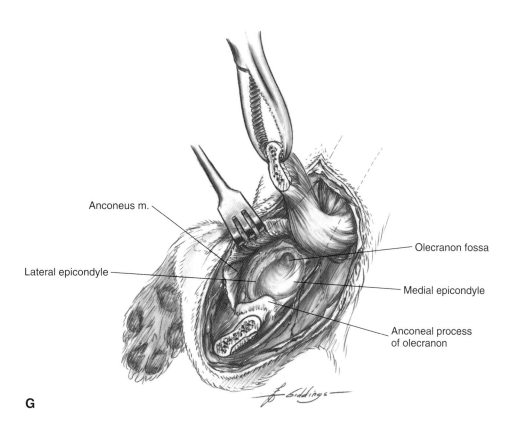

Anconeus m.

Lateral epicondyle

Olecranon fossa

Medial epicondyle

Anconeal process of olecranon

G

Approach to the Humeroulnar Part of the Elbow Joint by Tenotomy of the Triceps Tendon

Based on a Procedure of Dueland[13]

INDICATIONS

1. Open reduction of fractures of the condylar and supracondylar regions of the humerus.
2. Open reduction of chronic luxations of the elbow joint.
3. Exploration of the caudal compartment of the elbow joint.

ALTERNATIVE APPROACHES

The approach to the humeroulnar part of the elbow joint by olecranon osteotomy (see Plate 43) provides similar exposure. The choice between these two approaches is largely a matter of the surgeon's preference.

More limited exposure of fractures of the condylar and supracondylar regions of the humerus can be obtained with the medial approach (see Plate 38) in combination with one of the lateral approaches (see Plate 39, 41, or 42). Although this avoids ulnar osteotomy or triceps tenotomy, fracture reduction is generally more difficult.

The approach to the elbow by osteotomy of the proximal ulnar diaphysis (see Plate 45) provides total exposure of the humeral condyle and is more than needed for reduction of most condylar fractures.

PATIENT POSITIONING

Dorsal recumbency with the affected limb suspended for draping to allow access to both medial and lateral aspects of the elbow (see Plate 44A).

DESCRIPTION OF THE PROCEDURE

A, B. The skin incision commences over the proximal fourth of the ulna and crosses the elbow joint laterally to end on the distal third of the humeral shaft.

C. Subcutaneous fat and fascia are widely undermined and retracted caudally over the olecranon, exposing the triceps tendon. An incision is made in the brachial fascia along the cranial border of the lateral head of the triceps muscle.

PLATE 44

Approach to the Humeroulnar Part of the Elbow Joint by Tenotomy of the Triceps Tendon

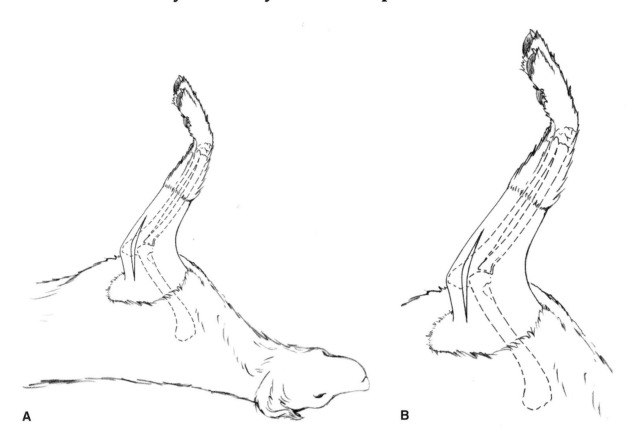

A

B

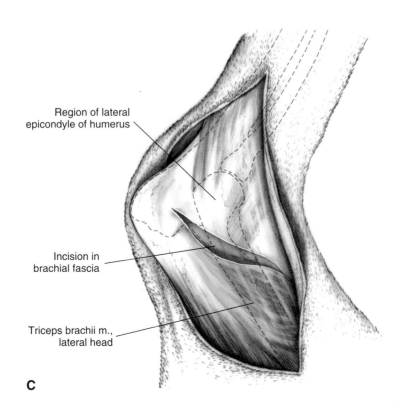

Region of lateral
epicondyle of humerus

Incision in
brachial fascia

Triceps brachii m.,
lateral head

C

Approach to the Humeroulnar Part of the Elbow Joint by Tenotomy of the Triceps Tendon *continued*

D.   The lateral head of the triceps muscle is undermined to allow elevation of the triceps tendon from the underlying extensor carpi radialis and anconeus muscles.

E.   The limb is abducted and the elbow flexed to allow dissection on the medial side of the joint.

PLATE 44

Approach to the Humeroulnar Part of the Elbow Joint by Tenotomy of the Triceps Tendon *continued*

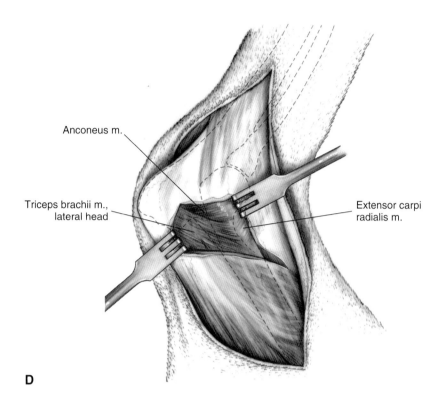

Anconeus m.

Triceps brachii m.,
lateral head

Extensor carpi
radialis m.

D

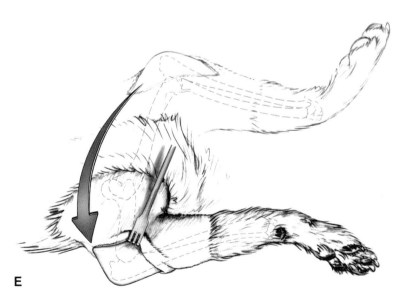

E

Approach to the Humeroulnar Part of the Elbow Joint by Tenotomy of the Triceps Tendon *continued*

F. Beginning at the medial epicondyle, subcutaneous fat and the triceps fascia are incised along the caudomedial margin of the humeral shaft. The ulnar nerve and collateral ulnar vessels lie parallel to the cranial border of the medial head of the triceps muscle and deep to it, under the antebrachial fascia (see Plate 38C). At the elbow, the nerve lies between the medial epicondyle and the olecranon when the joint is extended. The ulnar nerve and vessels should be identified and protected throughout the procedure by retracting them craniodistally.
When operating on the cat, refer at this point to Plate 38E.

G. The cranial border of the medial head of the triceps muscle is undermined and retracted caudally, beginning at the ulna and extending proximally to the midshaft of the humerus. Transection of the caudal cutaneous antebrachial nerve and vessels is unavoidable. However, care must be exercised at this point to be certain the ulnar nerve and collateral ulnar vessels are protected.

PLATE 44

Approach to the Humeroulnar Part of the Elbow Joint
by Tenotomy of the Triceps Tendon *continued*

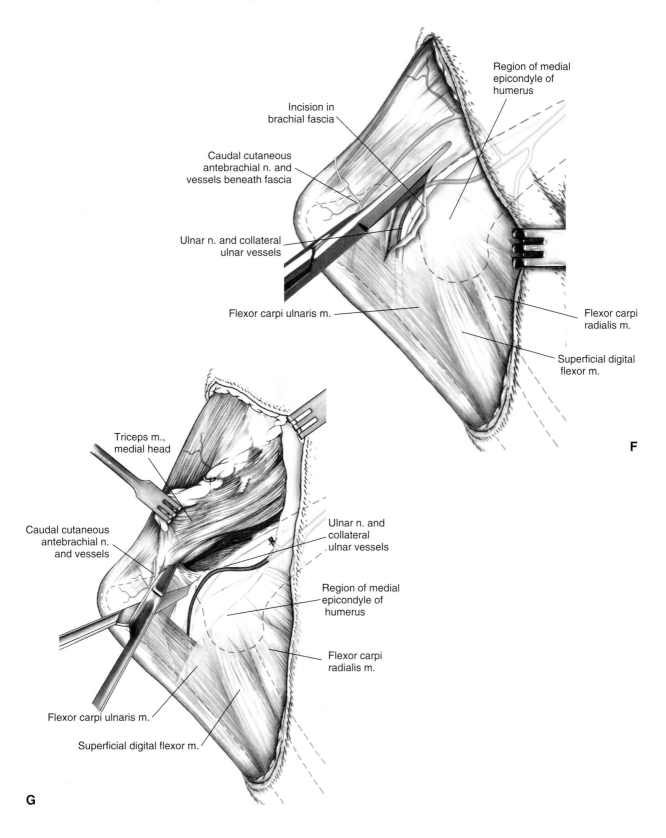

Incision in brachial fascia

Region of medial epicondyle of humerus

Caudal cutaneous antebrachial n. and vessels beneath fascia

Ulnar n. and collateral ulnar vessels

Flexor carpi ulnaris m.

Flexor carpi radialis m.

Superficial digital flexor m.

F

Triceps m., medial head

Caudal cutaneous antebrachial n. and vessels

Ulnar n. and collateral ulnar vessels

Region of medial epicondyle of humerus

Flexor carpi radialis m.

Flexor carpi ulnaris m.

Superficial digital flexor m.

G

Approach to the Humeroulnar Part of the Elbow Joint by Tenotomy of the Triceps Tendon *continued*

H. The triceps tendon is then transected near the olecranon process, leaving sufficient tendon for subsequent suture repair. It is important that the tenotomy be in tendon and not muscle to prevent suture pullout. Alternatively, the tendon may be cut close to the olecranon if direct attachment of the tendon to the bone is planned (see Closure).

I. The triceps brachii muscle group can now be reflected proximally to reveal the caudal surface of the distal shaft of the humerus and the humeroulnar joint. If the anconeus muscle is intact, an incision is made through the medial border of this muscle, beginning proximally and extending distally. The anconeus muscle is then reflected from the humerus with a periosteal elevator. At the elbow joint, both the anconeus muscle and the underlying joint capsule are incised along the medial aspect of the humeral condyle, then the incision continues distally onto the olecranon. Maximal exposure of the intra-articular area is gained by complete flexion of the joint and retraction of the anconeus muscle.

CLOSURE

No attempt is made to close the incision in the anconeus. The triceps tendon is repaired with one or two sutures inserted in a Kessler (see Figure 21C) or three-loop pulley (see Figure 21D) pattern. Alternatively, sutures may be anchored in one or two transverse, small-diameter drill holes in the olecranon (see Figure 22). The cranial borders of the triceps are sutured to the surrounding deep fascia, and subcutaneous sutures are used to pull the fat and fascia together and to take some of the tension off the skin sutures.

PRECAUTIONS

At the middle of the brachium, the ulnar nerve diverges from the median nerve and runs distally along the cranial border of the medial head of the triceps muscle. Medial to the elbow it is covered by heavy fascia. After crossing the medial epicondyle, it runs under the head of the flexor carpi ulnaris muscle.

Proximal retraction of the triceps muscles is limited by the radial nerve that emerges from the interval between the medial and long heads. It branches to innervate the medial, accessory, and long heads and passes distally across the lateral surface of the brachialis muscle (see Plate 44I).

ADDITIONAL EXPOSURE

Proximal extension of the approach medially is achieved in combination with the approaches to the distal shaft (see Plate 38) and midshaft (see Plate 35) of the humerus. However, these approaches are not continuous, and the ulnar nerve (see Plate 38C) and median and musculocutaneous nerves (see Plate 35F) must be identified and protected.

Proximal extension of the approach laterally is limited by the muscular branches of the radial nerve innervating the lateral and accessory heads of the triceps muscle (see Plate 44I).

PLATE 44

Approach to the Humeroulnar Part of the Elbow Joint by Tenotomy of the Triceps Tendon *continued*

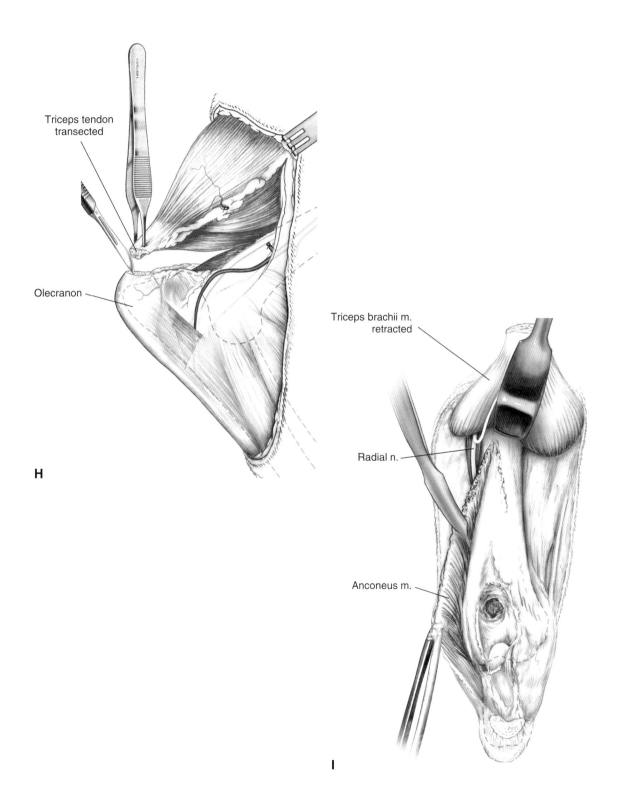

Triceps tendon transected

Olecranon

H

Triceps brachii m. retracted

Radial n.

Anconeus m.

I

Approach to the Elbow Joint by Osteotomy of the Proximal Ulnar Diaphysis

Based on a Procedure of Lenehan and Nunamaker[25]

INDICATIONS

1. Open reduction of multiple intra-articular fractures of the humeral condyle.
2. Open reduction of luxations of the elbow joint.
3. Exploration of multiple compartments of the elbow joint.

ALTERNATIVE APPROACHES

The approaches to the humeral condyle by olecranon osteotomy (see Plate 43) or triceps tenotomy (see Plate 44) provide adequate exposure for open reduction of intra-articular fractures of the humeral condyle in the majority of cases.

The approach to the lateral aspect of the humeral condyle (see Plate 39) provides adequate exposure for open reduction of simple fractures of the condyle.

The approach to the proximal shaft and trochlear notch of the ulna (see Plate 51) provides very limited access to the compartments of the elbow.

PATIENT POSITIONING

Dorsal recumbency with the affected limb abducted and suspended for draping.

DESCRIPTION OF THE PROCEDURE

A. The skin incision starts proximally at the level of the lateral epicondyle, halfway between it and the tuber olecrani. The incision curves distally following the lateral epicondylar crest, ending at the junction of the proximal and middle thirds of the antebrachium and lateral to the ulna.
B. Two incisions are made in the deep antebrachial fascia covering the muscles and ulna. The lateral incision runs between the ulna and the caudal border of the ulnaris lateralis muscle distally and through the insertion of the anconeus muscle on the tuber olecrani proximally. The medial incision is between the flexor carpi ulnaris and the ulna.

PLATE 45
Approach to the Elbow Joint by Osteotomy of the Proximal Ulnar Diaphysis

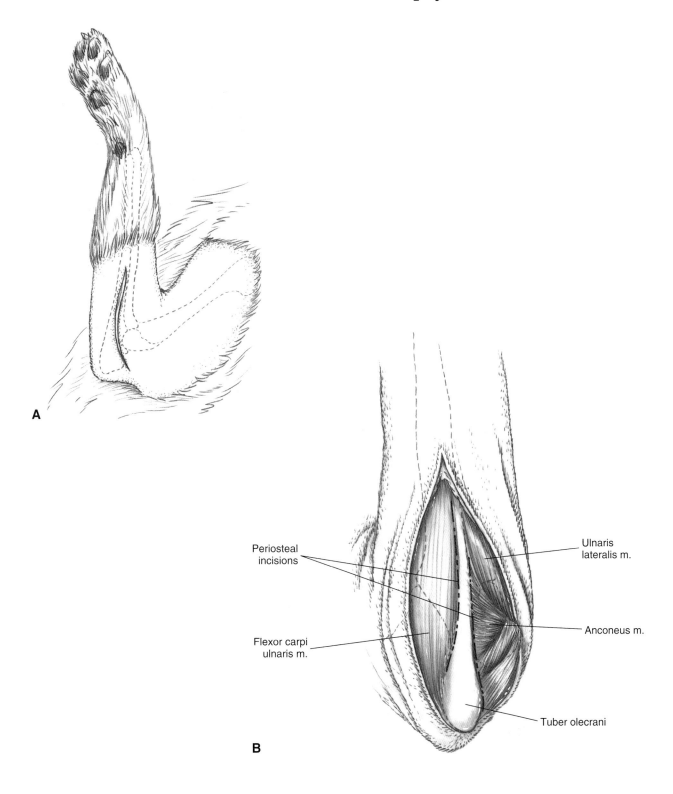

Periosteal
incisions

Ulnaris
lateralis m.

Anconeus m.

Flexor carpi
ulnaris m.

Tuber olecrani

A

B

Approach to the Elbow Joint by Osteotomy of the Proximal Ulnar Diaphysis *continued*

C. The anconeus and flexor carpi ulnaris muscles are subperiosteally elevated from the ulna. Retraction of the muscles will reveal the ulnar nerve and collateral ulnar vessels medially, running on the deep surface of the flexor muscles. The cranial interosseous vessels and interosseous nerve cross the field between the radius and ulna. The ulnar head of the deep digital flexor and the abductor pollicis longus muscles are subperiosteally elevated from the ulna to reveal the interosseous membrane and ligament. The lateral collateral ligament (caudal crus) and annular ligament are incised on the lateral aspect of the radioulnar joint.

D. Osteotomy of the ulna is performed just proximal to the interosseous ligament, taking care to protect the interosseous vessels and nerve. The osteotomy can be performed with a Gigli wire saw, as illustrated, or with a power saw. An osteotome should not be used because it tends to fragment the ulna.

PLATE 45

Approach to the Elbow Joint by Osteotomy of the Proximal Ulnar Diaphysis *continued*

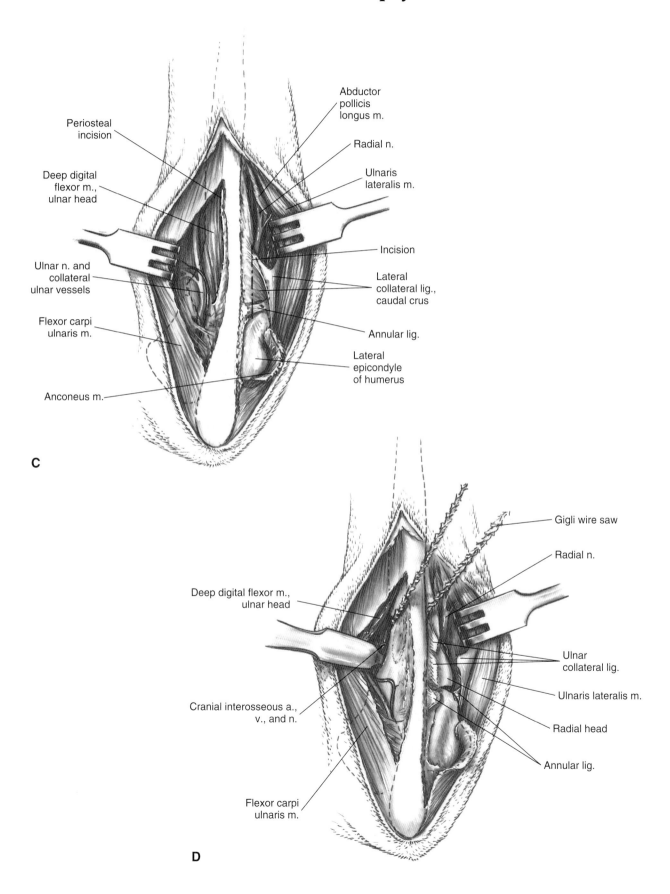

Periosteal incision

Deep digital flexor m., ulnar head

Ulnar n. and collateral ulnar vessels

Flexor carpi ulnaris m.

Anconeus m.

Abductor pollicis longus m.

Radial n.

Ulnaris lateralis m.

Incision

Lateral collateral lig., caudal crus

Annular lig.

Lateral epicondyle of humerus

C

Deep digital flexor m., ulnar head

Cranial interosseous a., v., and n.

Flexor carpi ulnaris m.

Gigli wire saw

Radial n.

Ulnar collateral lig.

Ulnaris lateralis m.

Radial head

Annular lig.

D

Approach to the Elbow Joint by Osteotomy of the Proximal Ulnar Diaphysis *continued*

E. Medial rotation of the proximal ulnar segment exposes the humeral condyle and radial head. Transection of the olecranon ligament will allow additional rotation of the ulna if required. Distraction of the humeroradial joint allows inspection of the articular surface of the radius, and extreme flexion of the joint exposes the humeral condyle fully.

CLOSURE

The proximal ulnar segment is reduced and fixed with one or two Steinmann pins or Kirschner wires driven from the tuber olecrani. Interfragmentary compression is supplied with a figure-of-8 wire (see Figure 23). No attempt is made to repair the lateral collateral or annular ligaments. Adequate stability of the elbow is afforded by the intact cranial crus of the collateral ligament and the muscles. The superficial fascia of the flexor carpi ulnaris is sutured to the fascia of the ulnaris lateralis and anconeus muscles. Proximally, the anconeus muscle is sutured to remnants of periosteum and fascia.

COMMENTS

Passive range of motion exercises and early weight bearing should be encouraged to restore function to the joint. Although this approach seems radical, it is less traumatic than combining approaches if generous exposure of the humeral condyle is needed.

PLATE 45

Approach to the Elbow Joint by Osteotomy of the Proximal Ulnar Diaphysis *continued*

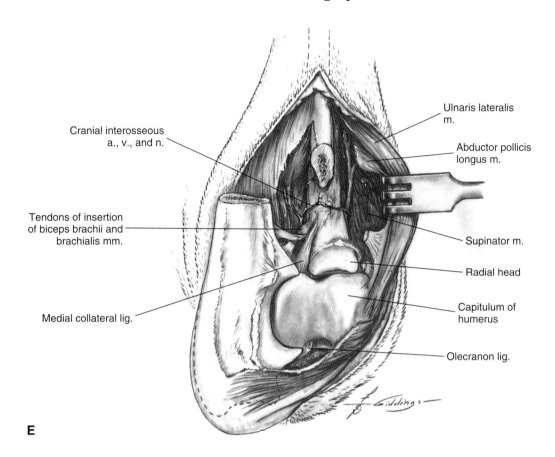

Cranial interosseous
a., v., and n.

Ulnaris lateralis
m.

Abductor pollicis
longus m.

Tendons of insertion
of biceps brachii and
brachialis mm.

Supinator m.

Radial head

Capitulum of
humerus

Medial collateral lig.

Olecranon lig.

E

Approach to the Head of the Radius and the Lateral Parts of the Elbow Joint

INDICATIONS

1. Open reduction of lateral luxations of the head of the radius.
2. Open reduction of fractures of the head of the radius.
3. Reconstruction of ruptures of the lateral collateral ligament of the elbow joint.

ALTERNATIVE APPROACHES

Slightly better exposure of the radial head is obtained by osteotomy of the lateral humeral epicondyle and retraction of the lateral collateral ligament and extensor muscles (see Plate 47).

For complete exposure of the cranial aspect of the radial head and the proximal metaphysis of the radius, the approach is made through the interval between the extensor carpi radialis and common digital extensor muscles (see Plate 54). However, exposure of the lateral aspect of the radial head is obscured by the radial nerve.

Exposure of the caudal compartment of the elbow joint by olecranon osteotomy (see Plate 43), triceps tenotomy (see Plate 44), or proximal ulna osteotomy (see Plate 45) may provide better exposure for reduction of chronic fractures and luxations.

PATIENT POSITIONING

Lateral recumbency with the affected limb uppermost.

DESCRIPTION OF THE PROCEDURE

A. The curved incision commences proximal to the lateral humeral epicondyle, crosses the joint following the lateral surface of the radius, and ends at the proximal fourth of the radius. Subcutaneous fascia is incised on the same line.
B. After retraction of the skin and subcutaneous fascia, the deeper-lying brachial and antebrachial fascia is incised on a similar line.
C. Incision and retraction of the fascia of the triceps brachii allows retraction of the lateral head of the triceps muscle and incision of the origin of the anconeus muscle along the lateral epicondylar crest. The tendon of origin and proximal portion of the ulnaris lateralis muscle are separated along the intermuscular septum with the lateral digital extensor muscle. The tendon of the ulnaris lateralis muscle is transected, leaving enough tendon proximally to allow suturing.

PLATE 46

Approach to the Head of the Radius and the Lateral Parts of the Elbow Joint

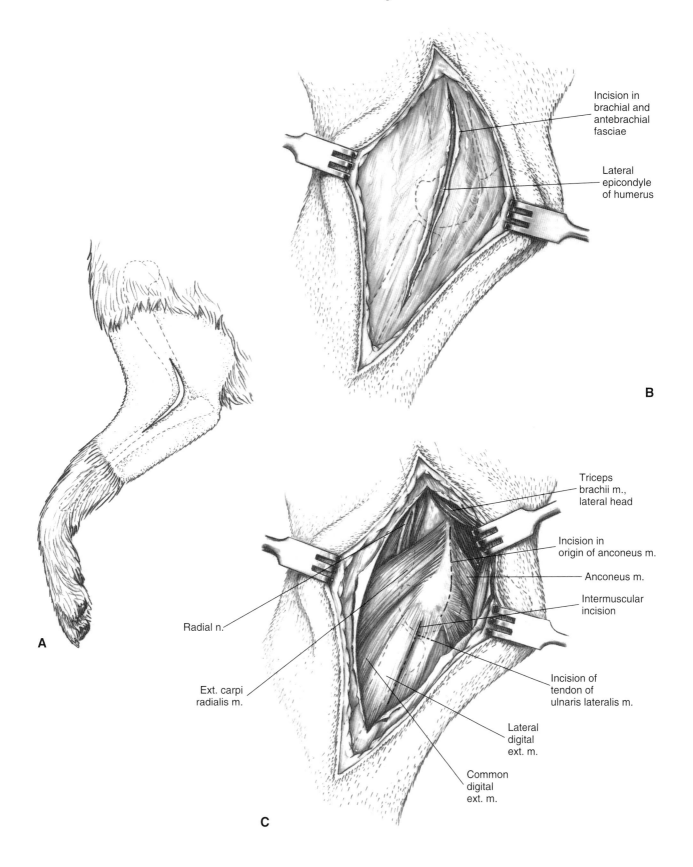

A

B

Incision in brachial and antebrachial fasciae

Lateral epicondyle of humerus

Triceps brachii m., lateral head

Incision in origin of anconeus m.

Anconeus m.

Intermuscular incision

Incision of tendon of ulnaris lateralis m.

Lateral digital ext. m.

Common digital ext. m.

Radial n.

Ext. carpi radialis m.

C

Approach to the Head of the Radius and the Lateral Parts of the Elbow Joint *continued*

D. Subperiosteal elevation of the anconeus muscle exposes the caudolateral humeroulnar joint compartment.

E. The remaining extensor muscles are elevated cranially with a Hohmann retractor. The tip of the retractor must be kept on the radius to avoid damage to the radial nerve. Transection of the collateral and annular ligaments may be necessary to gain adequate exposure of the head of the radius.

ADDITIONAL EXPOSURE

Further proximal exposure can be obtained in combination with the approach to the lateral (see Plate 41) or caudal (see Plate 42) humeroulnar part of the elbow joint.

CLOSURE

Transected portions of the lateral collateral ligament are sutured to the remaining portions of the ligament or a bone anchor (see Figure 22). The tendon of the ulnaris lateralis muscle is reattached with a modified Bunnell-Mayer or locking-loop suture (see Figure 21A,C). The origin of the anconeus muscle is sutured to the origins of the extensor muscles, and the cranial edge of the triceps brachii is attached to the brachial fascia. The two fascial layers and skin are closed routinely in separate layers.

PRECAUTIONS

The deep branch of the radial nerve supplies branches to the extensor carpi radialis muscle as it passes under this muscle on the flexor surface of the elbow. The remaining part of the nerve then continues under the supinator muscle, supplying branches to the joint capsule, supinator, and common and lateral digital extensor muscles as it continues distally in the interosseous space. Extension of this approach distally is prevented by these branches of the radial nerve.

PLATE 46

Approach to the Head of the Radius and the Lateral Parts of the Elbow Joint *continued*

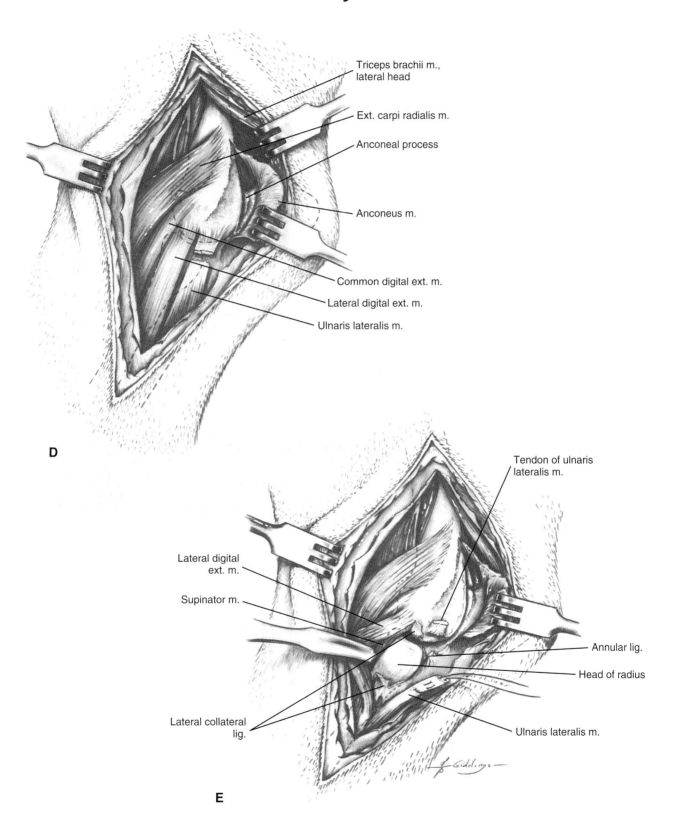

Triceps brachii m., lateral head

Ext. carpi radialis m.

Anconeal process

Anconeus m.

Common digital ext. m.

Lateral digital ext. m.

Ulnaris lateralis m.

D

Tendon of ulnaris lateralis m.

Lateral digital ext. m.

Supinator m.

Annular lig.

Head of radius

Lateral collateral lig.

Ulnaris lateralis m.

E

Approach to the Head of the Radius and Humeroradial Part of the Elbow Joint by Osteotomy of the Lateral Humeral Epicondyle

Based on a Procedure of Hohn[21]

INDICATIONS

1. Open reduction of lateral luxation of the head of the radius.
2. Open reduction of fractures of the head of the radius.

ALTERNATIVE APPROACHES

The alternative approach with tenotomy of the lateral collateral ligament (see Plate 46) provides less exposure of the radial head. The choice of tenotomy or osteotomy is primarily a matter of the surgeon's preference.

For complete exposure of the cranial aspect of the radial head and the proximal metaphysis of the radius, the approach is made through the interval between the extensor carpi radialis and common digital extensor muscles (see Plate 54). However, exposure of the lateral aspect of the radial head is obscured by the radial nerve.

Exposure of the caudal compartment of the elbow joint by olecranon osteotomy (see Plate 43), triceps tenotomy (see Plate 44), or proximal ulna osteotomy (see Plate 45) may provide better exposure for reduction of chronic fractures and luxations.

PATIENT POSITIONING

Lateral recumbency with the affected limb uppermost.

DESCRIPTION OF THE PROCEDURE

A. The curved incision commences proximal to the lateral humeral epicondyle, crosses the joint following the lateral surface of the radius, and ends at the proximal fourth of the radius. Subcutaneous and deep antebrachial fascia is incised on the same line.
B. Antebrachial and intermuscular fasciae are incised from the cranioventral borders of the lateral head of the triceps brachii distally, along a line that separates the extensor carpi radialis from the common digital extensor muscle. A similar incision is made between the anconeus and ulnaris lateralis muscles. These incisions are deepened to completely free the three enclosed extensor muscles from the underlying bone. If the epicondyle is to be reattached by a lag screw (see Plate 47C and Closure), a suitable glide and tap hole should be drilled now, just distal to the epicondyle.

PLATE 47

Approach to the Head of the Radius and Humeroradial Part of the Elbow Joint by Osteotomy of the Lateral Humeral Epicondyle

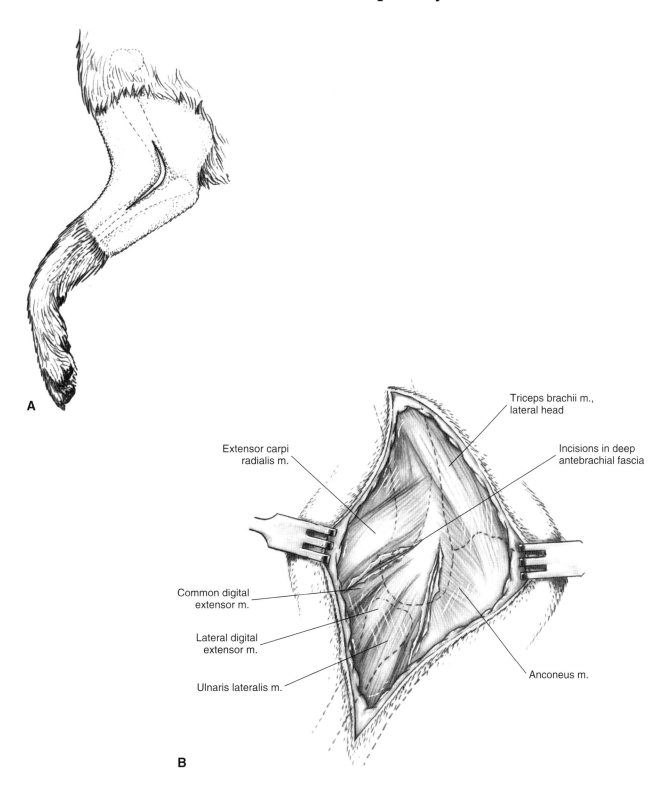

A

Triceps brachii m., lateral head

Extensor carpi radialis m.

Incisions in deep antebrachial fascia

Common digital extensor m.

Lateral digital extensor m.

Ulnaris lateralis m.

Anconeus m.

B

Approach to the Head of the Radius and Humeroradial Part of the Elbow Joint by Osteotomy of the Lateral Humeral Epicondyle *continued*

    C. The lateral humeral epicondyle is osteotomized so as to include the origins of the three extensor muscles. The orientation of the osteotomy from a cranial perspective is shown in Plate 47C1. No articular cartilage should be included in the osteotomy.

PLATE 47

Approach to the Head of the Radius and Humeroradial Part of the Elbow Joint by Osteotomy of the Lateral Humeral Epicondyle *continued*

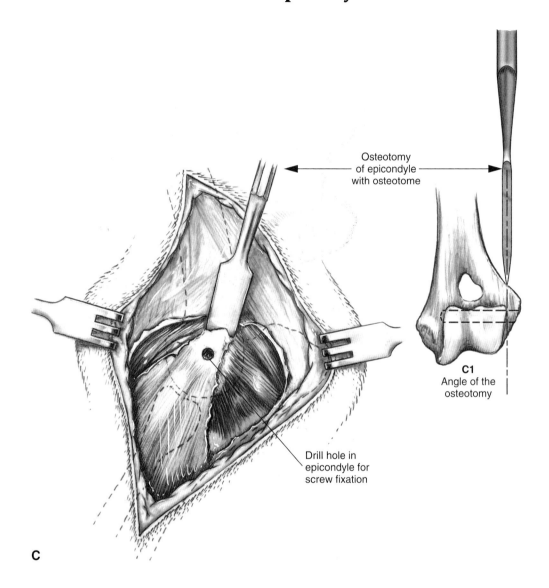

Osteotomy of epicondyle with osteotome

C1
Angle of the osteotomy

Drill hole in epicondyle for screw fixation

C

Approach to the Head of the Radius and Humeroradial Part of the Elbow Joint by Osteotomy of the Lateral Humeral Epicondyle *continued*

D. Retraction of the osteotomized epicondyle with attached collateral ligaments and extensor muscles is possible after incision of the joint capsule where necessary. Elevation of the supinator muscle will further expose the head of the radius. Care should be taken to protect the radial nerve, which crosses under the deep surface of the supinator muscle.

ADDITIONAL EXPOSURE

Additional proximal exposure is obtained in combination with the approach to the distal shaft of the humerus (see Plate 37E).

Access to the caudal compartment of the elbow and exposure of the anconeal process is gained by elevation of the anconeus muscle (see Plate 41).

CLOSURE

The humeral epicondyle is reattached to its origin by a lag screw or with pins and a tension band wire (see Figures 23 and 24). Incisions in the intermuscular septa, deep antebrachial fascia, subcutaneous fascia, and skin are each closed in separate layers.

PRECAUTIONS

The deep branch of the radial nerve supplies branches to the extensor carpi radialis muscle as it passes under this muscle on the flexor surface of the elbow. The remaining part of the nerve then continues under the supinator muscle, supplying branches to joint capsule, supinator, and common and lateral digital extensor muscles as it continues distally in the interosseous space. Extension of this approach distally is prevented by these branches of the radial nerve.

PLATE 47

Approach to the Head of the Radius and Humeroradial Part of the Elbow Joint by Osteotomy of the Lateral Humeral Epicondyle *continued*

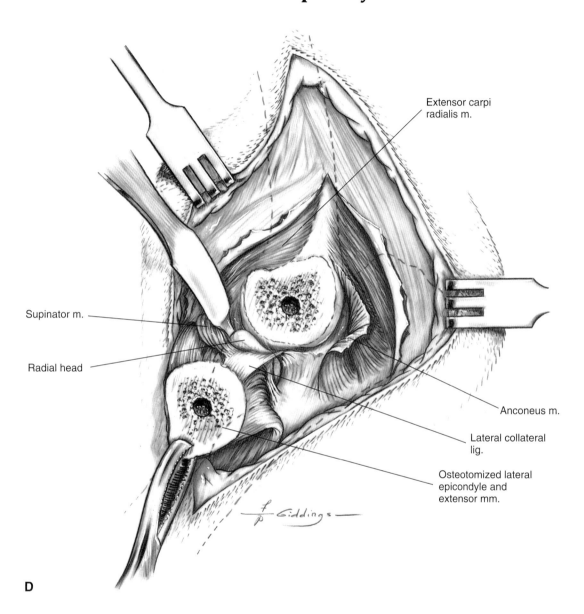

Extensor carpi radialis m.

Supinator m.

Radial head

Anconeus m.

Lateral collateral lig.

Osteotomized lateral epicondyle and extensor mm.

Giddings

D

Approach to the Medial Humeral Epicondyle

INDICATIONS

1. Reduction of fractures of the medial aspect of the humeral condyle.
2. Reduction of medial luxations of the elbow joint.
3. Insertion of an intramedullary pin into the humeral diaphysis using a retrograde technique.

PATIENT POSITIONING

Dorsal recumbency with the affected limb abducted and suspended for draping.

DESCRIPTION OF THE PROCEDURE

A. The skin incision is centered on the medial humeral epicondyle and follows the humeral shaft proximally and the ulnar shaft distally. It may be useful to lengthen the incision in some cases. The subcutaneous fat and fascia are incised on the same line and retracted with the skin.
B. The deep antebrachial fascia is incised in each direction from the epicondyle on the same line as the skin. Be aware of the neurovascular tissues deep to the fascia, as illustrated in Plate 48C.
C. Retraction of the deep fascia and clearing of areolar tissue will expose the epicondyle and the attached flexor muscle group. Dissection in the craniomedial direction must take into account the median nerve and brachial vessels, whereas the ulnar nerve and collateral ulnar vessels lie caudomedial to the epicondyle.

ADDITIONAL EXPOSURE

This approach forms the basis for several other approaches to the medial side of the elbow joint and will be cross-referenced to those approaches.

By reducing the magnitude of this approach (Plate 48), a limited exposure of the medial epicondyle is the starting point for the minimally invasive approach to the shaft of the humerus (see Plate 40).

Limited exposure of the medial compartment of the elbow joint is obtained in combination with the intermuscular approach (see Plate 49).

Greater exposure of the medial compartment of the elbow joint is obtained in combination with an osteotomy of the medial epicondyle (see Plate 50).

More proximal exposure of the medial aspect of the humerus is obtained in combination with the approach to the distal shaft and supracondylar region (see Plate 38) and midshaft (see Plate 35). However, these three approaches are not continuous, and the brachial artery and median and musculocutaneous nerves must be identified and protected (see Plate 35F).

CLOSURE

The deep antebrachial and brachial fascia is closed, followed by closure of the subcutaneous tissues and then closure of the skin.

PLATE 48

Approach to the Medial Humeral Epicondyle

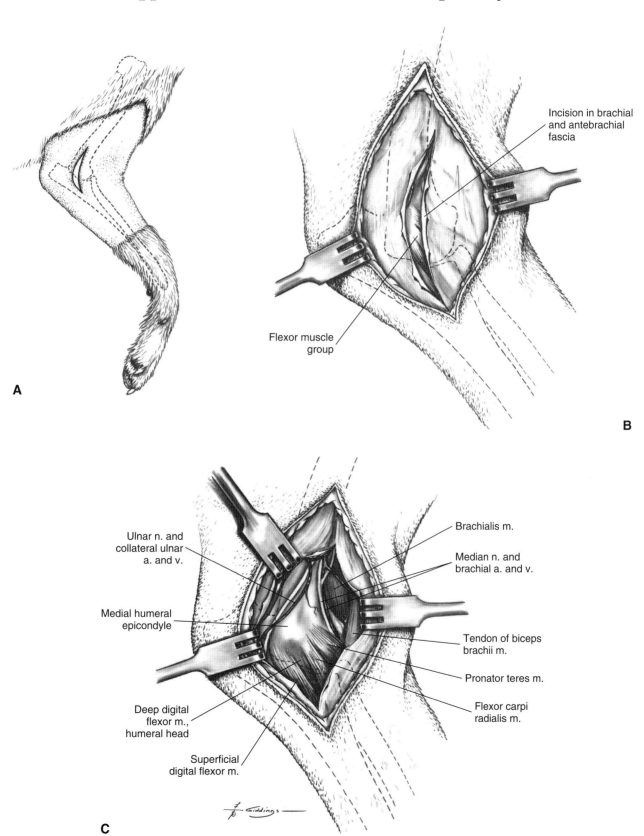

A

Incision in brachial
and antebrachial
fascia

Flexor muscle
group

B

Ulnar n. and
collateral ulnar
a. and v.

Medial humeral
epicondyle

Deep digital
flexor m.,
humeral head

Superficial
digital flexor m.

Brachialis m.

Median n. and
brachial a. and v.

Tendon of biceps
brachii m.

Pronator teres m.

Flexor carpi
radialis m.

C

Approach to the Medial Aspect of the Humeral Condyle and the Medial Coronoid Process of the Ulna by an Intermuscular Incision

Based on a Procedure of Probst, Flo, McLoughlin, and DeCamp[37]

INDICATION

Exploration of the medial elbow joint for osteochondritis dissecans and fragmented medial coronoid process.

ALTERNATIVE APPROACH

Slightly better exposure is gained with osteotomy of the medial epicondyle, but this is generally more exposure than is needed for exploration of fragmented medial coronoid process and humeral osteochondritis dissecans lesions (see Plate 50).

PATIENT POSITIONING

Dorsal recumbency with the affected limb abducted and suspended for draping. A sandbag bolster is placed on the table under the elbow.

DESCRIPTION OF THE PROCEDURE

A. This approach starts similarly to that shown in Plate 48, but the skin incision extends further distally. Deep antebrachial fascia is incised on the same line as the skin and retracted to expose the flexor muscle group, as in Plate 48B and C. Protect the ulnar nerve during the fascial incision and elevation.

PLATE 49

Approach to the Medial Aspect of the Humeral Condyle and the Medial Coronoid Process of the Ulna by an Intermuscular Incision

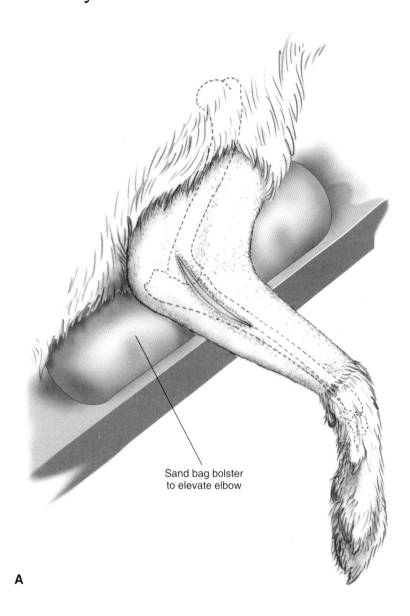

Sand bag bolster
to elevate elbow

A

Approach to the Medial Aspect of the Humeral Condyle and the Medial Coronoid Process of the Ulna by an Intermuscular Incision *continued*

B. The intermuscular septum between the flexor carpi radialis and deep digital flexor muscles is incised following ligation or coagulation of the intermuscular branches of the recurrent ulnar artery and vein. The division between these muscles is often not very distinct, but it can be found by blunt dissection in a longitudinal plane, distal to the medial epicondyle, which can be readily palpated. The intermuscular incision can alternatively be made between the pronator teres and flexor carpi radialis muscles (see Comments).

PLATE 49

Approach to the Medial Aspect of the Humeral Condyle and the Medial Coronoid Process of the Ulna by an Intermuscular Incision *continued*

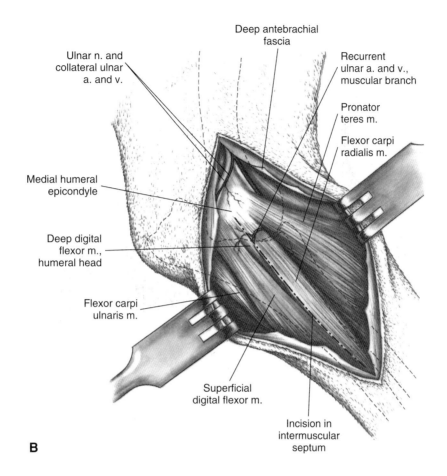

Deep antebrachial fascia

Ulnar n. and collateral ulnar a. and v.

Recurrent ulnar a. and v., muscular branch

Pronator teres m.

Flexor carpi radialis m.

Medial humeral epicondyle

Deep digital flexor m., humeral head

Flexor carpi ulnaris m.

Superficial digital flexor m.

Incision in intermuscular septum

B

Approach to the Medial Aspect of the Humeral Condyle and the Medial Coronoid Process of the Ulna by an Intermuscular Incision *continued*

C. Retraction of these muscles exposes the joint capsule distal to the medial epicondyle. *Although not required for arthrotomy of the elbow joint, a more liberal distal exposure is illustrated in this image to show the location of the median nerve and its muscular branches supplying the deep digital flexor muscle more distally.* The joint capsule is incised parallel to the muscles. Protect the underlying articular cartilage and medial collateral ligament when making this incision.

PLATE 49

Approach to the Medial Aspect of the Humeral Condyle and the Medial Coronoid Process of the Ulna by an Intermuscular Incision *continued*

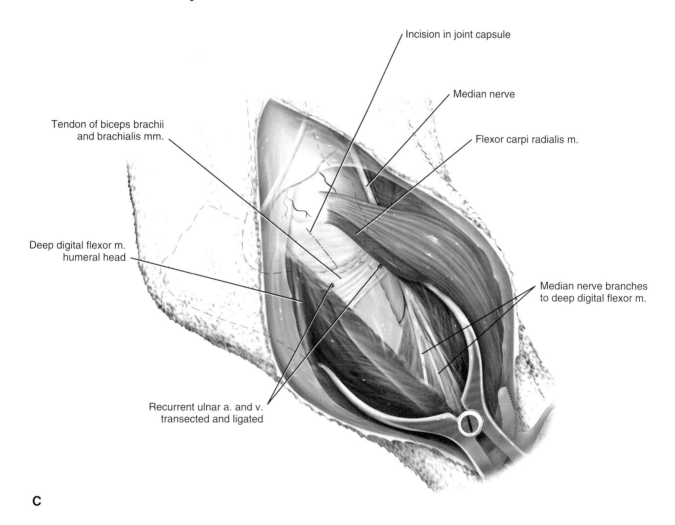

Incision in joint capsule

Median nerve

Tendon of biceps brachii and brachialis mm.

Flexor carpi radialis m.

Deep digital flexor m. humeral head

Median nerve branches to deep digital flexor m.

Recurrent ulnar a. and v. transected and ligated

C

Approach to the Medial Aspect of the Humeral Condyle and the Medial Coronoid Process of the Ulna by an Intermuscular Incision *continued*

D. Retraction of the joint capsule exposes the articular surfaces of the humeral condyle and the ulna. Osteochondritis dissecans lesions will be evident on the condyle at this point. Exposure of the medial coronoid process may require distal extension of the joint capsule incision. Just distal to the humeroulnar joint is the conjoined, broad flat tendon of the biceps brachii and brachialis muscles. Partial transection of this tendon along with the joint capsule provides greater exposure of the medial coronoid process.

PLATE 49

Approach to the Medial Aspect of the Humeral Condyle and the Medial Coronoid Process of the Ulna by an Intermuscular Incision *continued*

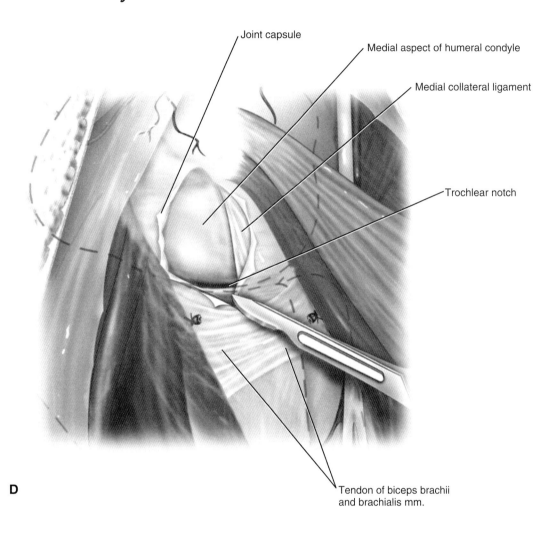

Joint capsule

Medial aspect of humeral condyle

Medial collateral ligament

Trochlear notch

Tendon of biceps brachii and brachialis mm.

D

Approach to the Medial Aspect of the Humeral Condyle and the Medial Coronoid Process of the Ulna by an Intermuscular Incision *continued*

E. Visualization of the medial coronoid process is facilitated by strong pronation and abduction of the antebrachium to open the joint on the medial side. A sandbag bolster or a folded towel under the drapes on the lateral side of the joint creates a fulcrum for this maneuver. A small Hohmann retractor hooked over the coronoid process is also useful for retraction of the medial collateral ligament. The medial collateral ligament inserts distally on the radius and also deep in the interosseous space. Therefore exposure of the medial coronoid process of the ulna can be achieved without significant disruption of the medial collateral ligament.

CLOSURE

Several interrupted sutures are placed in the joint capsule, followed by closure of the intermuscular fascia and the deep fascia. The subcutis and skin are closed in layers.

COMMENTS

This approach as described by Probst and his colleagues placed the intermuscular incision between the pronator teres and flexor carpi radialis muscles. There is little difference in our hands, but there seem to be fewer vascular branches in the intermuscular space used here, and the medial collateral ligament may be better protected.

PRECAUTIONS

Cranial to the medial epicondyle, the median nerve passes between the origins of the pronator teres and biceps brachii muscles. At the flexor surface of the elbow, it dips laterally under pronator teres and travels caudomedially, supplying muscular branches to pronator teres, pronator quadratus, flexor carpi radialis, superficial digital flexor, and the radial head of the deep digital flexor muscles. These branches limit distal dissection and separation of the intermuscular septum between the flexor carpi radialis and the digital flexor muscles (see Plate 49C).

PLATE 49

Approach to the Medial Aspect of the Humeral Condyle and the Medial Coronoid Process of the Ulna by an Intermuscular Incision *continued*

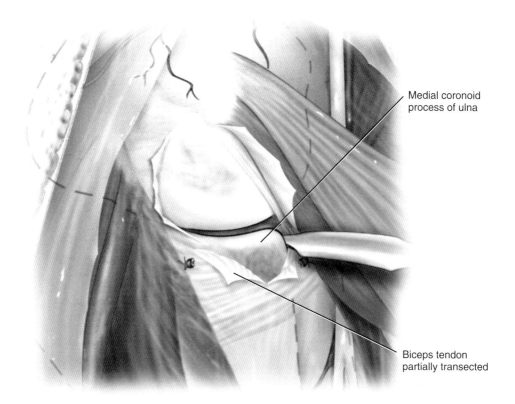

Medial coronoid
process of ulna

Biceps tendon
partially transected

E

Approach to the Medial Aspect of the Humeral Condyle and the Medial Coronoid Process of the Ulna by Osteotomy of the Medial Humeral Epicondyle

Based on a Procedure of Stoll[48]

INDICATIONS

1. Osteochondroplasty of the medial aspect of the humeral condyle for osteochondritis dissecans.
2. Excision of fragmented medial coronoid process of the ulna.
3. Open reduction of medial luxation of the head of the radius.

ALTERNATIVE APPROACH

The alternative approach by intermuscular separation provides less exposure of the medial compartment of the elbow (see Plate 49).

PATIENT POSITIONING

Dorsal recumbency with the affected limb abducted and suspended for draping. A sandbag bolster is placed on the table under the elbow (see Plate 49A).

DESCRIPTION OF THE PROCEDURE

This procedure is initiated as shown in Plate 48A-C.
A. After incising the deep antebrachial fascia and removing alveolar fat, the epicondylar osteotomy is planned. The osteotomy should include all of the origin of both the pronator teres and flexor carpi radialis muscles. Sharp dissection is necessary to separate fibers of the flexor carpi radialis from the adjacent digital flexor muscles. If the epicondyle is to be reattached with a lag screw (see Closure), a suitable glide and tap hole should be drilled at the medial epicondylar eminence before performing the osteotomy.
B. An osteotome of 10- to 12-mm width works well for a 50- to 70-lb (22- to 32-kg) dog. Osteotomies 1 and 2 are first made to a depth of approximately 5 mm, and then the third osteotomy is made in a parasagittal plane through the epicondyle, taking care to not include articular cartilage.

PLATE 50

Approach to the Medial Aspect of the Humeral Condyle and the Medial Coronoid Process of the Ulna by Osteotomy of the Medial Humeral Epicondyle

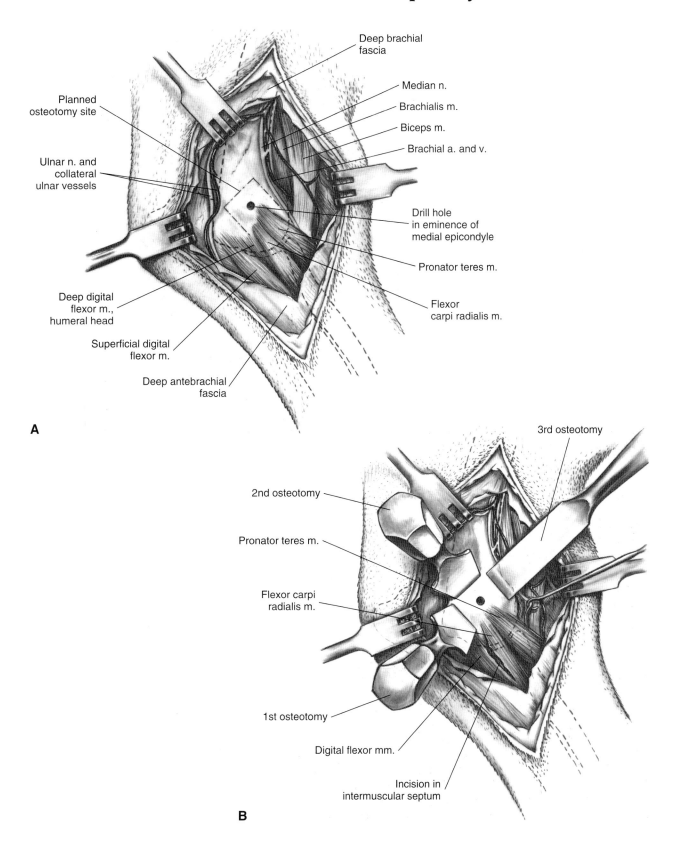

A

Planned osteotomy site

Ulnar n. and collateral ulnar vessels

Deep digital flexor m., humeral head

Superficial digital flexor m.

Deep antebrachial fascia

Deep brachial fascia

Median n.

Brachialis m.

Biceps m.

Brachial a. and v.

Drill hole in eminence of medial epicondyle

Pronator teres m.

Flexor carpi radialis m.

B

3rd osteotomy

2nd osteotomy

Pronator teres m.

Flexor carpi radialis m.

1st osteotomy

Digital flexor mm.

Incision in intermuscular septum

Approach to the Medial Aspect of the Humeral Condyle and the Medial Coronoid Process of the Ulna by Osteotomy of the Medial Humeral Epicondyle *continued*

C. The osteotomized bone with attached muscles and medial collateral ligament can be retracted distally after incising the joint capsule. Small Hohmann retractors are useful to expose the condyle and the medial coronoid process. The process is best visualized by abduction and pronation of the antebrachium.

CLOSURE

Interrupted sutures are placed in the joint capsule. The osteotomized epicondyle is reattached to its origin by a lag screw or with pins and a tension band wire (see Figures 23 and 24). Incisions in the intermuscular septa, deep antebrachial fascia, subcutaneous fascia, and skin are each closed in separate layers.

COMMENTS

The choice of osteotomy or muscle separation is primarily a matter of the surgeon's preference. Slightly better exposure is gained here than in the muscle separation approach. In young animals, the osteotomy approach carries a risk of growth plate damage and also epicondylar fixation failure due to the softness of the bone.

PRECAUTIONS

Cranial to the medial epicondyle, the median nerve passes between the origin of the pronator teres and biceps brachii muscles. At the flexor surface of the elbow, it dips laterally under the pronator teres and travels caudomedially, supplying muscular branches to the pronator teres, pronator quadratus, flexor carpi radialis, superficial digital flexor, and the radial head of the deep digital flexor muscles.

PLATE 50

Approach to the Medial Aspect of the Humeral Condyle and the Medial Coronoid Process of the Ulna by Osteotomy of the Medial Humeral Epicondyle *continued*

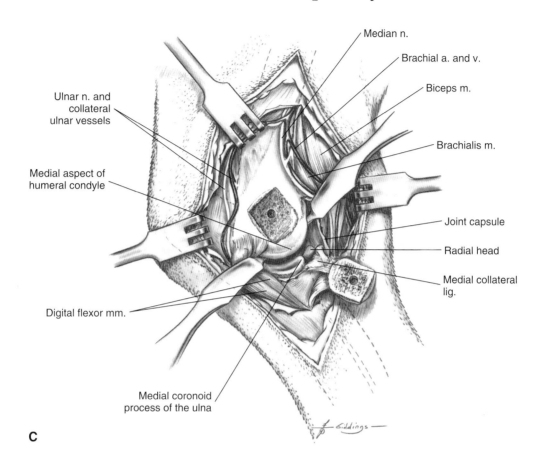

Median n.

Brachial a. and v.

Biceps m.

Ulnar n. and collateral ulnar vessels

Brachialis m.

Medial aspect of humeral condyle

Joint capsule

Radial head

Medial collateral lig.

Digital flexor mm.

Medial coronoid process of the ulna

C

Approach to the Proximal Shaft and Trochlear Notch of the Ulna

INDICATIONS

1. Open reduction of fractures in the region of the shaft or trochlear notch of the ulna.
2. Open reduction of fracture of the ulna and luxation of the head of the radius (Monteggia fracture).
3. Lengthening and shortening osteotomies of the proximal ulna.

ALTERNATIVE APPROACHES

The approach to the lateral humeroulnar part of the elbow provides better lateral exposure of the anconeal process (see Plate 41).

The lateral approaches to the elbow by collateral tenotomy (see Plate 46) or lateral epicondyle osteotomy (see Plate 47) provide better exposure of the lateral compartment of the elbow joint and radial head.

PATIENT POSITIONING

Dorsal recumbency with the affected limb suspended and retracted caudally for draping (see Plate 51A).

DESCRIPTION OF THE PROCEDURE

A. The caudal skin incision starts medial to the tuber olecrani and follows the shaft of the ulna distally to the midshaft region. The incision should be 5 to 10 mm medial to the ulnar midline. Subcutaneous and deep antebrachial fascia is incised on the same line.
B. A periosteal incision is made in the origin of the flexor carpi ulnaris muscle on the medial side of the tuber olecrani and shaft of the ulna. A short incision is also necessary in the insertion of the anconeus muscle on the lateral side. This incision continues distally through the fascia between the ulna and the ulnaris lateralis muscle.
C. Subperiosteal elevation and medial retraction of the flexor carpi ulnaris muscle and lateral retraction of the extensor carpi ulnaris muscle expose the ulna. Joint capsule incisions are made as necessary to expose the interior of the joint.

ADDITIONAL EXPOSURE

Greater exposure of the elbow joint is gained in combination with the olecranon osteotomy approach (see Plate 43) or the proximal ulnar diaphyseal osteotomy approach (see Plate 45).

More proximal exposure is gained laterally by elevation of the anconeus muscle (see Plate 52C).

Extension of the approach distally (see Plate 53) provides exposure of the entire ulnar shaft.

CLOSURE

External fasciae of the flexor and carpi ulnaris and ulnaris lateralis muscles are sutured over the caudal border of the ulna. Deep antebrachial fascia, subcutaneous tissues, and skin are closed in layers.

PLATE 51

Approach to the Proximal Shaft and Trochlear Notch of the Ulna

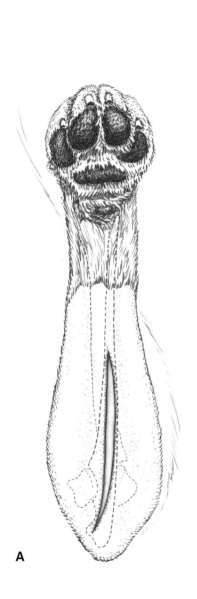

A

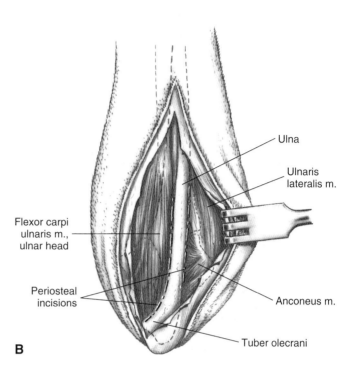

Ulna

Ulnaris
lateralis m.

Flexor carpi
ulnaris m.,
ulnar head

Periosteal
incisions

Anconeus m.

Tuber olecrani

B

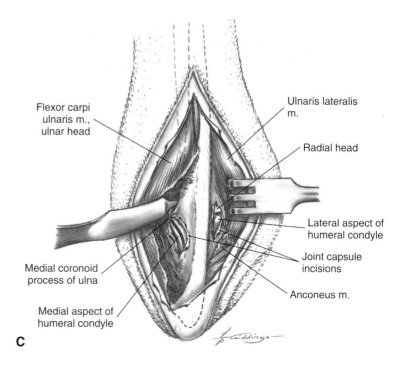

Flexor carpi
ulnaris m.,
ulnar head

Ulnaris lateralis
m.

Radial head

Lateral aspect of
humeral condyle

Joint capsule
incisions

Anconeus m.

Medial coronoid
process of ulna

Medial aspect of
humeral condyle

C

Approach to the Tuber Olecrani

INDICATIONS

1. Open reduction of fractures of the tuber olecrani.
2. Open reduction of fractures of the anconeal process.
3. Excision or fixation of an ununited anconeal process.

ALTERNATIVE APPROACHES

For excision or fixation of an ununited anconeal process, the choice between this approach and the lateral (see Plate 41) or caudal (see Plate 42) humeroulnar approaches is primarily a matter of the surgeon's personal preference.

PATIENT POSITIONING

Lateral recumbency with the affected limb uppermost.

DESCRIPTION OF THE PROCEDURE

A. The incision is centered between the lateral humeral epicondyle and the tuber olecrani and curves to follow the humeral condyle proximally and the olecranon distally. Subcutaneous fascia is incised on the same line and elevated with the skin.
B. Brachial fascia is incised parallel to the lateral head of the triceps brachii. A periosteal incision is made in the insertion of the anconeus muscle on the tuber olecrani. This incision continues proximally into the muscle, parallel to its fibers and near the edge of the lateral head of the triceps brachii muscle.
C. Elevation of the anconeus muscle exposes the humeral condyle, anconeal process, and tuber olecrani.

ADDITIONAL EXPOSURE

If the medial side of the tuber olecrani and trochlear notch must be exposed to allow for fracture reduction or placement of internal fixation, the flexor carpi ulnaris muscle can be elevated by incising fascia between the muscle and the bone. More proximal elevation of this muscle will require periosteal elevation, as in Plate 51C.

Extension of this approach distally (see Plate 53) provides exposure of the ulnar shaft.

Greater exposure of the elbow joint is gained in combination with the olecranon osteotomy (see Plate 43) or proximal ulnar osteotomy (see Plate 45) approach.

CLOSURE

The intramuscular incision in the anconeus is closed. The insertion of the muscle is sutured to remnants of its insertion or to fascia on the olecranon. The medial fascial incision is closed next, followed by closure of the brachial and subcutaneous fascia and then closure of the skin.

PLATE 52

Approach to the Tuber Olecrani

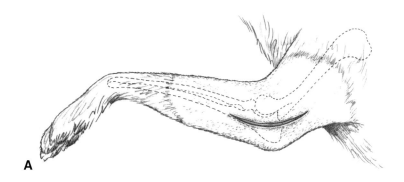

A

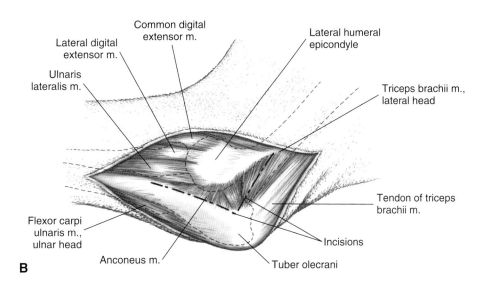

Common digital
extensor m.

Lateral digital
extensor m.

Ulnaris
lateralis m.

Lateral humeral
epicondyle

Triceps brachii m.,
lateral head

Tendon of triceps
brachii m.

Flexor carpi
ulnaris m.,
ulnar head

Incisions

Anconeus m.

Tuber olecrani

B

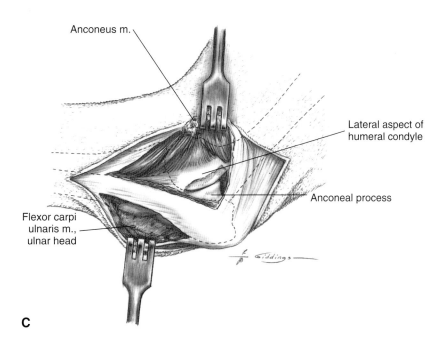

Anconeus m.

Lateral aspect of
humeral condyle

Anconeal process

Flexor carpi
ulnaris m.,
ulnar head

C

Approach to the Distal Shaft and Styloid Process of the Ulna

INDICATIONS

1. Ostectomy or osteotomy of the ulna for treatment of premature distal ulnar physeal closure.
2. Open reduction of fractures.

PATIENT POSITIONING

Lateral recumbency with the affected limb uppermost and suspended for draping.

DESCRIPTION OF THE PROCEDURE

A. The skin incision is made directly over the lateral surface of the bone, from the styloid to about the midshaft.
B. Incision of the subcutaneous tissues allows visualization beneath the antebrachial fascia of the tendon of the ulnaris lateralis muscle directly over, or slightly caudal to, the bone. Likewise, deep to the fascia is the tendon of the lateral digital extensor muscle cranial to the bone. The fascia is incised between the tendons.
C. Retraction of the tendons and fascia exposes the bone. If necessary, part of the origin of the abductor pollicis longus muscle can be elevated from its origin on the cranial border of the ulna and the interosseous ligament (see also Plate 56C and D).

ADDITIONAL EXPOSURE

For open reduction and internal fixation of fractures of the radius and ulna, this approach can be combined with the exposure of the radius laterally through the same skin incision (see Plate 56A and B) or medially through a separate skin incision (see Plate 55).

Distally the approach can be extended to gain exposure of the carpus and metacarpus (see Plate 57).

CLOSURE

Closure of the antebrachial fascia is followed by closure of the subcutis and the skin.

PLATE 53

Approach to the Distal Shaft and Styloid Process of the Ulna

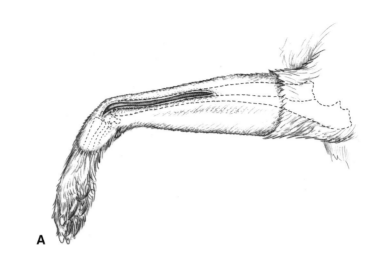

A

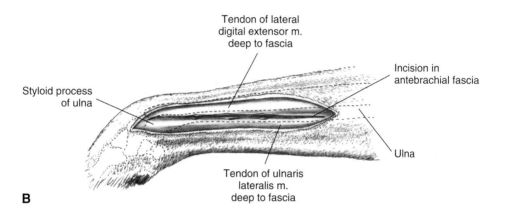

Tendon of lateral
digital extensor m.
deep to fascia

Incision in
antebrachial fascia

Styloid process
of ulna

Ulna

Tendon of ulnaris
lateralis m.
deep to fascia

B

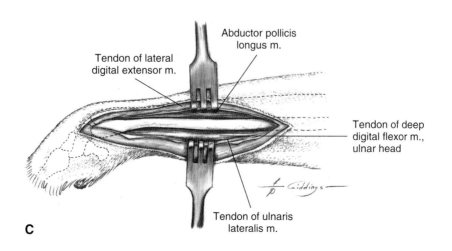

Abductor pollicis
longus m.

Tendon of lateral
digital extensor m.

Tendon of deep
digital flexor m.,
ulnar head

Tendon of ulnaris
lateralis m.

C

Approach to the Head and Proximal Metaphysis of the Radius

INDICATIONS

1. Open reduction of fractures.
2. Open reduction of luxation of the radial head.

ALTERNATIVE APPROACHES

The approaches to the head of the radius by lateral collateral tenotomy (see Plate 46) or lateral epicondyle osteotomy (see Plate 47) provide more limited exposure and cannot be extended distally because of the muscular branches of the radial nerve.

PATIENT POSITIONING

Lateral recumbency with the affected limb uppermost.

DESCRIPTION OF THE PROCEDURE

A. The skin is incised from the lateral epicondyle of the humerus on a line following the craniolateral border of the radius to the junction of the proximal and middle one third of the bone.
B. The deep antebrachial fascia is incised on the same line as the skin. The extensor muscles, collateral radial vessels, and a cutaneous branch of the radial nerve will be exposed. An incision is made in the intermuscular septum between the extensor carpi radialis and common digital extensor muscles. This incision starts just distal to the nerve. The vessels must be ligated.
C. Dissection between the extensor muscles allows their retraction and exposure of the supinator muscle. It is important that the deep ramus of the radial nerve be identified and protected throughout the rest of the procedure. Subperiosteal elevation of the supinator's insertion on the radius is begun distally.

PLATE 54

Approach to the Head and Proximal Metaphysis of the Radius

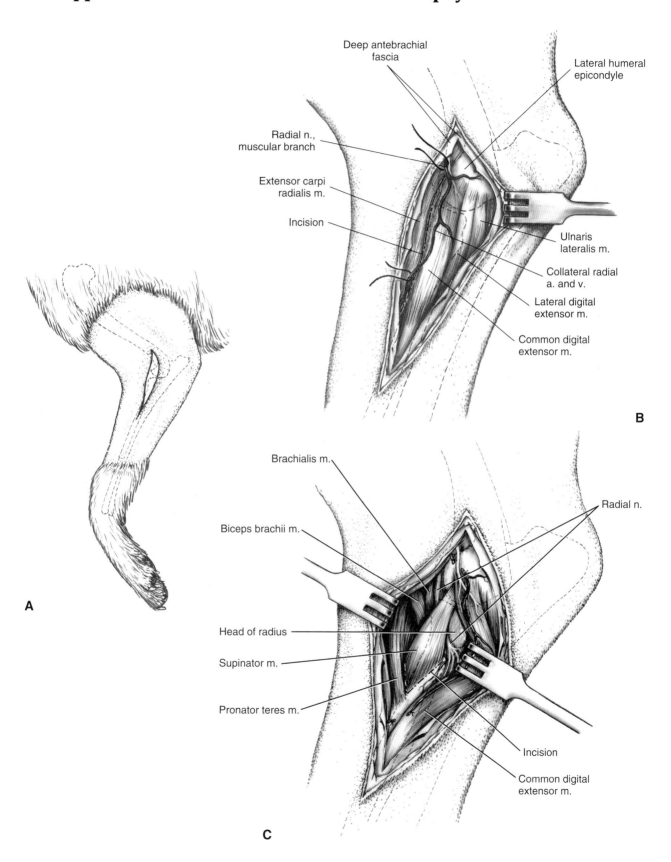

Approach to the Head and Proximal Metaphysis
of the Radius *continued*

D. Elevation of the proximal portion of the supinator muscle insertion must be done carefully to avoid injury of the radial nerve.

E. The radial nerve can be elevated and gently retracted with the supinator to expose the radius.

ADDITIONAL EXPOSURE

Proximal extension of the approach for exposure of the humeral condyle is gained in combination with the approach shown in Plate 39.

CLOSURE

There is usually very little of the supinator insertion left on the radius into which sutures can be placed. Sutures are placed in the external fascia of the supinator and attached to any other muscle fascia in the area, such as the pronator teres. The intermuscular septum is closed between the extensor muscles, followed by the deep antebrachial fascia, subcutaneous tissues, and skin.

PRECAUTIONS

The deep branch of the radial nerve supplies branches to the extensor carpi radialis muscle as it passes under this muscle on the flexor surface of the elbow. The remaining part of the nerve then continues under the supinator muscle, supplying branches to the joint capsule, supinator, and common and lateral digital extensor muscles as it continues distally in the interosseous space.

PLATE 54

Approach to the Head and Proximal Metaphysis of the Radius *continued*

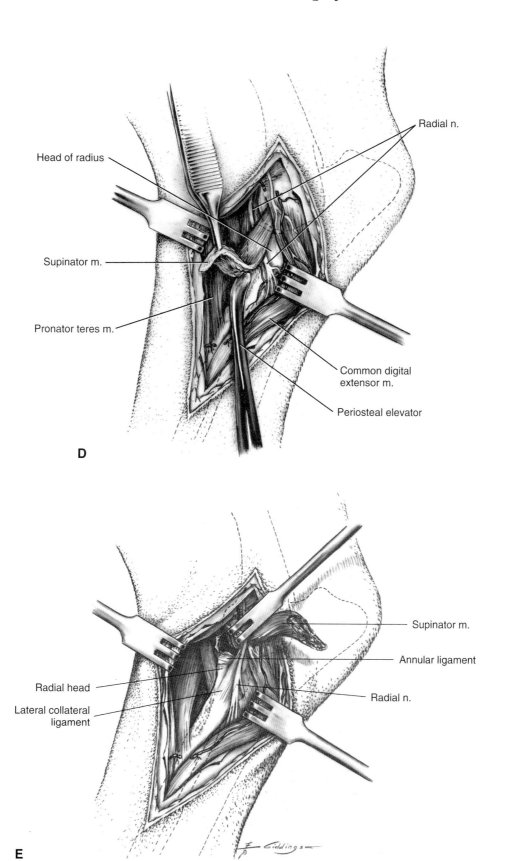

D

Head of radius

Radial n.

Supinator m.

Pronator teres m.

Common digital
extensor m.

Periosteal elevator

E

Supinator m.

Annular ligament

Radial head

Radial n.

Lateral collateral
ligament

Approach to the Shaft of the Radius Through a Medial Incision

INDICATIONS

1. Open reduction of fractures.
2. Osteotomy of the radius for treatment of growth deformities and malunion.

ALTERNATIVE APPROACH

The lateral approach to the shaft of the radius (see Plate 56) has the advantage that both the radius and ulna (see Plate 53) can be exposed through the same skin incision.

PATIENT POSITIONING

Dorsal recumbency with the affected limb abducted and suspended for draping.

DESCRIPTION OF THE PROCEDURE

A. The skin incision extends from the medial epicondyle of the humerus to the styloid process of the radius. The cephalic vein crosses beneath the distal portion of the incision and is protected during the incision.
B. Subcutaneous fascia is incised on the same line as the skin, and the skin edges are retracted to expose the underlying muscles. The deep antebrachial fascia is incised between the extensor carpi radialis and pronator muscles proximally, with the distal portion of the incision paralleling the extensor muscle. Note the proximity of the brachial artery and vein and median nerve at the proximal end of this incision (shown in more detail in Plate 50A).

PLATE 55

Approach to the Shaft of the Radius Through a Medial Incision

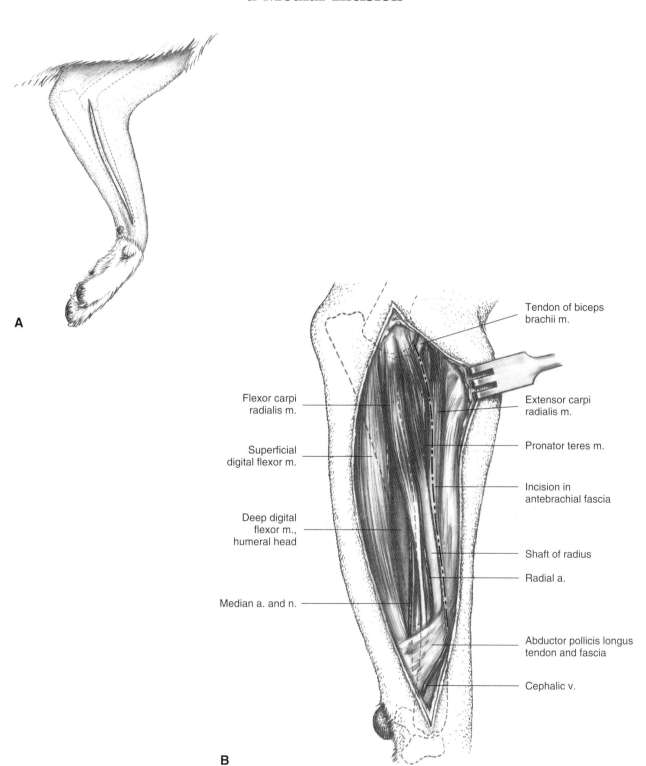

A

B

Tendon of biceps brachii m.

Flexor carpi radialis m.

Extensor carpi radialis m.

Pronator teres m.

Superficial digital flexor m.

Incision in antebrachial fascia

Deep digital flexor m., humeral head

Shaft of radius

Radial a.

Median a. and n.

Abductor pollicis longus tendon and fascia

Cephalic v.

Approach to the Shaft of the Radius Through a Medial Incision *continued*

C. Retraction of the extensor muscles laterally reveals the supinator muscle. If needed for exposure of the proximal radius, the insertions of the pronator and supinator muscles are incised on the radius.

D. Elevation of the pronator and supinator muscles completes the exposure of the proximal portion of the radius. The radial nerve lies deep to the proximal supinator and should be protected (see Plate 54C).

ADDITIONAL EXPOSURE

The flexor carpi radialis and deep digital flexor muscles can be elevated caudally for additional exposure of the radial shaft, but caution is needed to avoid severing the radial and caudal interosseous arteries that pass between the radius and these muscles.

Distally the skin incision can be curved toward the dorsal surface of the paw for additional exposure of the distal radius and carpus (see Plate 57).

CLOSURE

The pronator and supinator muscles are sutured to their insertions. If insufficient tissue remains at the insertion, these muscles are sutured to adjacent muscles: the pronator quadratus for the supinator and the medial edge of the extensor carpi radialis for the pronator. The deep antebrachial fascia and subcutaneous fascia are closed in separate layers.

PRECAUTIONS

During elevation of the pronator and supinator muscles, great care must be taken to protect the median and radial nerves. At the flexor surface of the elbow, the median nerve and brachial artery and vein dip laterally and pass deep to the pronator teres muscle. After emerging from under the pronator teres, the deep branch of the radial nerve gives off muscular branches innervating the flexor carpi radialis, superficial digital flexor, and the radial head of the deep digital flexor muscles. The deep branch of the radial nerve crosses the lateral surface of the elbow, then continues under the extensor carpi radialis and supinator muscles. On emerging from under the supinator, it immediately divides into branches that innervate the common and lateral digital extensor muscles.

PLATE 55

Approach to the Shaft of the Radius Through a Medial Incision *continued*

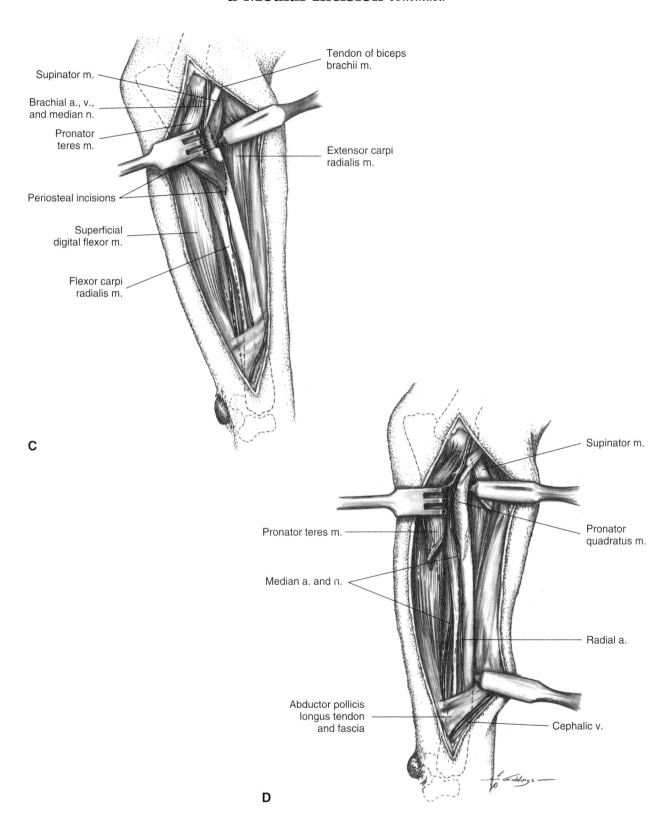

Supinator m.

Brachial a., v., and median n.

Pronator teres m.

Periosteal incisions

Superficial digital flexor m.

Flexor carpi radialis m.

Tendon of biceps brachii m.

Extensor carpi radialis m.

C

Pronator teres m.

Median a. and n.

Abductor pollicis longus tendon and fascia

Supinator m.

Pronator quadratus m.

Radial a.

Cephalic v.

D

Approach to the Shaft of the Radius Through a Lateral Incision

INDICATIONS

1. Open reduction and internal fixation of fractures of the shafts of the radius and ulna.
2. Osteotomy of the radius and ulna.

ALTERNATIVE APPROACH

The approach to the shaft of the radius through a medial incision (see Plate 55) is the alternative, but it does not permit simultaneous exposure of the ulna through the same skin incision.

PATIENT POSITIONING

Lateral recumbency with the affected limb uppermost and suspended for draping.

DESCRIPTION OF THE PROCEDURE

A. The incision is centered over the lateral edge of the radius, starting near the radial head and extending to the distal end of the bone. The subcutaneous fat and superficial antebrachial fascia are incised on the same line.
B. After retracting the skin margins, the shaft of the radius will come into view through the deep antebrachial fascia. This fascia is incised along the cranial border of the common digital extensor muscle to free this muscle for retraction.

PLATE 56

Approach to the Shaft of the Radius Through a Lateral Incision

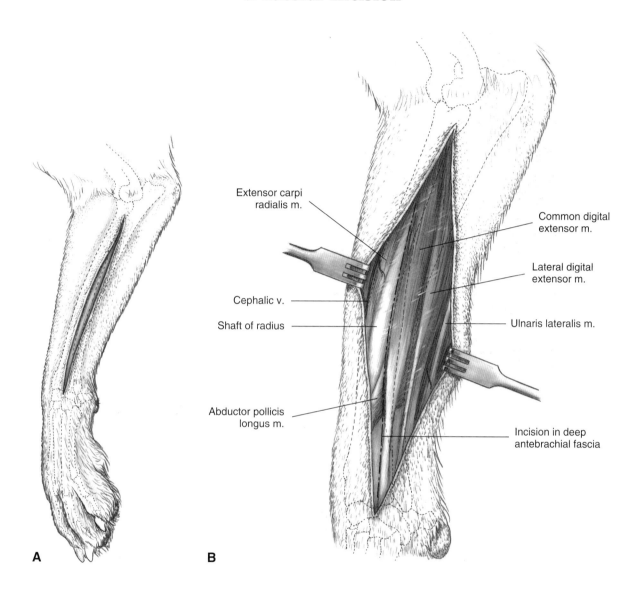

Extensor carpi radialis m.

Common digital extensor m.

Lateral digital extensor m.

Cephalic v.

Shaft of radius

Ulnaris lateralis m.

Abductor pollicis longus m.

Incision in deep antebrachial fascia

A

B

Approach to the Shaft of the Radius Through a Lateral Incision *continued*

C. Caudal retraction of the common and lateral digital extensor muscles exposes most of the shaft of the radius laterally. Better views of the cranial aspect are obtained by medial retraction of the extensor carpi radialis muscle. If more exposure of the caudolateral aspect of the radius and the ulna is needed, an incision is made through the abductor pollicis longus muscle near its origin on the ulna and parallel to the muscle extensor pollicis longus et indicis proprius.

D. Retraction of the extensor muscles provides complete exposure of the shafts of the radius and ulna.

ADDITIONAL EXPOSURE

For fractures and osteotomies, exposure of the ulna (see Plate 53) can be gained through the same skin incision.

Proximally, complete exposure of the radial head and proximal radius can be gained in combination with the approach shown in Plate 54.

Distally the skin incision can be curved toward the dorsal surface of the paw for additional exposure of the distal radius and carpus (see Plate 57).

CLOSURE

The abductor pollicis longus muscle is either reattached to its origin on the ulna or sutured to the cranial border of the extensor pollicis muscle. The deep antebrachial fascia is closed separately from the superficial fascia/subcutaneous fat layer. The skin is closed routinely.

COMMENTS

In the case of fractures, the choice between this lateral approach and the medial approach (see Plate 55) is often personal preference. However, if there is a need to reduce and apply fixation to the ulna in support of the radial fixation, this approach is superior to the medial approach. Soft-tissue injuries may also dictate which approach to choose.

PLATE 56
Approach to the Shaft of the Radius Through a Lateral Incision *continued*

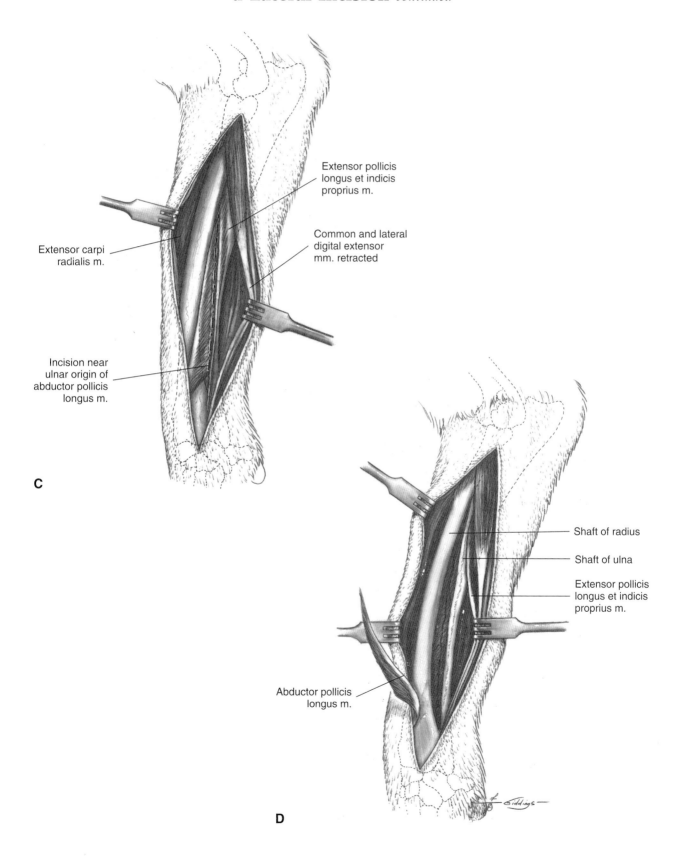

Extensor pollicis longus et indicis proprius m.

Common and lateral digital extensor mm. retracted

Extensor carpi radialis m.

Incision near ulnar origin of abductor pollicis longus m.

C

Shaft of radius

Shaft of ulna

Extensor pollicis longus et indicis proprius m.

Abductor pollicis longus m.

D

Approach to the Distal Radius and Carpus Through a Dorsal Incision

Based on a Procedure of Hurov, Lumb, Hankes, and Smith[24]

INDICATIONS

1. Open reduction of fractures of the distal radius or carpal bones.
2. Open reduction of luxations of the joint.
3. Arthrodesis of the carpus.

ALTERNATIVE APPROACHES

For pancarpal arthrodesis, the amount of exposure gained through a palmaromedial incision (see Plate 58) is inferior to that obtained with the dorsal approach.

The best exposure of fractures of the accessory carpal bone is obtained with the palmarolateral approach (see Plate 59).

PATIENT POSITIONING

Dorsal recumbency with the affected limb suspended for draping.

DESCRIPTION OF THE PROCEDURE

A. The skin incision is made on the mid-dorsal surface of the joint and extends from the juncture of the cephalic and accessory cephalic veins to the middle of the metacarpus. The incision is lateral to the accessory cephalic vein and curves laterally at its distal end to follow the vein.
   Subcutaneous fascia is likewise incised just lateral to the vein, with enough fascia being left on the vein to allow the placing of sutures in this tissue during closure. The vein and fascia are undermined and retracted medially with the skin.
B. The deep antebrachial fascia is incised midway between the tendon of the extensor carpi radialis and the tendon of the common digital extensor. The usual limits of incision are the abductor pollicis longus muscle proximally and the proximal metacarpal bones distally. The incision is then deepened to penetrate the periosteum on the distal end of the radius.
C. The periosteum is elevated medially and laterally to allow the retraction of the tendons without disturbing their sheaths. The fat pad attached to the extensor carpi radialis tendon may be trimmed, if necessary, to allow visualization of the joint cavity. The styloid process of the ulna may be exposed by continued lateral elevation of the periosteum and retraction of the lateral digital extensor tendon. Arthrotomy incisions are made as necessary.

PLATE 57

Approach to the Distal Radius and Carpus Through a Dorsal Incision

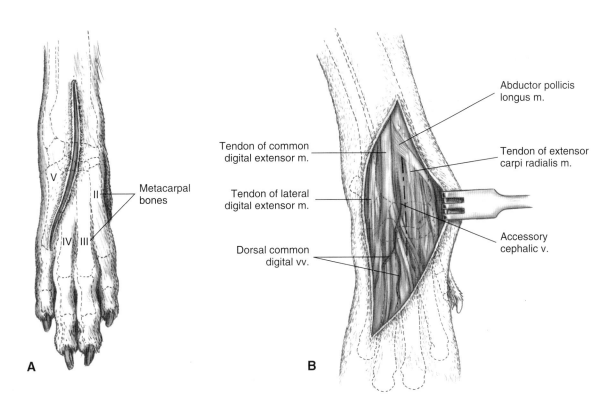

A

Metacarpal bones

Tendon of common digital extensor m.

Tendon of lateral digital extensor m.

Dorsal common digital vv.

Abductor pollicis longus m.

Tendon of extensor carpi radialis m.

Accessory cephalic v.

B

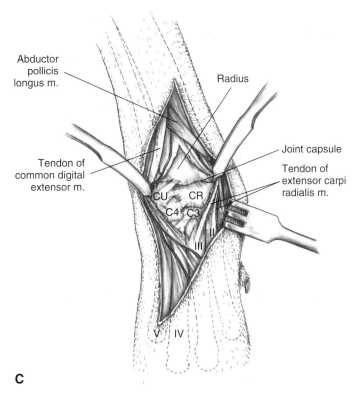

Abductor pollicis longus m.

Radius

Tendon of common digital extensor m.

Joint capsule

Tendon of extensor carpi radialis m.

C

Approach to the Distal Radius and Carpus Through a Dorsal Incision *continued*

  D. Because the synovium is adherent to the dorsal surfaces of individual carpal bones, the joint capsule must be incised around each bone to expose it. Exposure of the various joint spaces is enhanced by flexion of the carpus.

ADDITIONAL EXPOSURE

  E. Additional exposure of the distal third of the radial diaphysis can be obtained by extending the skin incision proximally; this will usually be necessary for bone plate application for pancarpal arthrodesis or fractures of the distal end of the radius. The skin incision should be located lateral to the cephalic vein, so that the vein and accompanying superficial branches of the radial nerve are all displaced medially with the skin margin. With separation of the skin margins using Gelpi retractors, the abductor pollicis longus muscle and tendon can be seen crossing the distal third of the radius obliquely. The common digital extensor tendon is lateral, and the tendons of extensor carpi radius are medial.

  F. After lateral retraction of the common digital extensor tendon, the origin of the abductor pollicis longus muscle is sharply incised from the periosteum of the radius along its lateral margin, and then elevated proximally using a periosteal elevator.

PLATE 57

Approach to the Distal Radius and Carpus Through a Dorsal Incision *continued*

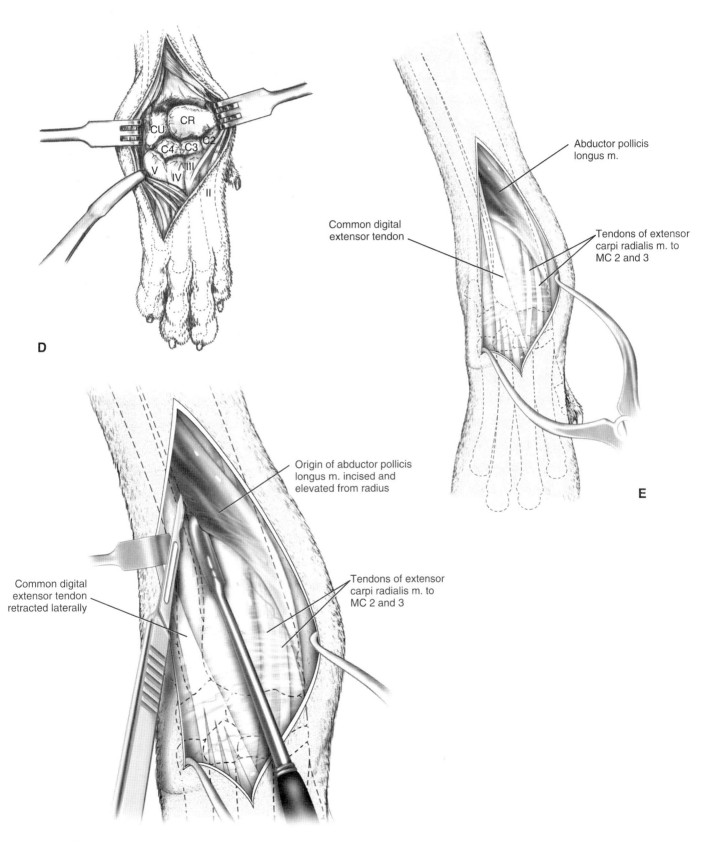

D

CR
CU
C2
C4 C3
V IV III
II

Abductor pollicis
longus m.

Common digital
extensor tendon

Tendons of extensor
carpi radialis m. to
MC 2 and 3

E

Origin of abductor pollicis
longus m. incised and
elevated from radius

Common digital
extensor tendon
retracted laterally

Tendons of extensor
carpi radialis m. to
MC 2 and 3

F

Approach to the Distal Radius and Carpus Through a Dorsal Incision *continued*

G. The abductor pollicis longus muscle is retracted medially. The synovial sheath surrounding the common digital extensor tendon is incised longitudinally all the way distally to the dorsal surface of the carpus. The tendon is displaced laterally out of the lateral sulcus on the distal end of the radius. Similarly the extensor carpi radialis tendon is released from the synovial sheath and middle sulcus on the distal radius.

PLATE 57

Approach to the Distal Radius and Carpus Through a Dorsal Incision *continued*

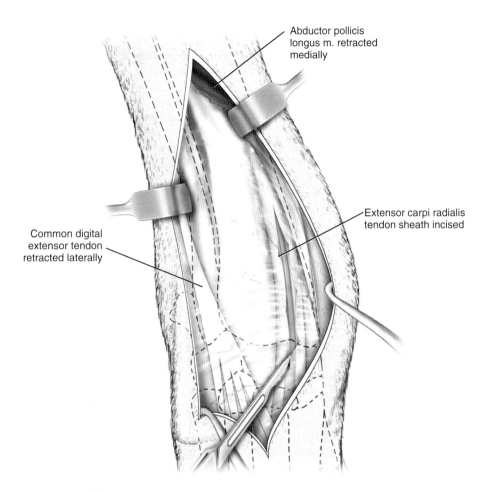

Abductor pollicis
longus m. retracted
medially

Extensor carpi radialis
tendon sheath incised

Common digital
extensor tendon
retracted laterally

G

Approach to the Distal Radius and Carpus Through a Dorsal Incision *continued*

H. Gelpi retractors are used to displace the extensor carpi radialis and abductor pollicis longus tendons medially. Greater exposure of the carpal joints can be achieved by transection of the insertions of the extensor carpi radialis tendons from the base of metacarpal bones II and III, respectively. The underlying joint capsule of the antebrachiocarpal joint is incised to expose the articular cartilage surfaces.

CLOSURE

There is usually little synovium available for closure. Simply close the deep and superficial fascial layers over the tendons before closing the skin.

PLATE 57

Approach to the Distal Radius and Carpus Through a Dorsal Incision *continued*

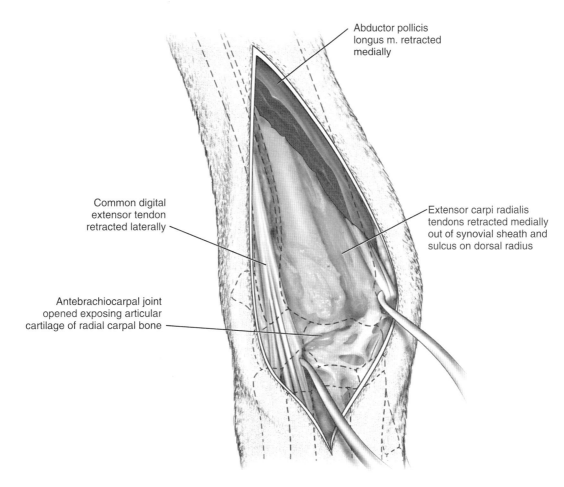

Abductor pollicis longus m. retracted medially

Common digital extensor tendon retracted laterally

Extensor carpi radialis tendons retracted medially out of synovial sheath and sulcus on dorsal radius

Antebrachiocarpal joint opened exposing articular cartilage of radial carpal bone

H

Approach to the Distal Radius and Carpus Through a Palmaromedial Incision

INDICATIONS

1. Panarthrodesis of the carpus with palmar bone plate.
2. Fixation of caudal fractures of the distal radius and palmar process fractures of the radial carpal bone.
3. Removal of bone fragments from carpal joints.

ALTERNATIVE APPROACH

For pancarpal arthrodesis, the amount of exposure gained through a dorsal incision (see Plate 57) is superior to that obtained with the palmaromedial approach.

The best exposure of fractures of the accessory carpal bone is obtained with the palmarolateral approach (see Plate 59).

PATIENT POSITIONING

Dorsal recumbency with the affected limb abducted and suspended for draping.

DESCRIPTION OF THE PROCEDURE

A. The longitudinal skin incision is equidistant between the radial styloid process and the carpal pad. A longer incision is needed for palmar bone plating.
B. The cephalic vein is double ligated and divided. An incision is made in the midportion of the flexor retinacular fascia and lengthened proximally into the antebrachial fascia as needed.
C. On retracting the retinacular fascia, the tendons of the flexor carpi radialis and the digital flexor muscles, as well as the median artery and nerve, will be visible. Branches of the vessels and nerves to the first digit are isolated and the vessels ligated. The flexor tendon can be divided, or simply retracted, depending on the exposure required. Because of the anatomic complexity of this region, considerable license has been taken with steps D and E. Omitted for clarity are the lumbricales, interosseus, adductor digiti secundi, and adductor/flexor pollicis muscles. Also omitted are the palmar carpal fibrocartilage and the palmar ligamentous structure. These tissues are incised and retracted as necessary to achieve the exposure depicted in Plate 58D and E.

PLATE 58

Approach to the Distal Radius and Carpus Through a Palmaromedial Incision

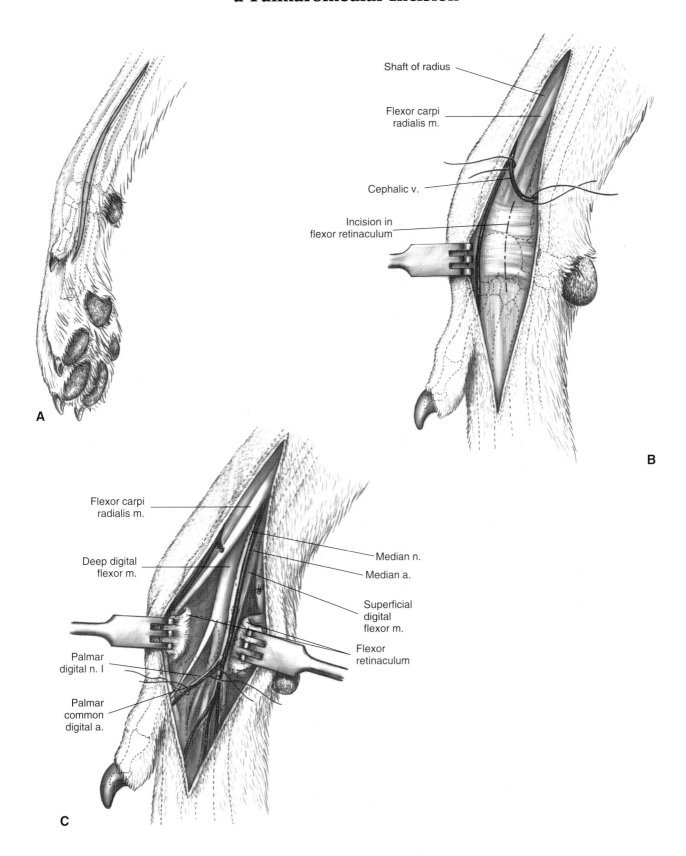

A

B

Shaft of radius

Flexor carpi radialis m.

Cephalic v.

Incision in flexor retinaculum

Flexor carpi radialis m.

Deep digital flexor m.

Median n.

Median a.

Superficial digital flexor m.

Flexor retinaculum

Palmar digital n. I

Palmar common digital a.

C

Approach to the Distal Radius and Carpus Through a Palmaromedial Incision *continued*

D. Retraction of the digital flexor tendons exposes the palmar carpal region superficially. The entire region will be covered by a combination of joint capsule, ligaments, and palmar carpal fibrocartilage. The desired joint spaces are identified by probing with a hypodermic needle. Incisions in the appropriate spaces are then made. Be aware of the deep palmar arch and palmar metacarpal arteries as these incisions are made.

E. Incisions in the joint capsules of the various joints are extended as needed.

CLOSURE

Unless an arthrodesis has been done, the joint capsule/ligament/fibrocartilage incisions are closed with interrupted sutures of nonabsorbable or polydioxanone materials. The flexor retinaculum and deep antebrachial fascia are similarly closed. There is usually not enough subcutaneous tissue to warrant suturing.

COMMENTS

External support by cast or splint is needed for several weeks to allow healing of the palmar carpal structures.

PLATE 58

Approach to the Distal Radius and Carpus Through a Palmaromedial Incision *continued*

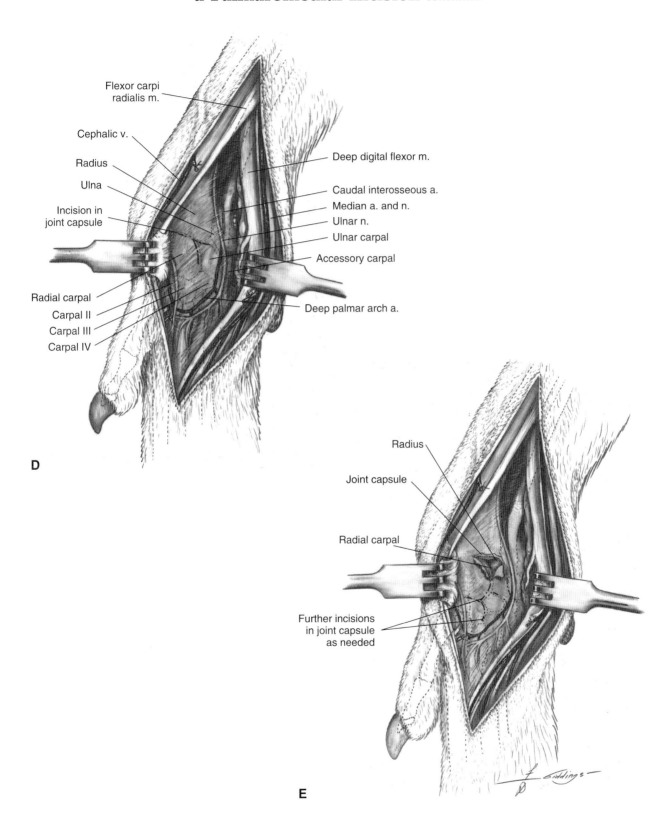

Flexor carpi radialis m.

Cephalic v.

Radius

Ulna

Incision in joint capsule

Radial carpal

Carpal II

Carpal III

Carpal IV

Deep digital flexor m.

Caudal interosseous a.

Median a. and n.

Ulnar n.

Ulnar carpal

Accessory carpal

Deep palmar arch a.

D

Radius

Joint capsule

Radial carpal

Further incisions in joint capsule as needed

E

Approach to the Accessory Carpal Bone and Palmarolateral Carpal Joints

INDICATIONS

1. Internal fixation of fractures of the accessory carpal bone.
2. Internal fixation of fractures of the palmar process of the ulnar carpal bone.
3. Ligamentous reconstructive procedures.

DESCRIPTION OF THE PROCEDURE

A.   The skin incision is made from the caudomedial border of the distal ulna, curving laterally around the accessory carpal bone and ending distally over the palmar side of the fifth metacarpal bone. Subcutaneous fascia is incised on the same line.

B.   Deep fascia intimately connects the carpal pad to the free end of the accessory carpal bone. This fascia is partially dissected to allow medial retraction of the skin and pad. Extending laterally from the free end of the accessory carpal and inserting on the tendon of the ulnaris lateralis is the lateral flexor retinaculum, which is incised near the accessory carpal bone. This will allow sharp dissection to free the abductor digiti quinti muscle from its origin on the accessory carpal bone. The muscle is freed from between the two accessory metacarpal ligaments and reflected distally (see Comments).

C.   Retraction of the accessory metacarpal ligaments will reveal the distomedial surface of the accessory carpal bone, the most common site of fractures.

PLATE 59

Approach to the Accessory Carpal Bone and Palmarolateral Carpal Joints

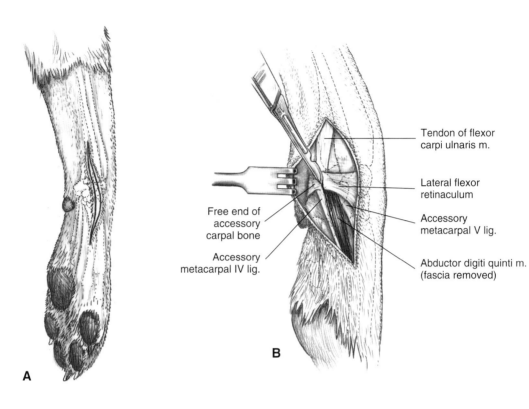

Tendon of flexor
carpi ulnaris m.

Lateral flexor
retinaculum

Accessory
metacarpal V lig.

Abductor digiti quinti m.
(fascia removed)

Free end of
accessory
carpal bone

Accessory
metacarpal IV lig.

A

B

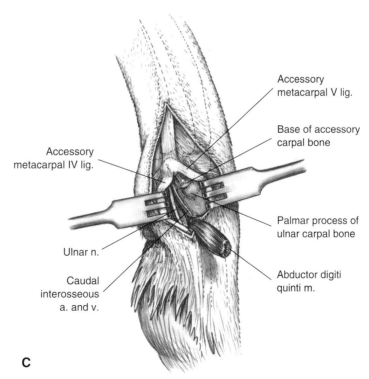

Accessory
metacarpal V lig.

Base of accessory
carpal bone

Palmar process of
ulnar carpal bone

Abductor digiti
quinti m.

Accessory
metacarpal IV lig.

Ulnar n.

Caudal
interosseous
a. and v.

C

Approach to the Accessory Carpal Bone and Palmarolateral Carpal Joints *continued*

D, E. To open the palmarolateral aspect of the antebrachiocarpal joint, the accessory carpal bone is retracted medially to help identify the joint space along its lateral border. This joint capsule is incised from the ulnar styloid process around the lateral side of the accessory carpal and onto the palmar process of the ulnar carpal bone. Try to leave some capsule tissue on the accessory carpal to allow for suturing. Strong medial and distal retraction of the free end of the accessory carpal bone will expose most of the articular surface and allow removal of small bone fragments.

CLOSURE

The joint capsule incision is closed with interrupted sutures. The abductor digiti quinti muscle is reattached to the accessory metacarpal ligaments; the flexor retinaculum is likewise closed with interrupted sutures, followed by closure of the skin.

COMMENTS

The abductor digiti quinti muscle does not need to be detached to make the joint capsule incision. The only purpose of reflecting the muscle is to allow inspection of the distomedial surface of the accessory carpal bone.

PLATE 59

Approach to the Accessory Carpal Bone and Palmarolateral Carpal Joints *continued*

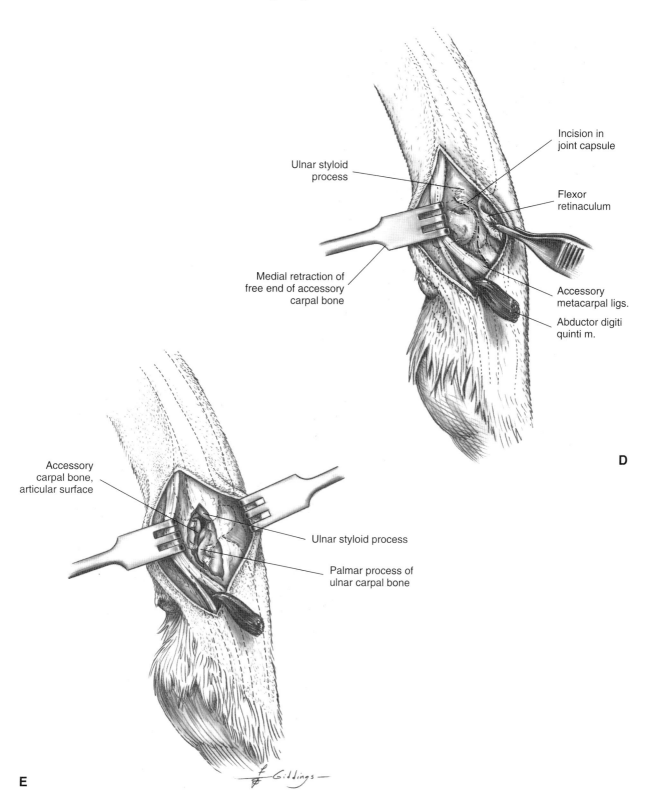

Incision in
joint capsule

Ulnar styloid
process

Flexor
retinaculum

Medial retraction of
free end of accessory
carpal bone

Accessory
metacarpal ligs.

Abductor digiti
quinti m.

D

Accessory
carpal bone,
articular surface

Ulnar styloid process

Palmar process of
ulnar carpal bone

E

Approaches to the Metacarpal Bones

INDICATION

Open reduction of fractures.

DESCRIPTION OF THE PROCEDURE

A. The anatomy shown in Plate 60A is considerably simplified compared with that in a live animal. Only the important structures are shown; other elements, such as small tendons and blood vessels, have been omitted. In an average-sized dog, these vestigial structures are so small that their identification and preservation are not practical during surgery.

PLATE 60

Approaches to the Metacarpal Bones

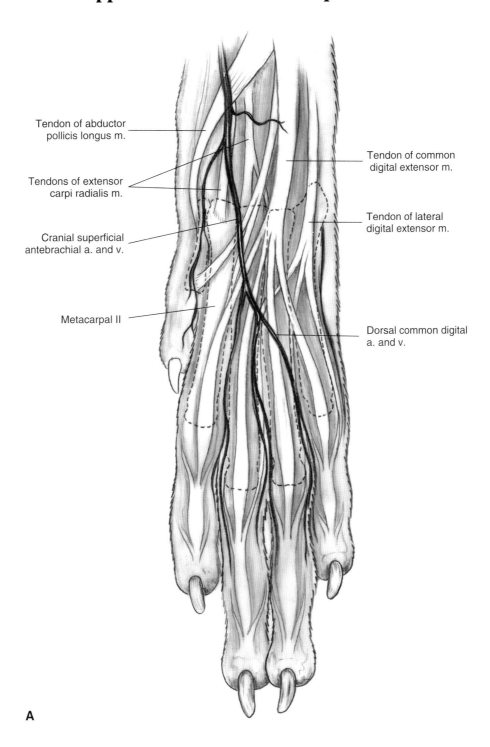

Tendon of abductor
pollicis longus m.

Tendons of extensor
carpi radialis m.

Cranial superficial
antebrachial a. and v.

Metacarpal II

Tendon of common
digital extensor m.

Tendon of lateral
digital extensor m.

Dorsal common digital
a. and v.

A

Approaches to the Metacarpal Bones *continued*

B, C. The incisional technique varies according to the bone or bones to be exposed. A single bone is approached by an incision directly over the bone, and two adjoining bones by an incision between them. If more than two bones need to be exposed, two parallel longitudinal incisions (see Plate 60B) or a single curved incision (see Plate 60C) can be used. The curved incision commences at the proximal end of metacarpal II, runs laterally to the midshaft of metacarpal V, and then curves medially again to end over the distal end of metacarpal II. The crescent-shaped skin flap can be elevated and retracted to expose a large part of all four bones.

To expose metacarpals II and III, the deep fascia is incised over bone II and the vessels and tendons are then undermined and retracted laterally. Deep fascia is incised over bone V to expose bones IV and V. Tendons and vessels are again undermined and retracted medially. Exposure of bone IV sometimes requires an incision between tendons, followed by sufficient dissection of the tendons from the surrounding fascia to allow their separation and retraction.

CLOSURE

Deep fascia is closed to ensure that tendons and vessels are held securely in their proper positions.

COMMENTS

A deep layer of small metacarpal blood vessels is found on and between the bones. These vessels are too small to avoid in most animals, and the resulting hemorrhage must be controlled by tamponade. Apply a snug bandage for 72 hours postoperatively to control oozing hemorrhage at the operative site.

PLATE 60

Approaches to the Metacarpal Bones *continued*

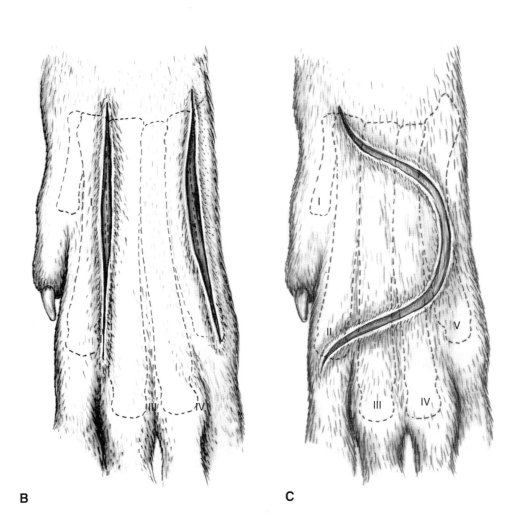

B

C

Approach to the Proximal Sesamoid Bones

INDICATION

Excision of fractured sesamoid bones.

DESCRIPTION OF THE PROCEDURE

A. The most commonly fractured sesamoid bones in both the fore and hind paws are those of metacarpal or metatarsal II and V. The skin incision curves around the metacarpal or metatarsal pad. A medial incision can be used for metacarpals/ metatarsals II and III, and a lateral incision for IV and V.

B. After reflection of the skin, the sesamoid bones are palpated at the metacarpophalangeal/metatarsophalangeal joint. A longitudinal incision is made in the manica flexoria and the sheath of the superficial digital flexor tendon directly over the sesamoids.

The Forelimb ■ 305

PLATE 61
Approach to the Proximal Sesamoid Bones

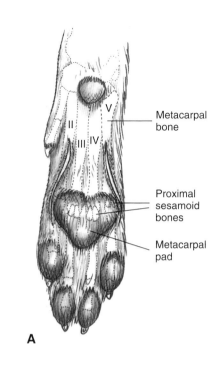

A

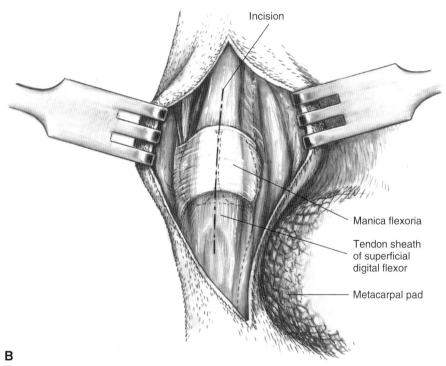

B

Approach to the Proximal Sesamoid Bones *continued*

    C. Retraction of the manica flexoria and sheath of the superficial digital flexor tendon reveals the paired sesamoid bones under the digital flexor tendons. Details of the cross-sectional anatomy are shown in Plate 61D. The tendons can be retracted in either direction to expose the sesamoid bones. If the bone is fractured at about the midportion, the entire bone is removed. If fractured toward the end of the bone, only the smaller fragment is removed. Removal consists of sharply dissecting away the intersesamoidean, lateral, medial, and cruciate ligaments of the sesamoid bones.

    D. A transverse section of the structures depicted in Part C is seen here.

CLOSURE

Interrupted sutures are placed in the manica flexoria superficial digital flexor tendon sheath incision. The skin is closed next, it being unnecessary to close the subcutaneous tissue.

COMMENT

A padded bandage should be worn for 10 days.

PLATE 61

Approach to the Proximal Sesamoid Bones *continued*

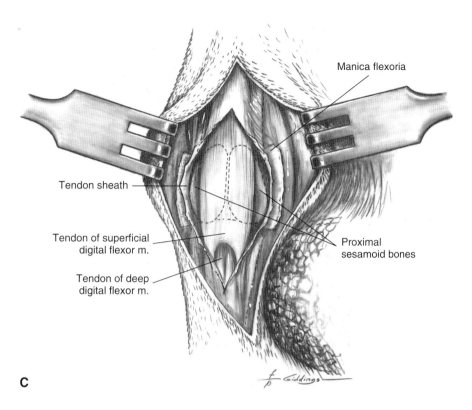

Manica flexoria

Tendon sheath

Tendon of superficial
digital flexor m.

Tendon of deep
digital flexor m.

Proximal
sesamoid bones

C

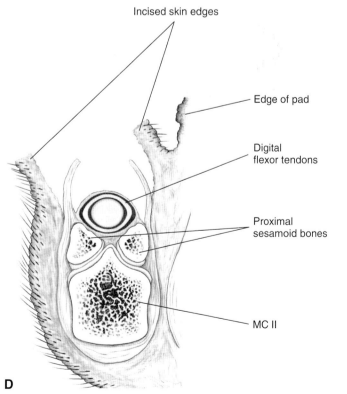

Incised skin edges

Edge of pad

Digital
flexor tendons

Proximal
sesamoid bones

MC II

D

Approaches to the Phalanges and Interphalangeal Joints

INDICATIONS

1. Open reduction of fractures of the phalanges.
2. Open reduction of luxations of the metatarsophalangeal, metacarpophalangeal, and interphalangeal joints.

DESCRIPTION OF THE PROCEDURE

A. The skin incision starts at the distal end of the appropriate metacarpal or metatarsal bone, proceeds distally over the dorsal surface of the phalanges, and ends over the distal phalanx. If the distal interphalangeal joint is to be exposed, a transverse incision can be made at the distal end of the longitudinal incision to form a T.
B. Sharp dissection is used to reflect skin flaps away from underlying bones and tendons.

CLOSURE

Because of the scarcity of subcutaneous tissues, the skin is often the only layer to be closed.

COMMENTS

A snug, padded bandage should be worn for 10 days, unless the foot is splinted.

PLATE 62
Approaches to the Phalanges and Interphalangeal Joints

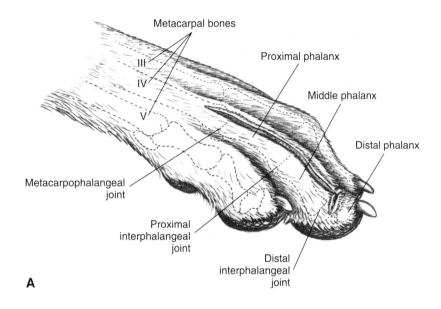

Metacarpal bones

III
IV
V

Proximal phalanx

Middle phalanx

Distal phalanx

Metacarpophalangeal joint

Proximal interphalangeal joint

Distal interphalangeal joint

A

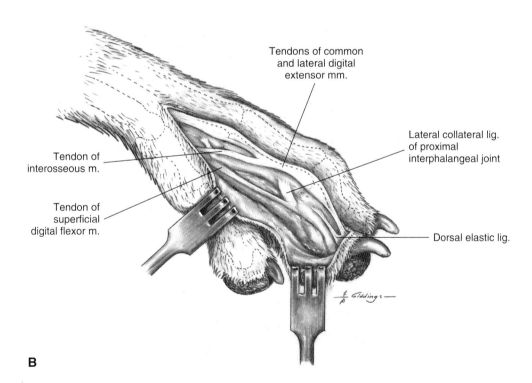

Tendons of common and lateral digital extensor mm.

Lateral collateral lig. of proximal interphalangeal joint

Tendon of interosseous m.

Tendon of superficial digital flexor m.

Dorsal elastic lig.

B

SECTION 6

The Pelvis and Hip Joint

- Approach to the Wing of the Ilium and Dorsal Aspect of the Sacrum

- Approach to the Ilium Through a Lateral Incision

- Approach to the Ventral Aspect of the Sacrum

- Approach to the Craniodorsal Aspect of the Hip Joint Through a Craniolateral Incision in the Dog

- Approach to the Craniodorsal Aspect of the Hip Joint Through a Craniolateral Incision in the Cat

- Approach to the Dorsal Aspect of the Hip Joint Through an Intergluteal Incision

- Approach to the Craniodorsal and Caudodorsal Aspects of the Hip Joint by Osteotomy of the Greater Trochanter

- Approach to the Craniodorsal and Caudodorsal Aspects of the Hip Joint by Tenotomy of the Gluteal Muscles

- Approach to the Caudal Aspect of the Hip Joint and Body of the Ischium

- Approach to the Lateral Aspect of the Hemipelvis

- Approach to the Ventral Aspect of the Hip Joint or the Ramus of the Pubis

- Approach to the Pubis and Pelvic Symphysis

- Approach to the Ischium

Approach to the Wing of the Ilium and Dorsal Aspect of the Sacrum

Based on a Procedure of Alexander, Archibald, and Cawley[2]

INDICATIONS

1. Open reduction of sacroiliac luxations and sacral fractures.
2. Open reduction of fractures of the wing of the ilium.
3. Collection of cancellous bone graft.

ALTERNATIVE APPROACHES

Dorsal midline exposure of fractures and luxations of lumbar vertebra 7 and the sacrum is obtained via the dorsal approach (see Plate 21).

To gain exposure of both the wing and shaft of the ilium, use the "gluteal roll-up" approach through a lateral incision (see Plate 64).

The ventral approach is an alternative means of gaining exposure of the sacroiliac joint (see Plate 65). An advantage of the ventral approach is that it can readily be combined with the lateral approach to the ilial shaft (see Plate 64).

PATIENT POSITIONING

Either lateral recumbency (illustrated) with the affected side uppermost or sternal recumbency when bilateral approaches are planned.

DESCRIPTION OF THE PROCEDURE

A. The skin incision starts cranially over the cranial dorsal iliac spine and continues caudally parallel to the midline to near the hip joint. Subcutaneous tissues and gluteal fascia and fat are incised on the same line to expose the cranial and caudal dorsal iliac spines.
B. If only the lateral (gluteal) surface of the wing of the ilium needs to be exposed, as for fractures or cancellous bone collection, an incision is made in the periosteal origin of the middle gluteal muscle on the lateral edge of the ilium near the cranial dorsal iliac spine and ending beyond the caudal dorsal spine. If the sacrum must also be exposed, a second incision is made in the periosteal origin of the sacrospinalis muscle, at the medial edge of the ilium. These incisions merge as they continue caudally, and it will be necessary to transect some fibers of the superficial gluteal muscle in this region.

PLATE 63

Approach to the Wing of the Ilium and Dorsal Aspect of the Sacrum

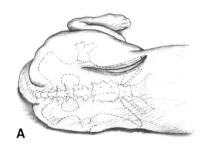

A

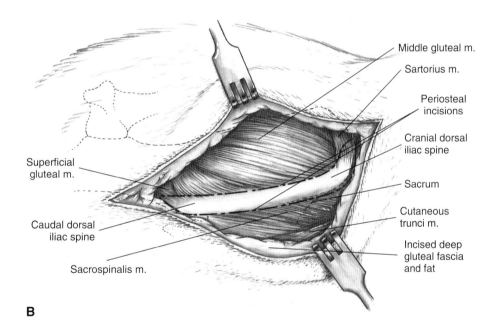

Middle gluteal m.

Sartorius m.

Periosteal incisions

Cranial dorsal iliac spine

Sacrum

Cutaneous trunci m.

Incised deep gluteal fascia and fat

Superficial gluteal m.

Caudal dorsal iliac spine

Sacrospinalis m.

B

Approach to the Wing of the Ilium and Dorsal Aspect of the Sacrum *continued*

C. The middle gluteal muscle is elevated subperiosteally in young animals, or simply scraped from its origin on the ilium in older animals. The elevation continues caudally to the caudal dorsal iliac spine. Continuing further, caudal dissection will result in severance of the cranial gluteal artery, vein, and nerve. Similar elevation of the sacrospinalis muscle on the medial side of the ilium gives limited exposure of the dorsal surface of the sacrum. Muscular elevation on the sacrum should be confined to the area lateral to the intermediate crests to avoid damage to dorsal nerve roots emerging through the dorsal foramina of the sacrum.

CLOSURE

Superficial fascia of the sacrospinalis and middle gluteal muscles is joined by a row of sutures crossing the wing of the ilium. Caudal to this, the fascia of the superficial gluteal muscle is sutured. This is followed by layer closure of the gluteal fascia, the gluteal fat and subcutaneous fascia, and the skin.

PRECAUTIONS

The approach should not be extended caudally beyond the caudal dorsal iliac spine. The cranial gluteal nerve arises as a branch of the lumbosacral trunk, just caudoventral to the sacroiliac joint. Accompanied by the cranial gluteal artery and vein, it then circles dorsally across the shaft of the ilium at the origin of the caudal bundle of the deep gluteal muscle.

PLATE 63

Approach to the Wing of the Ilium and Dorsal Aspect of the Sacrum *continued*

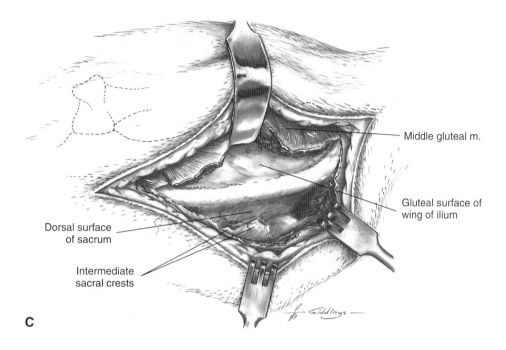

Middle gluteal m.

Gluteal surface of wing of ilium

Dorsal surface of sacrum

Intermediate sacral crests

C

Approach to the Ilium Through a Lateral Incision

Based on a Procedure of Hohn and Janes[22]

INDICATIONS

1. Open reduction of fractures of the wing and shaft of the ilium.
2. Osteotomy of the ilial shaft for the triple pelvic osteotomy procedure.

ALTERNATIVE APPROACH

The dorsal approach (see Plate 63) can be used if exposure of only the iliac wing is needed.

PATIENT POSITIONING

Lateral recumbency with the affected side uppermost.

DESCRIPTION OF THE PROCEDURE

A. The skin incision extends from the center of the iliac crest and ends just caudal and distal to the greater trochanter.
B. Subcutaneous tissues, gluteal fat, and superficial fascia are incised and elevated with the skin. Incision of the deep gluteal fascia on the same line as the skin allows incision of the intermuscular septum between the tensor fasciae latae and middle gluteal muscles. This incision extends from the ventral iliac spine to the cranial border of the biceps femoris muscle. Fascia is also incised along the cranial border of the biceps femoris muscle to create a T-shaped fascial incision.
C. Retraction of the middle gluteal muscle exposes the deep gluteal muscle and a portion of the iliac shaft.

PLATE 64

Approach to the Ilium Through a Lateral Incision

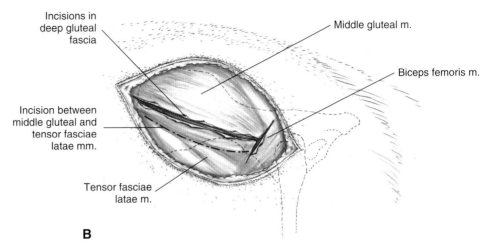

Incisions in deep gluteal fascia

Middle gluteal m.

Biceps femoris m.

Incision between middle gluteal and tensor fasciae latae mm.

Tensor fasciae latae m.

B

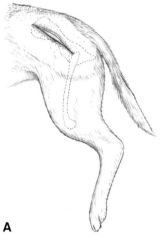

A

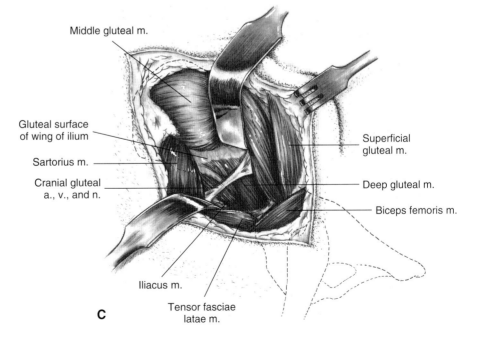

Middle gluteal m.

Gluteal surface of wing of ilium

Sartorius m.

Cranial gluteal a., v., and n.

Superficial gluteal m.

Deep gluteal m.

Biceps femoris m.

Iliacus m.

Tensor fasciae latae m.

C

Approach to the Ilium Through a Lateral Incision *continued*

D. An incision is made in the origin of the middle gluteal muscle on the ilium, starting at the caudal ventral iliac spine and continuing cranially and dorsally as needed. Some sharp dissection may be needed between the middle gluteal and sartorius muscles, the fibers of which blend together. The iliolumbar vessels are ligated at the ventral edge of the ilium. An incision is started in the origin of the deep gluteal muscle to allow caudal retraction of this muscle.

E. Subperiosteal elevation of the gluteal muscles exposes the crest, wing, and shaft of the ilium.

Maximal exposure of the shaft of the ilium, cranial to the acetabulum, may necessitate sacrificing branches of the cranial gluteal artery, vein, and nerve that supply the tensor fasciae latae muscle. Elevation of the iliacus muscle along the ventral border of the iliac shaft (see Plate 65) usually results in severing a nutrient artery on the ventral aspect of the shaft. The severed artery must then be cauterized or plugged with bone wax.

ADDITIONAL EXPOSURE

Extension of this approach cranioventrally provides exposure of the ventral aspect of the sacrum and sacroiliac joint (see Plate 65).

Additional exposure of the cranial margin of the acetabulum and femoral head and neck is obtained in combination with the craniolateral exposure of the hip joint (see Plate 66).

For exposure of both the ilial shaft and dorsal rim of the acetabulum, this lateral approach can be combined with the dorsal approaches to the hip joint by osteotomy of the greater trochanter (see Plate 69) or gluteal tenotomy (see Plate 70).

Total exposure of the hemipelvis is shown in Plate 72.

CLOSURE

Sutures are placed between fasciae of the middle gluteal muscle and the sartorius muscle. This suture line continues caudally between middle gluteal and tensor fasciae latae muscles. Deep gluteal fat and fascia, subcutaneous tissues, and skin are approximated in layers.

PRECAUTIONS

Consideration must be given to the sciatic nerve when retracting the gluteal muscles (see Plate 64E) or using bone-holding forceps on the ilium. The nerve lies close to the dorsomedial aspect of the iliac shaft. With care in retracting, the cranial gluteal vessels and nerve can usually be preserved.

PLATE 64

Approach to the Ilium Through a Lateral Incision *continued*

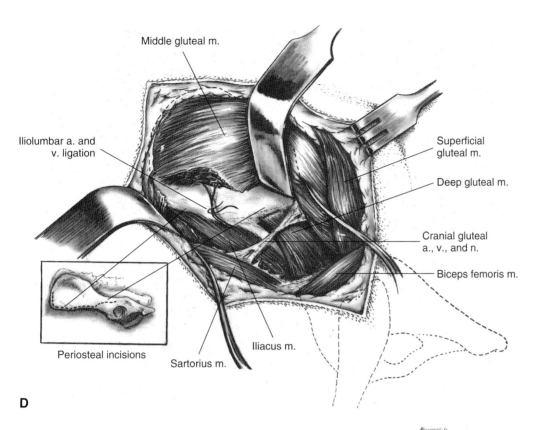

Middle gluteal m.

Iliolumbar a. and v. ligation

Superficial gluteal m.

Deep gluteal m.

Cranial gluteal a., v., and n.

Biceps femoris m.

Periosteal incisions

Sartorius m.

Iliacus m.

D

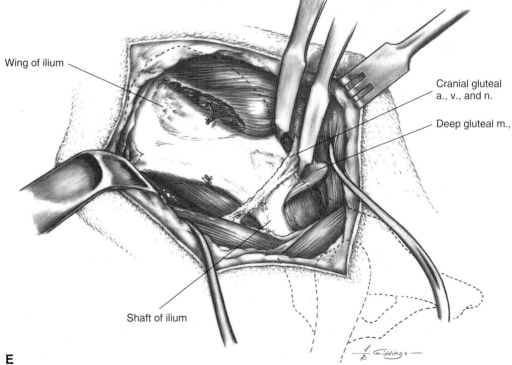

Wing of ilium

Cranial gluteal a., v., and n.

Deep gluteal m.,

Shaft of ilium

E

Approach to the Ventral Aspect of the Sacrum

Based on a Procedure of Montavon, Boudrieau, and Hohn[27]

INDICATION

Internal fixation of sacroiliac joint fracture/luxation.

ALTERNATIVE APPROACH

The approach to the sacroiliac joint through a dorsal incision (see Plate 63) allows superior visualization of the sacral wing in sacroiliac luxation. However, a disadvantage of the dorsal approach is that it cannot be extended caudally for a combined exposure of the ilial shaft and hip joint.

PATIENT POSITIONING

Lateral recumbency with the affected side uppermost.

DESCRIPTION OF THE PROCEDURE

This approach is an extension of Approach to the Ilium Through a Lateral Incision and should be performed as shown in Plate 64A-C. Elevation of the deep gluteal muscle, as shown in Plate 64D and E, is unnecessary.

A. The iliacus muscle is incised at its origin along the ventromedial border of the ilium and is subperiosteally elevated sufficiently to allow insertion of a finger into the pelvic canal. The nutrient artery of the ilium may be disrupted during elevation of the iliacus muscle and is best controlled by cautery or bone wax.

B. The body of the sacrum is palpable now; in the case of a sacroiliac luxation, the whole ilial body and wing are mobile enough that the region of the synchondrosis can be palpated on the medial side of the ilium, and the smooth articular surface can be felt on the sacral wing.

ADDITIONAL EXPOSURE

Complete exposure of the sacroiliac joint and ilial shaft is obtained by combining this approach with the lateral approach (see Plate 64).

By extending the muscle elevation craniodorsally around the iliac crest, the approach can be combined with the approach to the wing of the ilium and dorsal aspect of the sacrum (see Plate 63). This allows direct visualization of the sacroiliac joint, which is useful when fractures are present. However, this combined approach may result in significant disruption of the origin of the middle gluteal muscle.

CLOSURE

Sutures are placed between the fasciae of the middle gluteal and sartorius muscles, and this suture line is continued caudally between the middle gluteal and tensor fasciae latae muscles. Deep gluteal fascia and fat, subcutis, and skin are closed in layers.

PRECAUTIONS

The lumbosacral trunk, arising from the ventral branches of the sixth and seventh lumbar nerves and the first sacral nerve, originates ventral to the sacroiliac joint. It passes medial to the ilial shaft and at the greater ischiatic foramen receives a branch from the second sacral nerve, at which point it becomes the sciatic nerve.

PLATE 65

Approach to the Ventral Aspect of the Sacrum

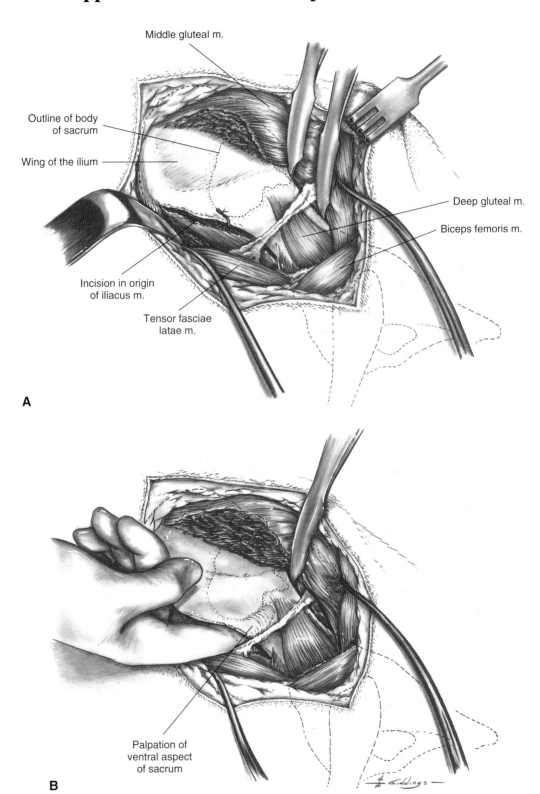

Middle gluteal m.

Outline of body of sacrum

Wing of the ilium

Deep gluteal m.

Biceps femoris m.

Incision in origin of iliacus m.

Tensor fasciae latae m.

A

Palpation of ventral aspect of sacrum

B

Approach to the Craniodorsal Aspect of the Hip Joint Through a Craniolateral Incision in the Dog

Based on Procedures of Archibald, Brown, Nasti, and Medway[3] and Brown and Rosen[6]

INDICATIONS

1. Femoral head and neck resection.
2. Open reduction of fractures of the femoral head and neck.
3. Open reduction of coxofemoral luxations.
4. Installation of total hip prosthesis.

ALTERNATIVE APPROACHES

Greater exposure of the hip joint and dorsum of the acetabulum is provided by the dorsal approach with osteotomy of the greater trochanter (see Plate 69) or with gluteal tenotomy (see Plate 70).

The approach to the ventral aspect of the hip joint (see Plate 73) is an alternative for femoral head and neck resection, but the amount of exposure gained is very limited.

The approach to the caudal aspect of the hip joint is an alternative for open reduction of craniodorsal coxofemoral luxation (see Plate 71).

Total exposure of the hemipelvis is shown in Plate 72.

PATIENT POSITIONING

Lateral recumbency with the affected side uppermost.

DESCRIPTION OF THE PROCEDURE

A. The skin incision is centered at the level of the greater trochanter and lies over the cranial border of the shaft of the femur. Distally, it extends one third to one half the length of the femur; proximally, it curves slightly cranially to end just short of the dorsal midline. When performing the total hip replacement procedure, the skin incision is modified to facilitate femoral reaming; proximally it curves caudally over the trochanter and toward the base of the tail.
B. The skin margins are undermined and retracted. An incision is made through the superficial leaf of the fascia lata, along the cranial border of the biceps femoris muscle.
C. The biceps femoris muscle is retracted caudally to allow incision in the deep leaf of the fascia lata to free the insertion of the tensor fasciae latae muscle. The incision continues proximally through the intermuscular septum between the cranial border of the superficial gluteal muscle and the tensor fasciae latae muscle.

PLATE 66

Approach to the Craniodorsal Aspect of the Hip Joint Through a Craniolateral Incision in the Dog

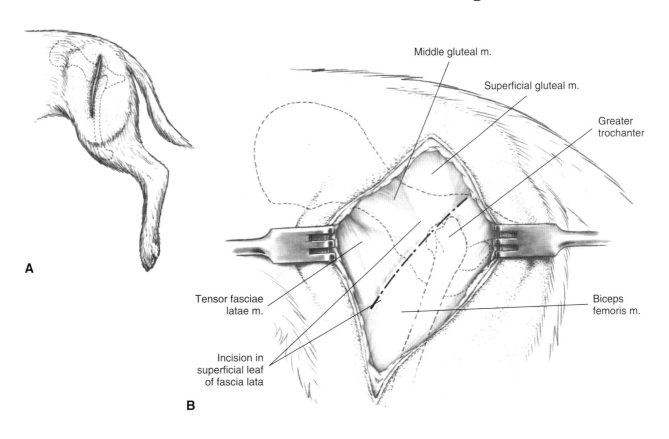

A

Middle gluteal m.

Superficial gluteal m.

Greater trochanter

Tensor fasciae latae m.

Biceps femoris m.

Incision in superficial leaf of fascia lata

B

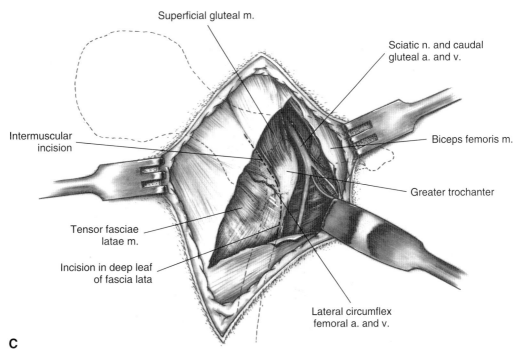

Superficial gluteal m.

Sciatic n. and caudal gluteal a. and v.

Intermuscular incision

Biceps femoris m.

Greater trochanter

Tensor fasciae latae m.

Incision in deep leaf of fascia lata

Lateral circumflex femoral a. and v.

C

Approach to the Craniodorsal Aspect of the Hip Joint Through a Craniolateral Incision in the Dog *continued*

D. The fascia lata and the attached tensor fasciae latae muscle are retracted cranially and the biceps caudally. Blunt dissection and separation along the neck of the femur with the fingertip allows visualization of a triangle bounded dorsally by the middle and deep gluteal muscles, laterally by the vastus lateralis muscle, and medially by the rectus femoris muscle.

E. The joint capsule is covered by areolar tissue, which must be cleared away by blunt dissection. An incision is then made in the joint capsule and continued laterally along the femoral neck through the origin of the vastus lateralis muscle on the neck and lesser trochanter. Exposure can be improved by tenotomy of a portion of the deep gluteal tendon close to the trochanter, leaving enough tendon on the bone to allow suturing. The muscle is split proximally, parallel to its fibers, and the pedicle is allowed to retract.

PLATE 66

Approach to the Craniodorsal Aspect of the Hip Joint Through a Craniolateral Incision in the Dog *continued*

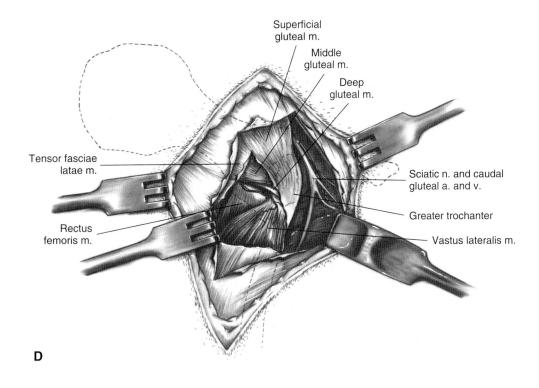

Superficial gluteal m.

Middle gluteal m.

Deep gluteal m.

Tensor fasciae latae m.

Sciatic n. and caudal gluteal a. and v.

Greater trochanter

Rectus femoris m.

Vastus lateralis m.

D

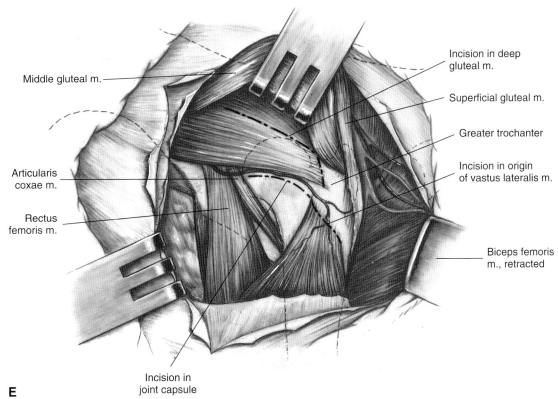

Middle gluteal m.

Incision in deep gluteal m.

Superficial gluteal m.

Greater trochanter

Incision in origin of vastus lateralis m.

Articularis coxae m.

Rectus femoris m.

Biceps femoris m., retracted

Incision in joint capsule

E

Approach to the Craniodorsal Aspect of the Hip Joint
Through a Craniolateral Incision in the Dog *continued*

F. The origin of the vastus lateralis muscle is elevated from the femoral neck and reflected distally. The muscle comes free most easily if the elevation proceeds from distal to proximal. This elevation can be subperiosteal in the immature animal or extraperiosteal in the mature animal. Hohmann retractors are placed intracapsularly ventral and caudal to the femoral neck to allow visualization of the femoral head. Caution is needed to be certain that the caudal retractor is intracapsular, or at least between the deep gluteal muscle and the femoral neck, to avoid entrapping the sciatic nerve on the caudodorsal surface of the deep gluteal muscle.

ADDITIONAL EXPOSURE

Extension of this approach cranially to gain exposure of the ilial shaft is possible by combining with the approach to the ilium through a lateral incision (see Plate 64).

Distally, exposure of the femur can be obtained in combination with the approach to the greater trochanter and subtrochanteric region of the femur (see Plate 76) or the approach to the shaft of the femur (see Plate 77).

CLOSURE

One or two mattress sutures (see Figure 21B) or a pulley suture (see Figure 21D) are placed in the deep gluteal tendon incision, and the origin of the vastus lateralis muscle is sutured to the cranial edge of the deep gluteal muscle. Continuous sutures are placed in the insertion of the tensor fasciae latae muscle distally and are continued proximally along the cranial border of the superficial gluteal muscle. The superficial leaf of the fascia lata distally and the gluteal fascia proximally are closed to the cranial border of the biceps femoris with a continuous pattern. The rest of the incision is closed routinely in layers.

PRECAUTIONS

Dorsal to the hip joint, the sciatic nerve emerges from the ischiatic foramen under the superficial gluteal muscle. It passes caudal to the deep gluteal muscle, across the gemelli and internal obturator muscles, then passes down the thigh deep to the biceps femoris muscle. To reduce the risk of damage to the sciatic nerve, sharp retractors such as the Meyerding should not be used to retract the biceps femoris muscle.

PLATE 66

Approach to the Craniodorsal Aspect of the Hip Joint Through a Craniolateral Incision in the Dog *continued*

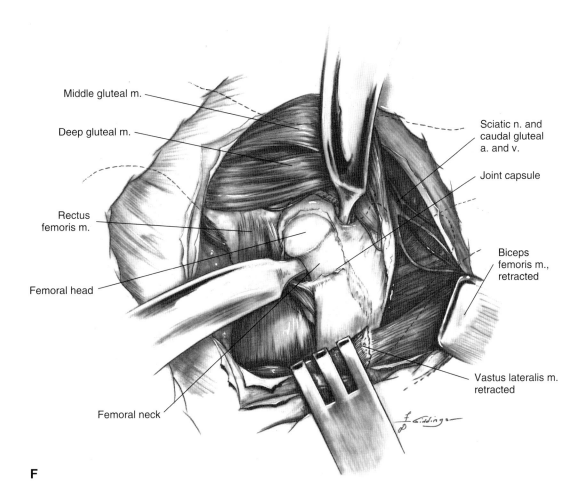

Middle gluteal m.

Deep gluteal m.

Rectus femoris m.

Femoral head

Femoral neck

Sciatic n. and caudal gluteal a. and v.

Joint capsule

Biceps femoris m., retracted

Vastus lateralis m. retracted

F

Approach to the Craniodorsal Aspect of the Hip Joint Through a Craniolateral Incision in the Cat

INDICATIONS

1. Femoral head and neck resection.
2. Open reduction of fractures of the femoral head and neck.
3. Open reduction of coxofemoral luxations.
4. Installation of total hip prosthesis.

PATIENT POSITIONING

Lateral recumbency with the affected side uppermost.

DESCRIPTION OF THE PROCEDURE

A. The skin incision is centered at the level of the greater trochanter and lies over the cranial border of the shaft of the femur. Distally, it extends one third to one half the length of the femur; proximally, it curves slightly cranially to end just short of the dorsal midline.

B. The musculature surrounding the hip joint in the cat is similar to the dog. However, the gluteal muscles may be relatively larger in the cat, making the exposure of the hip joint more difficult. Also, care is taken not to mistake the caudofemoralis muscle for the superficial gluteal muscle.

PLATE 67

Approach to the Craniodorsal Aspect of the Hip Joint Through a Craniolateral Incision in the Cat

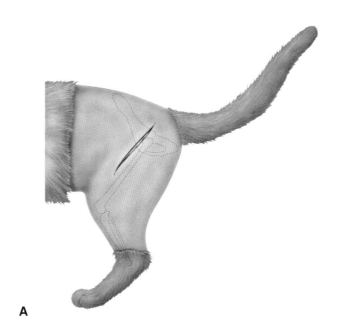

A

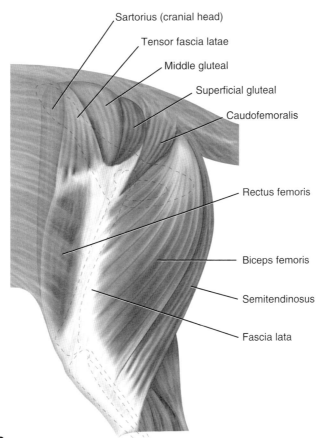

Sartorius (cranial head)

Tensor fascia latae

Middle gluteal

Superficial gluteal

Caudofemoralis

Rectus femoris

Biceps femoris

Semitendinosus

Fascia lata

B

Approach to the Craniodorsal Aspect of the Hip Joint Through a Craniolateral Incision in the Cat *continued*

C. The skin margins are undermined and retracted. An incision is made through the superficial leaf of the fascia lata, along the cranial border of the caudofemoralis and biceps femoris muscles.

D. With blunt dissection using Metzenbaum scissors, the fascial plane underlying the tensor fasciae latae and superficial gluteal muscles is identified and opened.

E. The incision in the deep leaf of the fascia lata continues proximally through the intermuscular septum between the cranial border of the gluteal muscles and the tensor fasciae latae muscle.

PLATE 67

Approach to the Craniodorsal Aspect of the Hip Joint Through a Craniolateral Incision in the Cat *continued*

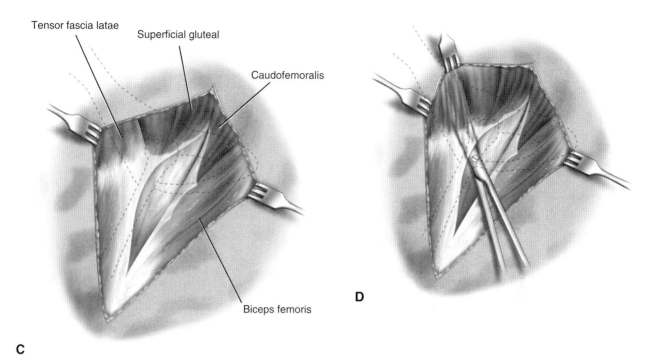

Tensor fascia latae

Superficial gluteal

Caudofemoralis

Biceps femoris

C

D

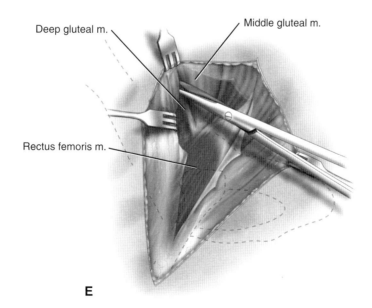

Deep gluteal m.

Middle gluteal m.

Rectus femoris m.

E

Approach to the Craniodorsal Aspect of the Hip Joint Through a Craniolateral Incision in the Cat *continued*

F. The cranial edge of the middle gluteal muscle is identified and separated along the intermuscular septum from the underlying deep gluteal muscle. The middle gluteal muscle is retracted caudoproximally. The deep gluteal muscle is separated and elevated from the underlying joint capsule.

G. Exposure can be improved by tenotomy of a portion of the deep gluteal tendon close to the trochanter, leaving enough tendon on the bone to allow suturing. The muscle is split proximally, parallel to its fibers, and the pedicle is allowed to retract. The articularis coxae muscle overlying the joint capsule is well developed and covers the joint capsule in the cat.

PLATE 67

Approach to the Craniodorsal Aspect of the Hip Joint Through a Craniolateral Incision in the Cat *continued*

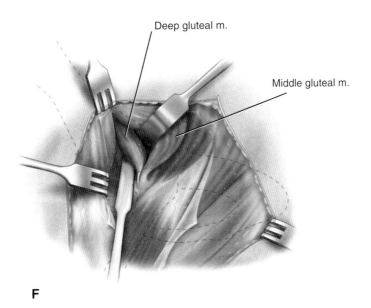

Deep gluteal m.

Middle gluteal m.

F

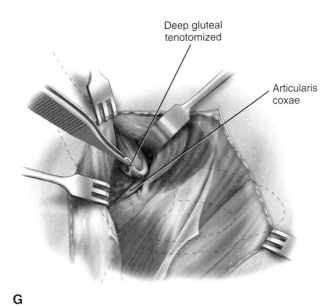

Deep gluteal
tenotomized

Articularis
coxae

G

Approach to the Craniodorsal Aspect of the Hip Joint Through a Craniolateral Incision in the Cat *continued*

H. An incision is then made, transecting the articularis coxae muscle and then continuing through the underlying joint capsule. It is continued laterally along the femoral neck through the origin of the vastus lateralis muscle on the neck and lesser trochanter.

I. The origin of the vastus lateralis muscle is elevated from the femoral neck and reflected distally. Hohmann retractors are placed intracapsularly ventral and caudal to the femoral neck to allow visualization of the femoral head (see Plate 66F). Caution is needed to be certain that the caudal retractor is intracapsular, or at least between the deep gluteal muscle and the femoral neck, to avoid entrapping the sciatic nerve on the caudodorsal surface of the deep gluteal muscle.

CLOSURE

One or two mattress sutures (see Figure 21B) or a pulley suture (see Figure 21D) are placed in the deep gluteal tendon incision, and the origin of the vastus lateralis muscle is sutured to the cranial edge of the deep gluteal muscle. Continuous sutures are placed in the insertion of the tensor fasciae latae muscle distally and are continued proximally along the cranial border of the superficial gluteal muscle. The superficial leaf of the fascia lata distally and the gluteal fascia proximally are closed to the cranial border of the caudofemoralis and biceps femoris muscles with a continuous pattern. The rest of the incision is closed routinely in layers.

PRECAUTIONS

Dorsal to the hip joint, the sciatic nerve emerges from the ischiatic foramen under the superficial gluteal muscle. It passes caudal to the deep gluteal muscle, across the gemelli and internal obturator muscles, then passes down the thigh deep to the caudofemoralis and biceps femoris muscles. To reduce the risk of damage to the sciatic nerve, sharp retractors such as the Meyerding should not be used to retract these muscles.

PLATE 67

Approach to the Craniodorsal Aspect of the Hip Joint Through a Craniolateral Incision in the Cat *continued*

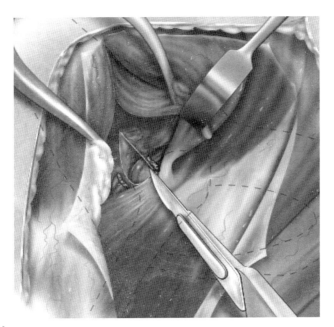

H

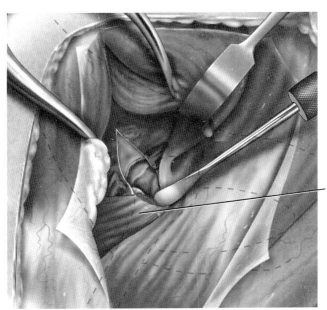

I

Vastus
lateralis
elevated
from femur

Approach to the Dorsal Aspect of the Hip Joint Through an Intergluteal Incision

Based on a Procedure of Wadsworth and Henry[50]

INDICATION

Internal fixation of noncomminuted fractures in the central part of the acetabulum (see Comments).

ALTERNATIVE APPROACHES

Greater exposure of the hip joint and dorsum of the acetabulum is provided by the dorsal approaches with osteotomy of the greater trochanter (see Plate 69) or with gluteal tenotomy (see Plate 70).

Total exposure of the hemipelvis is shown in Plate 72.

PATIENT POSITIONING

Lateral recumbency with the affected side uppermost.

DESCRIPTION OF THE PROCEDURE

A. Commencing distal to the greater trochanter of the femur, the skin incision crosses the trochanter and curves in a craniomedial direction proximally, ending about halfway between the trochanter and the dorsal midline.
B. Skin and subcutaneous fat are undermined and retracted to allow visualization of the gluteal fascia, which is incised along the cranial border of the biceps femoris and superficial gluteal muscles. These two incisions meet in the region of the greater trochanter.
C. The belly of the superficial gluteal muscle is elevated preparatory to tenotomizing it near its insertion on the third trochanter of the femur. The sciatic nerve will be visualized as this muscle is elevated. Cranial retraction of the middle gluteal muscle results in a separation developing between it and the piriformis muscle (as illustrated), or they may remain attached and be retracted as a single muscle.

PLATE 68

Approach to the Dorsal Aspect of the Hip Joint Through an Intergluteal Incision

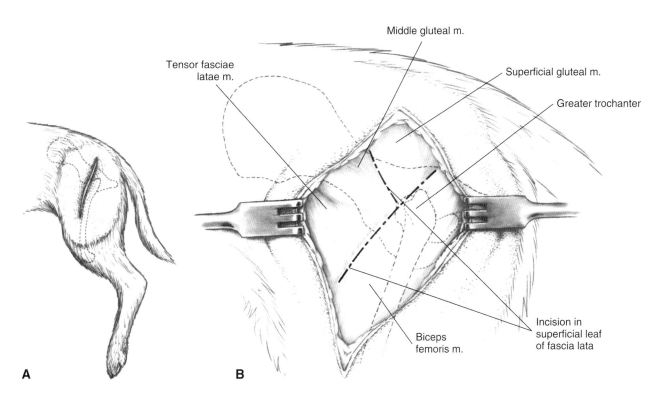

Middle gluteal m.

Superficial gluteal m.

Greater trochanter

Tensor fasciae latae m.

Biceps femoris m.

Incision in superficial leaf of fascia lata

A

B

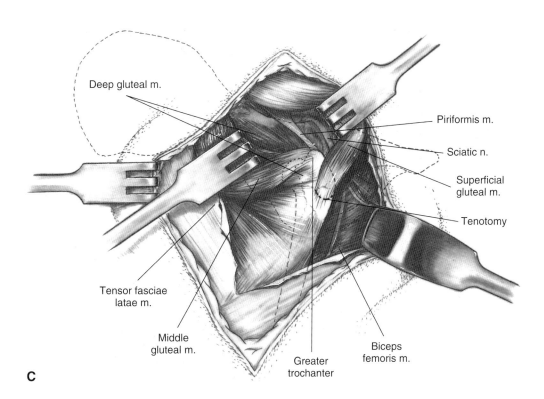

Deep gluteal m.

Piriformis m.

Sciatic n.

Superficial gluteal m.

Tenotomy

Tensor fasciae latae m.

Middle gluteal m.

Greater trochanter

Biceps femoris m.

C

Approach to the Dorsal Aspect of the Hip Joint Through an Intergluteal Incision *continued*

D. Elevation and retraction of the superficial gluteal muscle will allow retraction of the sciatic nerve with a Penrose rubber drain (see Additional Exposure). The origin of the deep gluteal muscle on the shaft of the ilium is incised, starting at its caudal border near the ischiatic spine. This incision continues cranially as needed to allow elevation and retraction of the muscle belly in a craniolateral direction to expose the dorsal rim of the acetabulum. Pointed Hohmann retractors are placed cranial and caudal to the femoral head, the latter serving to retract the internal obturator and gemelli muscles. The joint capsule can be incised to aid in inspection of the articular surface.

ADDITIONAL EXPOSURE

Greater exposure of the caudal part of the acetabulum can be obtained by transection of the combined tendons of the internal obturator and gemelli muscles in the trochanteric fossa (see Plate 71D). As these muscles are retracted, they retract and protect the sciatic nerve (see Plate 71E).

CLOSURE

Interrupted absorbable sutures are placed in the joint capsule. The deep gluteal muscle is reattached to its origin if any tissue is available for suturing; otherwise, the muscle is simply placed back in position and allowed to heal by fibrosis. Mattress sutures are used in the superficial gluteal tendon; fascia, subcutaneous tissues, and skin are closed routinely in layers.

COMMENTS

Although relatively speedy to perform, this approach gives limited exposure, especially in large, heavily muscled dogs. The fracture must be in the center of the joint and noncomminuted.

PRECAUTIONS

Dorsal to the hip joint, the sciatic nerve emerges from the ischiatic foramen under the superficial gluteal muscle. It passes caudal to the deep gluteal muscle, across the gemelli and internal obturator muscles, then passes down the thigh deep to the biceps femoris muscle. To reduce the risk of damage to the sciatic nerve, sharp retractors such as the Meyerding should not be used to retract the biceps femoris muscle.

PLATE 68

Approach to the Dorsal Aspect of the Hip Joint Through an Intergluteal Incision *continued*

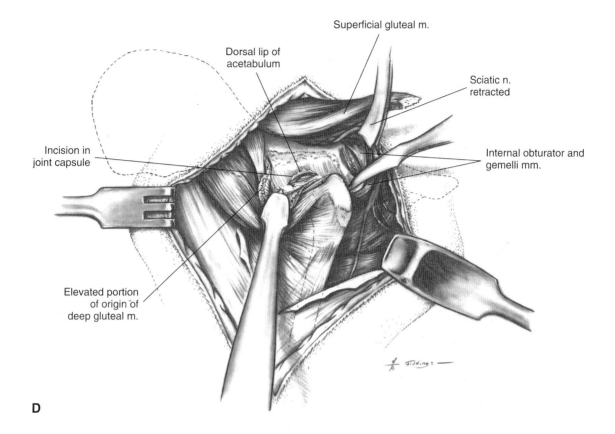

Dorsal lip of
acetabulum

Superficial gluteal m.

Sciatic n.
retracted

Incision in
joint capsule

Internal obturator and
gemelli mm.

Elevated portion
of origin of
deep gluteal m.

D

Approach to the Craniodorsal and Caudodorsal Aspects of the Hip Joint by Osteotomy of the Greater Trochanter

Based on a Procedure of Gorman[17]

INDICATIONS

1. Open reduction of coxofemoral luxations.
2. Open reduction of fractures in the cranial half of the acetabulum or the caudal shaft of the ilium.
3. Open reduction of fractures of the femoral head and neck (see Alternative Approaches).
4. Installation of total hip prostheses (see Alternative Approaches).

ALTERNATIVE APPROACHES

Although this approach is popular for fractures of the acetabulum and femoral neck, adequate exposure for reduction of coxofemoral luxation and total hip replacement usually can be obtained by the approach to the craniodorsal aspect of the hip joint through a craniolateral incision (see Plate 66), a somewhat quicker procedure.

The choice between this approach and the approach to the craniodorsal and caudodorsal aspects of the hip joint by tenotomy of the gluteal muscles (see Plate 70) is primarily one of surgeon's preference. There is little difference in the exposure obtained.

The approach to the dorsal aspect of the hip joint through an intergluteal incision (see Plate 68) gives limited exposure, especially in large, heavily muscled dogs. It is best for noncomminuted, central acetabular fractures.

Total exposure of the hemipelvis is shown in Plate 72.

PATIENT POSITIONING

Lateral recumbency with the affected side uppermost.

DESCRIPTION OF THE PROCEDURE

A. The skin incision is centered on the cranial aspect of the greater trochanter of the femur, curving craniomedially to near the midline and following the cranial border of the femur distally to near midshaft. The alternative curved flap incision is preferred by some surgeons.
B. Subcutaneous tissues are reflected with the skin. An incision is made in the superficial leaf of the fascia lata along the cranial border of the biceps femoris muscle for the entire length of the exposure.

PLATE 69

Approach to the Craniodorsal and Caudodorsal Aspects of the Hip Joint by Osteotomy of the Greater Trochanter

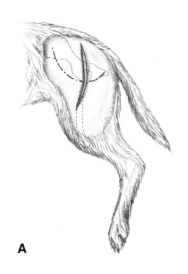

A

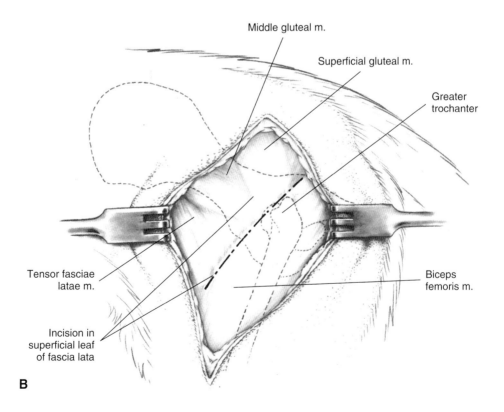

Middle gluteal m.

Superficial gluteal m.

Greater trochanter

Tensor fasciae latae m.

Biceps femoris m.

Incision in superficial leaf of fascia lata

B

Approach to the Craniodorsal and Caudodorsal Aspects of the Hip Joint by Osteotomy of the Greater Trochanter *continued*

C. The biceps femoris muscle is retracted caudally and the sciatic nerve identified. An incision is made in the deep leaf of the fascia lata to free the insertion of the tensor fasciae latae muscle. This incision is continued proximally along the cranial border of the superficial gluteal muscle. The tendon of insertion of this muscle is transected close to the third trochanter, leaving enough tissue on the bone to allow suturing.

D. The superficial gluteal muscle is retracted craniodorsally. The greater trochanter is osteotomized by placing the osteotome on the lateral surface of the greater trochanter, just proximal to the superficial gluteal muscle insertion on the third trochanter.

PLATE 69

Approach to the Craniodorsal and Caudodorsal Aspects of the Hip Joint by Osteotomy of the Greater Trochanter *continued*

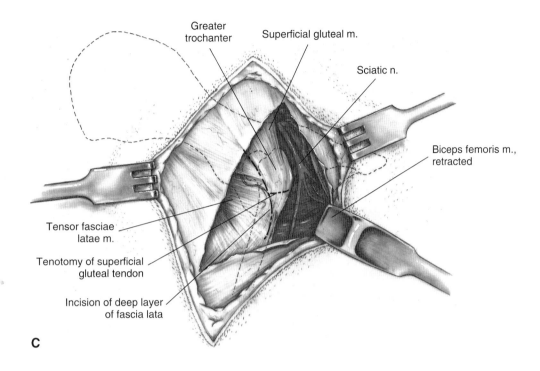

Greater trochanter

Superficial gluteal m.

Sciatic n.

Biceps femoris m., retracted

Tensor fasciae latae m.

Tenotomy of superficial gluteal tendon

Incision of deep layer of fascia lata

C

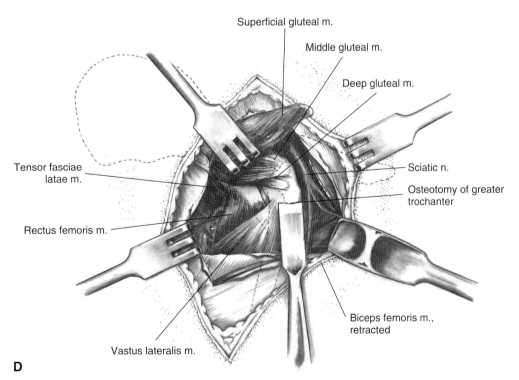

Superficial gluteal m.

Middle gluteal m.

Deep gluteal m.

Tensor fasciae latae m.

Sciatic n.

Osteotomy of greater trochanter

Rectus femoris m.

Biceps femoris m., retracted

Vastus lateralis m.

D

Approach to the Craniodorsal and Caudodorsal Aspects of the Hip Joint by Osteotomy of the Greater Trochanter *continued*

E. The osteotome is directed to form a 45-degree angle with the long axis of the femur so as to cut the trochanter flush with the femoral neck, beneath the insertions of the middle and deep gluteal muscles. Alternatively, a Gigli wire saw can be used for the osteotomy.

F. The middle and deep gluteal muscles are reflected dorsomedially as a unit with the greater trochanter. The deep gluteal muscle must be sharply dissected from the underlying joint capsule and it can then be subperiosteally elevated from the ilium as desired for exposure. The sciatic nerve must be protected during this dissection.

ADDITIONAL EXPOSURE

Extension of this approach cranially to gain exposure of the ilial shaft is possible by combining with the approach to the ilium through a lateral incision (see Plate 64).

For additional exposure of fractures involving the caudal part of the acetabulum or ischium, this approach is combined with the approach to the caudal aspect of the hip joint and body of the ischium (see Plate 71).

CLOSURE

The greater trochanter is reattached by two Kirschner wires and a tension band wire (see Figure 23A). Mattress or pulley (see Figure 21B,D) sutures are placed in the insertion of the superficial gluteal muscle, and continuous sutures are placed in the insertion of the tensor fasciae latae muscle. The superficial leaf of the fascia lata distally and the gluteal fascia proximally are closed to the cranial border of the biceps femoris with a continuous pattern. Subcutaneous tissues and skin are closed in separate layers.

PRECAUTIONS

Dorsal to the hip joint, the sciatic nerve emerges from the ischiatic foramen under the superficial gluteal muscle. It passes caudal to the deep gluteal muscle, across the gemelli and internal obturator muscles, then passes down the thigh deep to the biceps femoris muscle. To reduce the risk of damage to the sciatic nerve, sharp retractors such as the Meyerding should not be used to retract the biceps femoris muscle.

PLATE 69

Approach to the Craniodorsal and Caudodorsal Aspects of the Hip Joint by Osteotomy of the Greater Trochanter *continued*

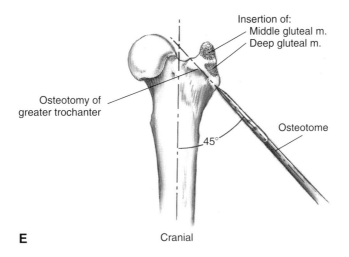

Insertion of:
Middle gluteal m.
Deep gluteal m.

Osteotomy of
greater trochanter

Osteotome

45°

E

Cranial

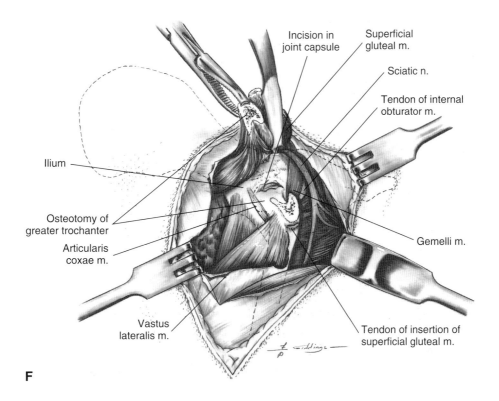

Incision in
joint capsule

Superficial
gluteal m.

Sciatic n.

Tendon of internal
obturator m.

Ilium

Osteotomy of
greater trochanter

Articularis
coxae m.

Gemelli m.

Vastus
lateralis m.

Tendon of insertion of
superficial gluteal m.

F

Approach to the Craniodorsal and Caudodorsal Aspects of the Hip Joint by Tenotomy of the Gluteal Muscles

Based on a Procedure of Brown[5]

INDICATIONS

1. Open reduction of fractures of the cranial half of the acetabulum or the caudal shaft of the ilium (see Comments).
2. Open reduction of fractures of the femoral head and neck (see Comments).

ALTERNATIVE APPROACHES

Although this approach is popular for fractures of the acetabulum and femoral neck, adequate exposure for reduction of coxofemoral luxation and total hip replacement can usually be obtained by the approach to the craniodorsal aspect of the hip joint through a craniolateral incision (see Plate 66), a somewhat quicker procedure.

The choice between this approach and the approach to the craniodorsal and caudodorsal aspects of the hip joint by osteotomy of the greater trochanter (see Plate 69) is primarily one of surgeon's preference. There is little difference in the exposure obtained, but because of the tenotomies, function may be regained faster with the osteotomy approach.

The approach to the dorsal aspect of the hip joint through an intergluteal incision (see Plate 68) gives limited exposure, especially in large, heavily muscled dogs. It is best for non-comminuted, central acetabular fractures.

Total exposure of the hemipelvis is shown in Plate 72.

PATIENT POSITIONING

Lateral recumbency with the affected side uppermost.

DESCRIPTION OF THE PROCEDURE

This approach is started as depicted in Plate 69A-C.

A. The superficial gluteal muscle is retracted proximally to expose the middle gluteal muscle, and the belly of this muscle is undermined near its insertion on the trochanter. The tendinous insertion is transected as close as possible to the bone. Protect the sciatic nerve during these procedures.

The freed middle gluteal and attached piriformis muscles are retracted dorsally to allow the deep gluteal muscle to be undermined similarly to the middle gluteal muscle. The insertion of the deep gluteal extends more cranially and distally on the trochanter than does the middle gluteal. A tenotomy is performed close to the bone.

B. Sharp dissection is required to free the deep gluteal muscle from the underlying joint capsule, following which it can be subperiosteally elevated from the ilium as desired for exposure.

PLATE 70

Approach to the Craniodorsal and Caudodorsal Aspects of the Hip Joint by Tenotomy of the Gluteal Muscles

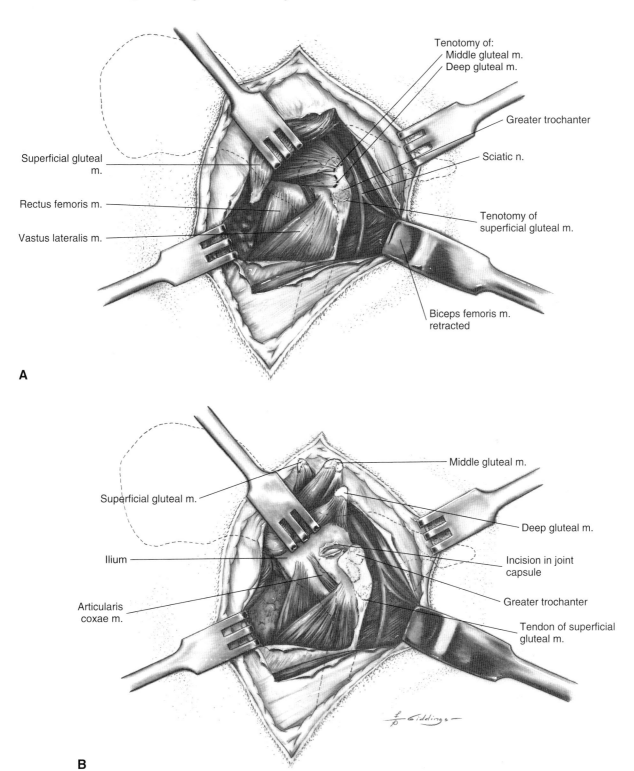

A

B

Approach to the Craniodorsal and Caudodorsal Aspects of the Hip Joint by Tenotomy of the Gluteal Muscles *continued*

CLOSURE

Interrupted sutures are placed in the joint capsule. The tendons of the deep and middle gluteal muscles are reattached to the trochanter by passing suture through holes drilled in the trochanter, as illustrated in Figure 22. Mattress (see Figure 21B) or pulley (see Figure 21D) sutures are placed in the tendon of the superficial gluteal muscle, and a continuous layer is used in the insertion of the tensor fasciae latae muscle. The superficial leaf of the tensor fasciae latae distally and the gluteal fascia proximally are closed to the cranial border of the biceps femoris with a continuous pattern.

ADDITIONAL EXPOSURE

Extension of this approach cranially to gain exposure of the ilial shaft is possible by combining with the approach to the ilium through a lateral incision (see Plate 64). With this combination of approaches, the deep gluteal muscle may become devitalized, particularly if there is accompanying trauma with an ilial fracture. In these instances, the muscle may need to be partially resected.

For additional exposure of fractures involving the caudal part of the acetabulum or ischium, this approach is combined with the approach to the caudal aspect of the hip joint and body of the ischium (see Plate 71).

Distally, additional exposure of the subtrochanteric region of the femur is gained by elevation of the origin of the vastus lateralis muscle (see Plate 76D and E).

Approach to the Craniodorsal and Caudodorsal Aspects of the Hip Joint by Tenotomy of the Gluteal Muscles *continued*

COMMENTS

This approach may be preferable to osteotomy in the skeletally immature animal because there is no disruption of the physis of the greater trochanter.

PRECAUTIONS

Dorsal to the hip joint, the sciatic nerve emerges from the ischiatic foramen under the superficial gluteal muscle. It passes caudal to the deep gluteal muscle, across the gemelli and internal obturator muscles, then passes down the thigh deep to the biceps femoris muscle. To reduce the risk of damage to the sciatic nerve, sharp retractors such as the Meyerding should not be used to retract the biceps femoris muscle.

Approach to the Caudal Aspect of the Hip Joint and Body of the Ischium

Based on Procedures of Hohn[19] and Slocum and Hohn[45]

INDICATIONS

1. Femoral head and neck resection.
2. Open reduction of fractures of the caudal region of the acetabulum and of the cranial body of the ischium.
3. Open reduction of craniodorsal coxofemoral luxations (see Comments).

ALTERNATIVE APPROACHES

An alternative approach that is equally suitable for the reduction of craniodorsal coxofemoral luxation and femoral head and neck resection is the approach to the craniodorsal aspect of the hip joint through a craniolateral incision (see Plate 66).

The approach to the craniodorsal and caudodorsal aspects of the hip joint by osteotomy of the greater trochanter (see Plate 69) provides better exposure for fractures of the dorsal region of the acetabulum, particularly if they are comminuted.

The approach to the dorsal aspect of the hip joint through an intergluteal incision (see Plate 68) gives limited exposure, especially in large, heavily muscled dogs. It is best for noncomminuted, central acetabular fractures.

Total exposure of the hemipelvis is shown in Plate 72.

PATIENT POSITIONING

Lateral recumbency with the affected side uppermost.

DESCRIPTION OF THE PROCEDURE

A. The curved incision is centered on the caudal surface of the greater trochanter. It starts near the dorsal midline, continues caudal to the trochanter, and extends through the proximal one fourth to one third of the femur.
B. The subcutaneous fat is undermined and retracted with the skin. The fascia of the biceps muscle is incised along the cranial border of this muscle, beginning proximally at the sacrotuberous ligament, and extending distally to the end of the skin incision.
C. The tendinous insertion of the superficial gluteal muscle is transected near its attachment on the third trochanter, and the incision is continued into the deep leaf of the fascia lata. The tensor fasciae latae muscle is now retracted craniodorsally and the biceps femoris caudally to expose the external rotator muscles of the hip.
D. With the femur internally rotated, the combined tendon of insertion of the internal obturator and gemelli muscles is cut close to its attachment in the trochanteric fossa.
E. A stay suture in the tendon of the internal obturator and gemelli muscles will aid in its retraction. As it is retracted, it also retracts and protects the sciatic nerve as the obturator fossa of the ischium is exposed. A Hohmann retractor placed ventral to the femoral head will help retract the external obturator and quadratus muscles. Care must be taken to protect the sciatic nerve and circumflex femoral vessels. For improved local

PLATE 71

Approach to the Caudal Aspect of the Hip Joint and Body of the Ischium

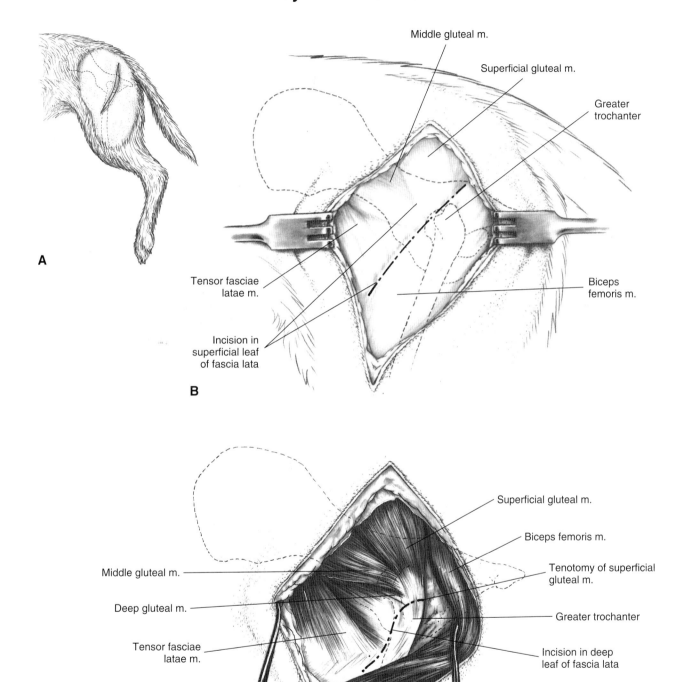

A

B

Middle gluteal m.

Superficial gluteal m.

Greater trochanter

Biceps femoris m.

Tensor fasciae latae m.

Incision in superficial leaf of fascia lata

C

Superficial gluteal m.

Biceps femoris m.

Tenotomy of superficial gluteal m.

Greater trochanter

Incision in deep leaf of fascia lata

Middle gluteal m.

Deep gluteal m.

Tensor fasciae latae m.

Approach to the Caudal Aspect of the Hip Joint and
Body of the Ischium *continued*

exposure of the ischium, the cranial portion of the origin of the gemelli muscles is elevated from the bone, all the way to the ischiatic spine dorsally. Where the tendon of internal obturator muscle crosses the ischiatic spine, there is a thin-walled bursa that is 1 to 2 cm wide surrounding this tendon. Incision of this bursa allows the internal obturator muscle to be retracted further caudally. For caudal acetabular fractures, this increased exposure allows for the application of a bone plate that extends caudally to a point halfway along the body of the ischium. To avoid undue retraction of the sciatic nerve, the nerve is moved cranially during plate application. Screws can be inserted through the interval between the gemelli and internal obturator muscles dorsally, and the external obturator and quadratus femoris muscles ventrally. For local enhancement of the exposure of the acetabular labrum more cranially, a portion of the origin of the deep gluteal muscle is elevated.

ADDITIONAL EXPOSURE

In large, heavily muscled dogs, additional local exposure can be obtained by transection of the cranial third of the origin of the biceps femoris muscle on the sacrotuberous ligament. Also, the tendon of the external obturator muscle is transected in the trochanteric fossa and retracted along with the gemelli and internal obturator muscles. This increases exposure of the most caudoventral region of the acetabulum and the body of the ischium.

For additional exposure of fractures involving the dorsal or cranial regions of the acetabulum, this approach is commonly combined with the approach to the craniodorsal and caudodorsal aspects of the hip joint by osteotomy of the greater trochanter (see Plate 69) or by gluteal tenotomy (see Plate 70).

CLOSURE

Nonabsorbable suture is used to place a modified Bunnell-Mayer or locking-loop suture (see Figure 21A, C) in the tendon of the internal obturator and gemelli muscles. It is usually impossible to suture to the small portion of the insertion that remains in the trochanteric fossa; therefore the suture is attached to the insertions of the deep and middle gluteal muscles at the trochanter. Alternatively, twin holes can be drilled through the femoral neck as illustrated in Plate 72D, and the suture is passed through these holes and tied.

COMMENTS

When used in the open reduction of a craniodorsal coxofemoral luxation, this approach provides good exposure of the acetabulum, allowing it to be easily cleaned of debris before reduction is attempted.

PRECAUTIONS

Dorsal to the hip joint, the sciatic nerve emerges from the ischiatic foramen under the superficial gluteal muscle. It passes caudal to the deep gluteal muscle, across the gemelli and internal obturator muscles, then passes down the thigh deep to the biceps femoris muscle. To reduce the risk of damage to the sciatic nerve, sharp retractors such as the Meyerding should not be used to retract the biceps femoris muscle.

PLATE 71

Approach to the Caudal Aspect of the Hip Joint and Body of the Ischium *continued*

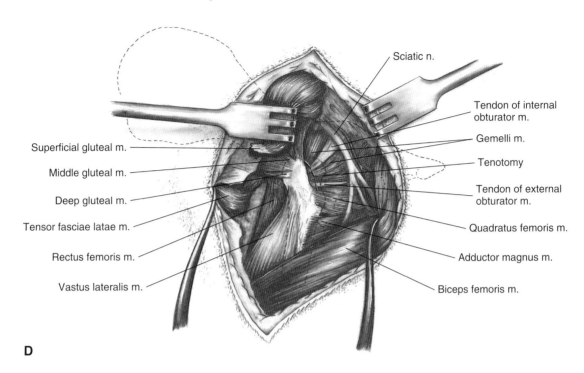

Sciatic n.

Tendon of internal obturator m.

Gemelli m.

Tenotomy

Tendon of external obturator m.

Quadratus femoris m.

Adductor magnus m.

Biceps femoris m.

Superficial gluteal m.

Middle gluteal m.

Deep gluteal m.

Tensor fasciae latae m.

Rectus femoris m.

Vastus lateralis m.

D

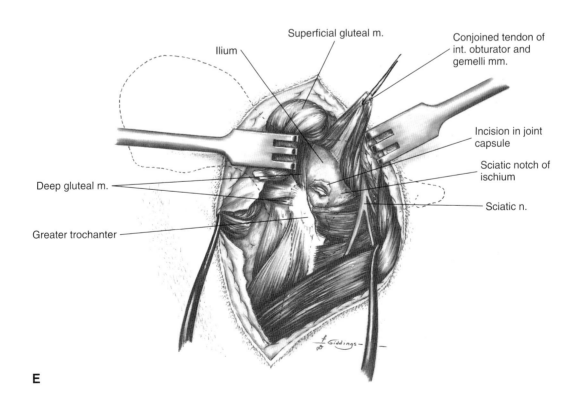

Superficial gluteal m.

Ilium

Conjoined tendon of int. obturator and gemelli mm.

Incision in joint capsule

Sciatic notch of ischium

Sciatic n.

Deep gluteal m.

Greater trochanter

E

Approach to the Lateral Aspect of the Hemipelvis

INDICATION

Open reduction and internal fixation of multiple fractures of the hemipelvis.

EXPLANATORY NOTE

This procedure combines elements of three approaches: Approach to the Ilium Through a Lateral Incision (see Plate 64), Approach to the Craniodorsal and Caudodorsal Aspects of the Hip Joint by Osteotomy of the Greater Trochanter (see Plate 69), and Approach to the Caudal Aspect of the Hip Joint and Body of the Ischium (see Plate 71). They should be studied before proceeding.

PATIENT POSITIONING

Lateral recumbency with the affected side uppermost (illustrated).

DESCRIPTION OF THE PROCEDURE

A. The skin incision begins near the center of the iliac crest, runs caudally to a point distal to the greater trochanter of the femur, and then curves dorsally to end near the ischiatic tuberosity. Subcutaneous tissues and gluteal fascia are incised along the same line as the skin. Additional gluteal fascial incisions are made as shown in Plate 64B and Plate 69B and C. The superficial gluteal muscle is tenotomized near its insertion and the greater trochanter is osteotomized as in Plate 69D and E.

B. Middle and deep gluteal muscles are elevated from the wing and shaft of the ilium and reflected dorsomedially with the trochanter. This is sufficient exposure for the iliac shaft and cranial acetabular areas.

C, D. For exposure of the caudal acetabular and ischial regions, the combined tendon of the internal obturator and gemelli muscles is cut at its insertion in the trochanteric fossa. Caudomedial retraction of these muscles protects the sciatic nerve and exposes the region of the ischiatic notch. Note that the modified Bunnell-Mayer suture to be used in closure has been inserted in the tendon to aid in retraction of these muscles.

CLOSURE

Plate 72D shows how the conjoined tendon of the internal obturator and gemelli muscles is attached to the femoral neck. Two holes drilled through the femoral neck allow the tendon to be securely approximated. The greater trochanter is attached to the femur by means of Kirschner wires and tension band wire (see Figure 23A). The tendon of the superficial gluteal muscle is sutured to its insertion of the third trochanter. Fascial incisions, subcutaneous tissues, and skin are closed in separate layers.

PRECAUTIONS

Dorsal to the hip joint, the sciatic nerve emerges from the ischiatic foramen under the superficial gluteal muscle. It passes caudal to the deep gluteal muscle, across the gemelli and internal obturator muscles, then passes down the thigh deep to the biceps femoris muscle. To reduce the risk of damage to the sciatic nerve, sharp retractors such as the Meyerding should not be used to retract the biceps femoris muscle.

PLATE 72

Approach to the Lateral Aspect of the Hemipelvis

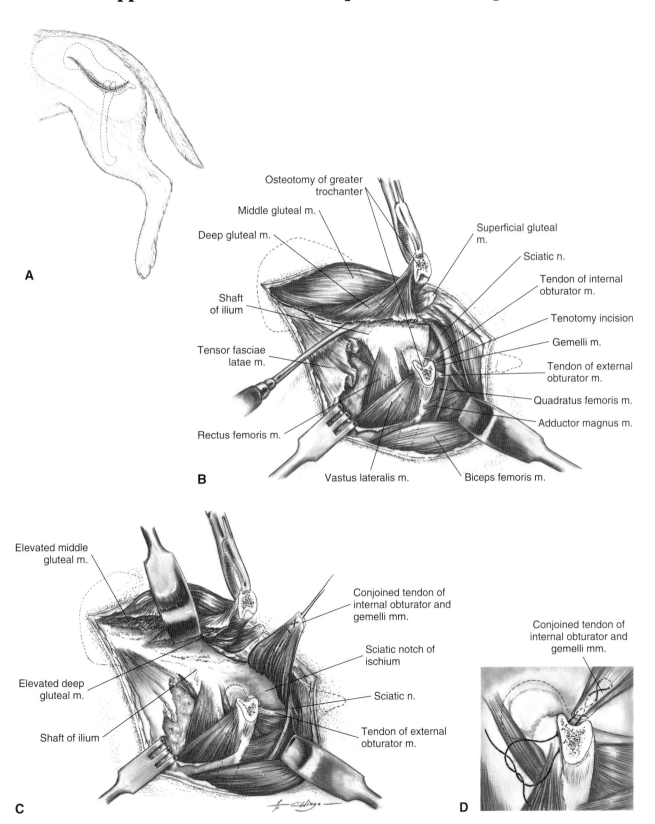

A

Osteotomy of greater trochanter

Middle gluteal m.

Deep gluteal m.

Superficial gluteal m.

Sciatic n.

Tendon of internal obturator m.

Shaft of ilium

Tenotomy incision

Gemelli m.

Tensor fasciae latae m.

Tendon of external obturator m.

Quadratus femoris m.

Adductor magnus m.

Rectus femoris m.

B

Vastus lateralis m.

Biceps femoris m.

Elevated middle gluteal m.

Conjoined tendon of internal obturator and gemelli mm.

Sciatic notch of ischium

Sciatic n.

Elevated deep gluteal m.

Tendon of external obturator m.

Shaft of ilium

C

Conjoined tendon of internal obturator and gemelli mm.

D

Approach to the Ventral Aspect of the Hip Joint or the Ramus of the Pubis

Based on Procedures of Hohn[19] and Slocum and Devine[43]

INDICATIONS

1. Open reduction of ventral luxations of the femoral head.
2. Open reduction of fractures of the ventral aspect of the acetabulum.
3. Femoral head and neck resection (see Comments).
4. Ostectomy of the ramus of the pubis for triple pelvic osteotomy.

ALTERNATIVE APPROACHES

Alternative approaches that are equally suitable for femoral head and neck resection are the approach to the craniodorsal aspect of the hip joint through a craniolateral incision (see Plate 66) and the approach to the caudal aspect of the hip joint and body of the ischium (see Plate 71).

PATIENT POSITIONING

Dorsolateral recumbency with the affected side down (illustrated), except when performing multiple approaches to the pelvis, such as the triple pelvic osteotomy procedure; then, lateral recumbency with the affected limb uppermost and suspended for draping.

DESCRIPTION OF THE PROCEDURE

A. The skin incision is made over the cranial border of the pectineus muscle, starting at the ventral lip of the acetabulum. The incision runs distally along the pectineus for a distance of one third the length of the femur.
B. The fascia is opened in line with the skin incision and the skin undermined and retracted. The belly of the pectineus muscle is mobilized by blunt dissection, with care being taken to protect the femoral artery, vein, and saphenous nerve that run along the cranial border of the muscle. The pectineus is transected at its origin on the prepubic tendon and iliopubic eminence of the pelvis.
C. The pectineus muscle is reflected distally to reveal the iliopsoas muscle and the medial circumflex femoral artery and vein that run caudally and medially to the acetabular portion of the pelvis. It may be necessary to free these vessels from the surrounding fascia and to retract them proximally. Small branches from these vessels may be disrupted during retraction.

PLATE 73

Approach to the Ventral Aspect of the Hip Joint or the Ramus of the Pubis

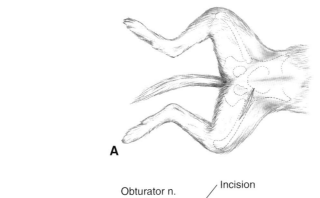

A

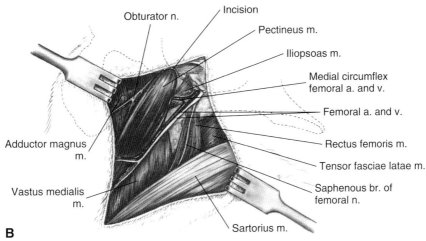

Obturator n.

Incision

Pectineus m.

Iliopsoas m.

Medial circumflex
femoral a. and v.

Femoral a. and v.

Rectus femoris m.

Tensor fasciae latae m.

Saphenous br. of
femoral n.

Adductor magnus
m.

Vastus medialis
m.

Sartorius m.

B

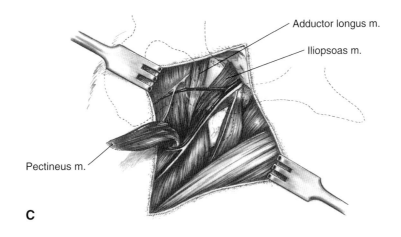

Adductor longus m.

Iliopsoas m.

Pectineus m.

C

Approach to the Ventral Aspect of the Hip Joint or the Ramus of the Pubis *continued*

    D. If only the pubic ramus is to be exposed, go directly to step E. An interval between the iliopsoas and the adductor longus muscle is developed by blunt dissection. Retraction of the iliopsoas cranially and the adductor caudally exposes the rim of the acetabulum. The joint capsule is shown incised so as to reveal the femoral head. Best exposure of the neck of the femur can be developed by placing Hohmann retractors cranial and caudal to the femoral neck.

    E. Exposure of the ramus of the pubis is accomplished by retraction of the iliopsoas muscle with a Hohmann retractor placed craniomedial to the iliopectineal eminence. Some of the origin of the adductor longus muscle is elevated from the ramus and another retractor is placed in the obturator foramen. Care must be taken to prevent trapping the obturator nerve between the retractor and the bone.

ADDITIONAL EXPOSURE

For reduction and internal fixation of comminuted fractures of the acetabulum in which there is fragmentation of the ventral and medial bone, this ventral approach can be performed in combination with one of the dorsal approaches (see Plates 69 and 70). Note that the dorsal and ventral approaches are not continuous because of the femoral artery and vein and the rectus femoris and iliopsoas muscles that intervene.

CLOSURE

Mattress sutures may be used to attach the pectineus muscle to the prepubic tendon. In the triple pelvic osteotomy procedure, the pectineus muscle is left unsutured or transected distally and discarded. A layered closure follows, taking care to avoid suturing the femoral artery and vein.

COMMENTS

Exposure of the joint by this approach is quite restricted, and its use is therefore quite limited, although some consider it the approach of choice for femoral head excision because the integrity of the structures dorsal to the joint is maintained.

PLATE 73

Approach to the Ventral Aspect of the Hip Joint or the Ramus of the Pubis *continued*

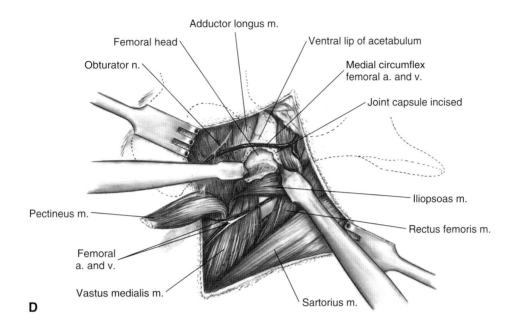

Adductor longus m.

Femoral head

Ventral lip of acetabulum

Obturator n.

Medial circumflex femoral a. and v.

Joint capsule incised

Iliopsoas m.

Pectineus m.

Rectus femoris m.

Femoral a. and v.

Vastus medialis m.

Sartorius m.

D

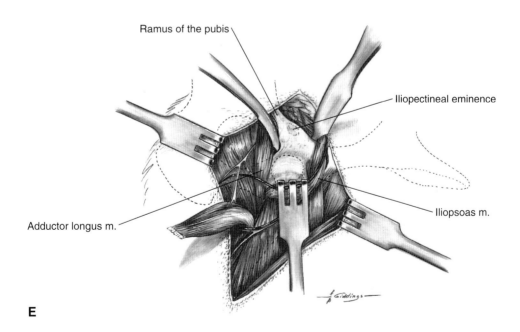

Ramus of the pubis

Iliopectineal eminence

Iliopsoas m.

Adductor longus m.

E

Approach to the Pubis and Pelvic Symphysis

INDICATIONS

1. Open reduction of fractures of the pubis.
2. Pubic symphysiotomy.
3. Juvenile pubic symphysiodesis.

PATIENT POSITIONING

Ventral recumbency (illustrated) with hindlimbs abducted.

DESCRIPTION OF THE PROCEDURE

A. The skin incision on a male dog is made alongside the penis and extends from the scrotum to a point 1 inch (2.5 cm) cranial to the pubis. In the female dog and cat, the incision is made from the vulva cranially on the midline. The latter technique can also be applied to the male cat.
B. The penis is retracted past the midline, following the incision of the fascia alongside the penis and blunt dissection under the organ. A large branch of the external pudendal artery must be ligated to make the fascial incision.
C. Deep fascia and fat are incised and retracted.

PLATE 74
Approach to the Pubis and Pelvic Symphysis

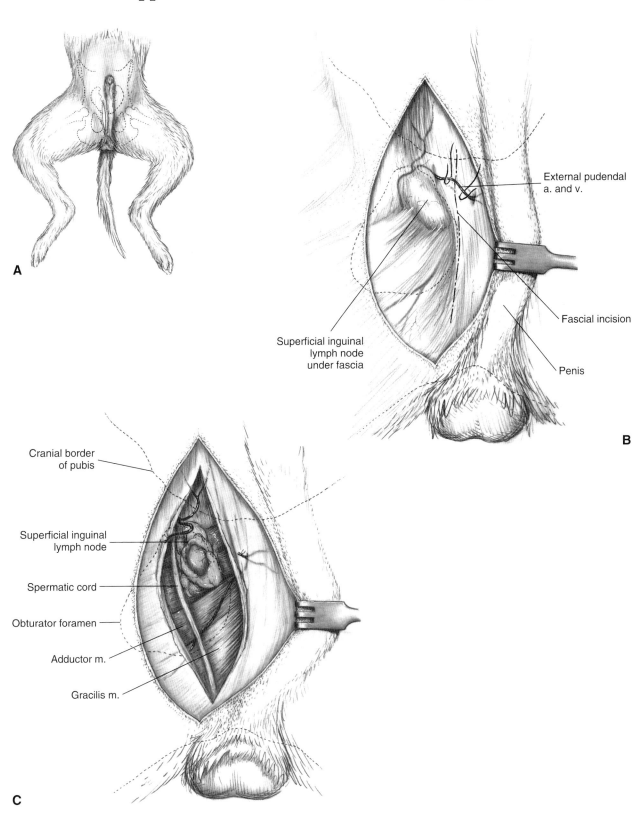

A

External pudendal
a. and v.

Fascial incision

Penis

Superficial inguinal
lymph node
under fascia

B

Cranial border
of pubis

Superficial inguinal
lymph node

Spermatic cord

Obturator foramen

Adductor m.

Gracilis m.

C

Approach to the Pubis and Pelvic Symphysis *continued*

D. A midline incision commencing just cranial to the pubis is made through the linea alba and continued caudally through the subpelvic tendon to the surface of the pubic symphysis.

E. The gracilis and adductor muscles are elevated from the pubic symphysis. Avoid opening the peritoneum if possible.

CLOSURE

The gracilis and adductor muscles are joined at the symphysis by sutures. Any disruption of the insertion of the prepubic tendons must be securely sutured. Attachment to the fascia of the adductor and gracilis muscles is satisfactory. Care must be taken to ensure closure of the peritoneum cranially to the pubis if the peritoneum has been disrupted.

COMMENTS

Excessive abduction of the hindlimbs should be prevented for several days by loosely hobbling the legs together.

PLATE 74

Approach to the Pubis and Pelvic Symphysis *continued*

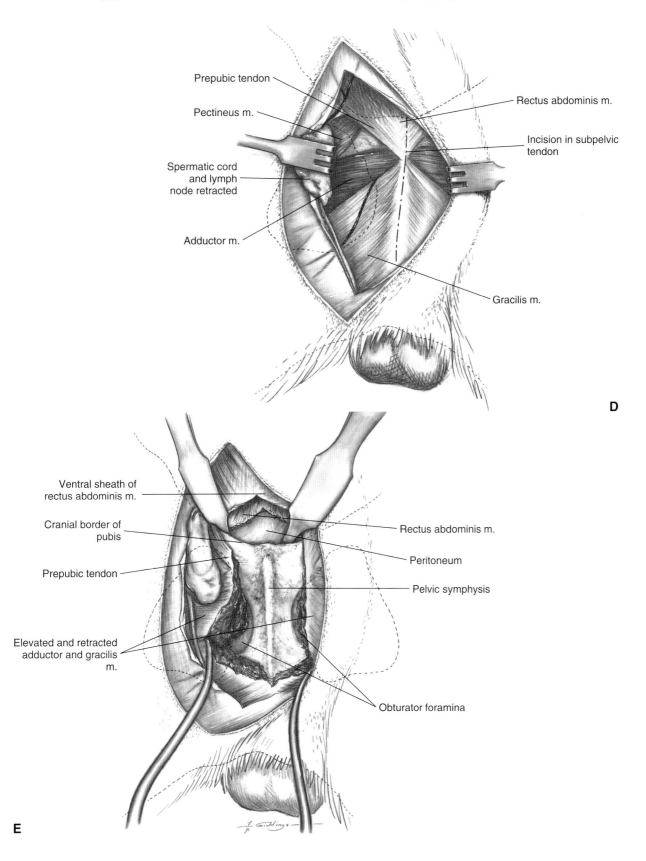

Prepubic tendon

Pectineus m.

Spermatic cord
and lymph
node retracted

Adductor m.

Rectus abdominis m.

Incision in subpelvic
tendon

Gracilis m.

D

Ventral sheath of
rectus abdominis m.

Cranial border of
pubis

Prepubic tendon

Elevated and retracted
adductor and gracilis
m.

Rectus abdominis m.

Peritoneum

Pelvic symphysis

Obturator foramina

E

Approach to the Ischium

INDICATIONS

1. Open reduction of fractures of the ischium.
2. Osteotomy of the ramus for triple pelvic osteotomy.

DESCRIPTION OF THE PROCEDURE

A. For exposure of fractures, the skin incision is made over the sacrotuberous ligament (absent in cats), which is located by palpation. The incision extends from the level of the greater trochanter to the ischiatic tuberosity. For osteotomy of the ramus, the incision is parallel to the midline, starting caudally at the medial angle of the ischiatic tuberosity and extending cranially only half the distance to the level of the greater trochanter (for osteotomy only, go directly to step D).

B. For exposure of the cranial aspect of the spine of the ischium and visualization of the sciatic nerve, an intermuscular incision is made between the superficial gluteal muscle and the biceps femoris muscle.

C. Caudal retraction of the biceps femoris muscle and cranial retraction of the superficial gluteal muscle provide good exposure of the spine of the ischium and the sciatic nerve.

D. To expose the entire ramus of the ischium, the caudal edge of the origin of the internal obturator muscle is elevated cranially from the table surface until the obturator foramen is visible.

ADDITIONAL EXPOSURE

For additional exposure of the body of the ischium, the approach can be performed in combination with the approach to the caudal aspect of the hip joint and body of the ischium (see Plate 71).

For reduction and internal fixation of multiple pelvic fractures, other separate approaches to the ilium (see Plate 64), hip joint (see Plates 66, 68, 69, 70, and 71), or entire hemipelvis (see Plate 72) may be necessary.

CLOSURE

The elevated internal obturator muscle is sutured to fascia and remnants of periosteum along the ramus. The rest of the incisions are closed in layers.

PLATE 75

Approach to the Ischium

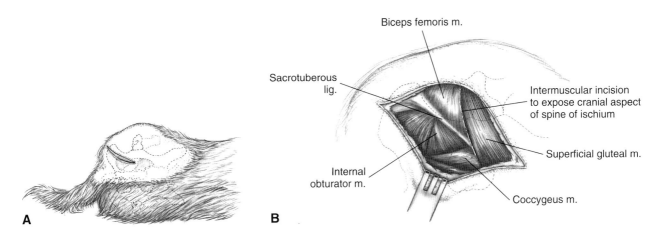

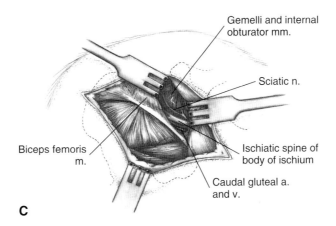

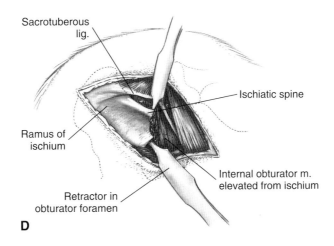

SECTION 7

The Hindlimb

Approach to the Greater Trochanter and Subtrochanteric Region of the Femur

INDICATION

Open reduction of fractures in the trochanteric and subtrochanteric regions of the femur.

PATIENT POSITIONING

Lateral recumbency with the affected limb uppermost.

DESCRIPTION OF THE PROCEDURE

A. The skin incision runs from a point dorsal and slightly cranial to the trochanter, extends over the lateral surface of the trochanter, and ends distally at the proximal one third of the shaft of the femur.
B. The subcutaneous fat and fascia are incised and cleared from the area so that the superficial leaf of the fascia lata can be clearly visualized. An incision is made through the fascia lata along the cranial border of the biceps femoris muscle.
C. The biceps is reflected caudally and the skin and fascia lata cranially. The borders of the superficial gluteal muscle are developed by dissection from the surrounding fascia, and the tendon of insertion of this muscle is cut near the femur. Sufficient tendon is left distally to allow suturing at closure.

PLATE 76

Approach to the Greater Trochanter and Subtrochanteric Region of the Femur

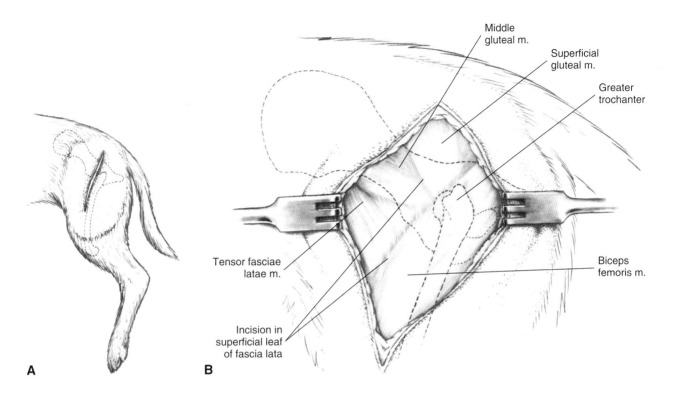

Middle gluteal m.

Superficial gluteal m.

Greater trochanter

Tensor fasciae latae m.

Biceps femoris m.

Incision in superficial leaf of fascia lata

A

B

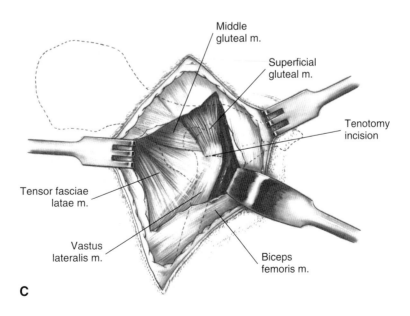

Middle gluteal m.

Superficial gluteal m.

Tenotomy incision

Tensor fasciae latae m.

Vastus lateralis m.

Biceps femoris m.

C

Approach to the Greater Trochanter and Subtrochanteric Region of the Femur *continued*

D. The superficial gluteal muscle is retracted proximally to expose the greater trochanter and the middle gluteal muscle. An incision is now made through the fibers of origin of the vastus lateralis muscle along the ridge of the third trochanter of the femur. This incision is deepened to include the periosteum in young animals.

E. Subperiosteal elevation of this proximal lateral portion of the vastus lateralis muscle exposes the proximal shaft of the femur. The adductor muscle on the caudal side of the bone can also be elevated from the bone to give additional exposure.

ADDITIONAL EXPOSURE

Proximally this approach can be extended to combine with either the approach to the craniodorsal aspect of the hip joint through a craniolateral incision (see Plate 66) or the dorsal exposure of the acetabulum using a trochanteric osteotomy (see Plate 69) or gluteal tenotomy (see Plate 70).

Distally this approach can be extended to expose the entire shaft of the femur (see Plate 77).

CLOSURE

The vastus lateralis muscle is reattached medially to the middle or deep gluteal tendons and laterally to the superficial gluteal tendon. Interrupted mattress sutures are used in the tendon of the superficial gluteal muscle. The fascia lata is then sutured to the biceps femoris, followed by subcutis and skin.

PRECAUTIONS

The sciatic nerve emerges from the pelvis under the superficial gluteal muscle, caudal to the deep gluteal muscle. It then passes across the gemelli and internal obturator muscles and down the thigh, under the biceps femoris muscle. To reduce risk of damage to the sciatic nerve, sharp retractors such as the Meyerding should not be used to retract the biceps femoris muscle.

PLATE 76

Approach to the Greater Trochanter and Subtrochanteric Region of the Femur *continued*

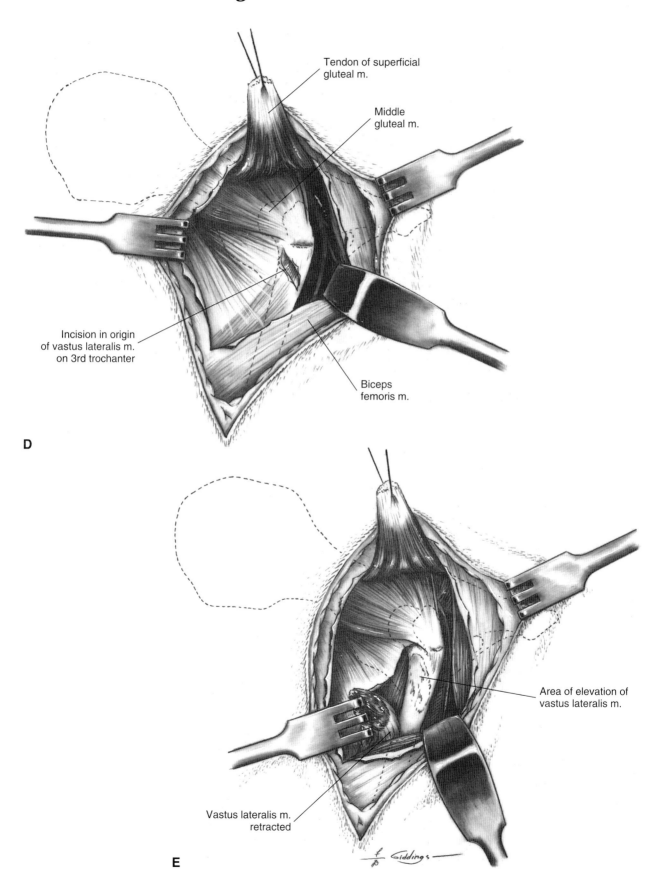

Tendon of superficial gluteal m.

Middle gluteal m.

Incision in origin of vastus lateralis m. on 3rd trochanter

Biceps femoris m.

D

Area of elevation of vastus lateralis m.

Vastus lateralis m. retracted

E

Approach to the Shaft of the Femur in the Dog

Based on a Procedure of Brinker[4]

INDICATION

Open reduction of fractures of the femoral shaft proximal to the supracondylar region.

PATIENT POSITIONING

Lateral recumbency with the hindlimb suspended for draping.

DESCRIPTION OF THE PROCEDURE

A. The skin incision is made along the craniolateral border of the shaft of the bone from the level of the greater trochanter to the level of the patella. The subcutaneous fat and superficial fascia are incised directly under the skin incision.

B. The skin margins are undermined and retracted and the superficial leaf of the fascia lata is incised along the cranial border of the biceps femoris muscle. This incision extends the entire length of the skin incision. If muscle fibers are encountered, the incision should be directed more cranially.

C. Caudal retraction of the biceps femoris reveals the shaft of the femur. It is necessary to incise the fascial aponeurotic septum on the lateral shaft of the bone to adequately retract the vastus lateralis.

D. The vastus lateralis and intermedius muscles on the cranial surface of the shaft are retracted by freeing the loose fascia between the muscle and the bone.

ADDITIONAL EXPOSURE

Proximally this approach can be extended to combine with the approach to the greater trochanter and subtrochanteric region of the femur (see Plate 76).

Distally this approach can be extended to combine with the approach to the distal femur and stifle joint through a lateral incision (see Plate 80).

CLOSURE

Closure consists of suturing the fascia lata to the cranial border of the biceps muscle in one tier and the subcutaneous fat and fascia in a second tier.

COMMENTS

Limit elevation of the adductor muscle on the caudal one third of the shaft to the extent necessary for visualization of fracture lines. This muscle is a valuable source of periosteal blood supply to the healing fracture.

PRECAUTIONS

Caudal to the hip joint the sciatic nerve passes across the gemelli and internal obturator muscles. Passing down the caudal thigh under the biceps femoris muscle, it crosses over the quadratus femoris, adductor, and semimembranosus muscles. At about midthigh it branches into tibial and peroneal nerves. To reduce the risk of damage to the sciatic nerve, care should be taken during retraction of the biceps femoris muscle.

PLATE 77

Approach to the Shaft of the Femur in the Dog

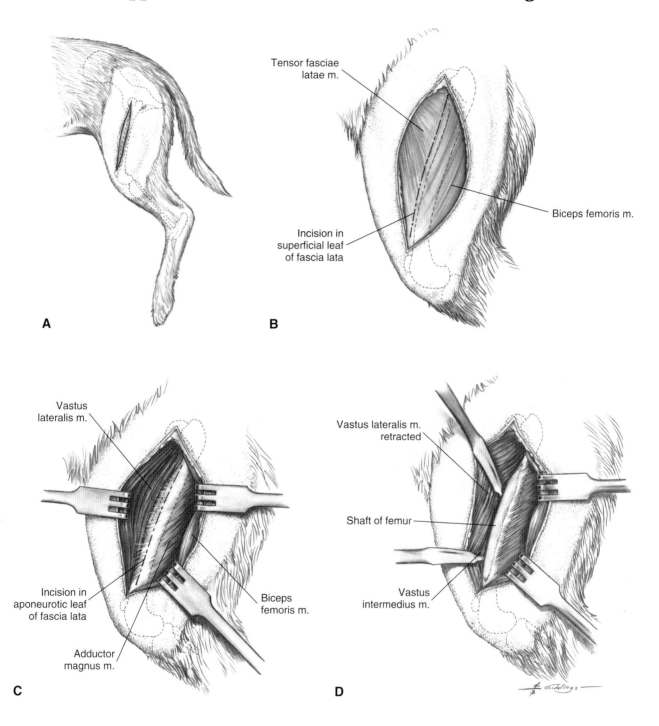

A

B

Tensor fasciae latae m.

Biceps femoris m.

Incision in superficial leaf of fascia lata

Vastus lateralis m.

Incision in aponeurotic leaf of fascia lata

Adductor magnus m.

Biceps femoris m.

C

Vastus lateralis m. retracted

Shaft of femur

Vastus intermedius m.

D

Approach to the Shaft of the Femur in the Cat

INDICATION

Open reduction of fractures of the femoral shaft.

PATIENT POSITIONING

Lateral recumbency with the hindlimb suspended for draping.

DESCRIPTION OF THE PROCEDURE

A. The skin incision is made along the craniolateral border of the shaft of the bone from the level of the greater trochanter to the level of the patella. The subcutaneous fat and superficial fascia are incised directly under the skin incision.

B. There are several anatomic differences in the musculature surrounding the hip joint and femur in the cat with which the surgeon must be familiar. The gluteal muscles may be relatively larger in the cat than in the dog. Also, the caudofemoralis muscle, a muscle not present in the dog, is interposed between the superficial gluteal and biceps femoris muscles.

PLATE 78

Approach to the Shaft of the Femur in the Cat

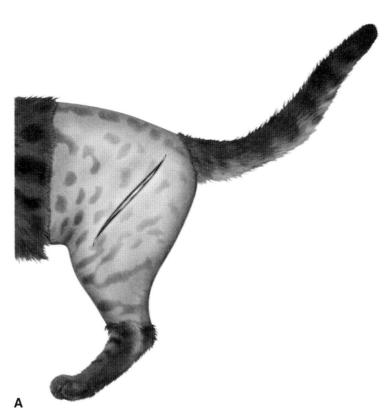

A

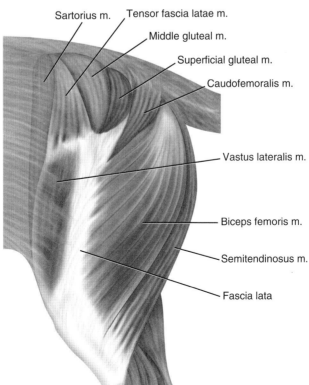

Sartorius m.   Tensor fascia latae m.

Middle gluteal m.

Superficial gluteal m.

Caudofemoralis m.

Vastus lateralis m.

Biceps femoris m.

Semitendinosus m.

Fascia lata

B

Approach to the Shaft of the Femur in the Cat *continued*

C. The skin margins are undermined and retracted. An incision is made through the superficial leaf of the fascia lata, along the cranial border of the caudofemoralis and biceps femoris muscles. This incision extends the entire length of the skin incision. If muscle fibers are encountered, the incision should be directed more cranially.

D. Caudal retraction of the biceps femoris muscle using an atraumatic retractor, such as a Senn or Langenbeck, reveals the shaft of the femur and the sciatic nerve. It is necessary to incise the fascial aponeurotic septum on the lateral shaft of the bone to adequately expose the vastus lateralis.

PLATE 78

Approach to the Shaft of the Femur in the Cat *continued*

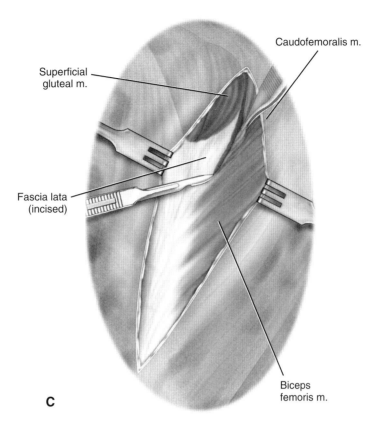

Superficial
gluteal m.

Caudofemoralis m.

Fascia lata
(incised)

Biceps
femoris m.

C

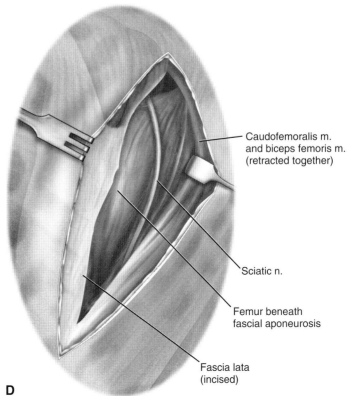

Caudofemoralis m.
and biceps femoris m.
(retracted together)

Sciatic n.

Femur beneath
fascial aponeurosis

Fascia lata
(incised)

D

Approach to the Shaft of the Femur in the Cat *continued*

    E. The origin of the vastus lateralis muscle has a firm insertion along most of the shaft of the femur. To gain exposure of the lateral surface of the femur, the lateral margin of the vastus lateralis muscle is sharply incised.

    F. Using a periosteal elevator, the vastus lateralis muscle is elevated from the shaft of the femur, progressing in a distal-to-proximal direction. For additional exposure proximally, the origin of the vastus lateralis muscle is transected at the third trochanter.

    G. The vastus lateralis and intermedius muscles on the cranial surface of the shaft are retracted to expose the femoral shaft.

ADDITIONAL EXPOSURE

Proximally this approach can be extended to combine with the approach to the greater trochanter and subtrochanteric region of the femur (see Plate 76) or the craniodorsal approach to the hip joint (Plate 67D-I).

    Distally this approach can be extended to combine with the approach to the distal femur and stifle joint through a lateral incision (see Plate 80).

CLOSURE

Closure consists of suturing the fascia lata to the cranial border of the biceps muscle in one tier and the subcutaneous fat and fascia in a second tier.

PLATE 78

Approach to the Shaft of the Femur in the Cat *continued*

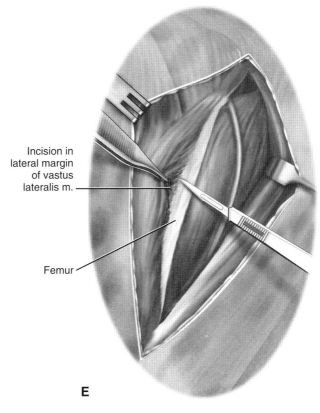

Incision in lateral margin of vastus lateralis m.

Femur

E

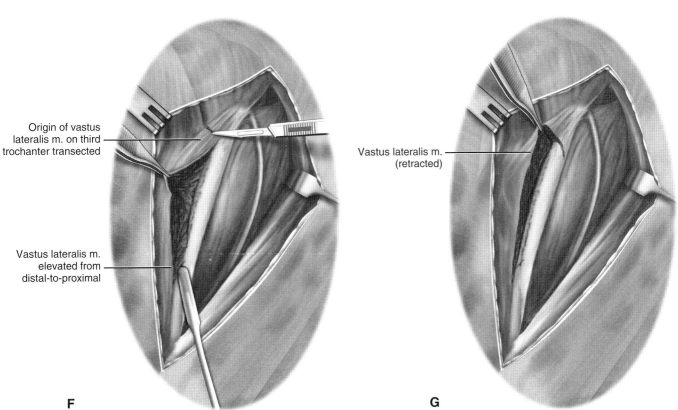

Origin of vastus lateralis m. on third trochanter transected

Vastus lateralis m. elevated from distal-to-proximal

F

Vastus lateralis m. (retracted)

G

Minimally Invasive Approach to the Shaft of the Femur

Based on a Procedure of Pozzi and Lewis[36]

INDICATION

Minimally invasive plate osteosynthesis or interlocking nailing of fractures involving the femoral shaft.

PATIENT POSITIONING

Lateral recumbency with the hindlimb suspended for draping.

DESCRIPTION OF THE PROCEDURE

The magnitude of exposure has been intentionally enlarged in the following descriptive illustrations, to highlight the relevant features of the surgical anatomy. Once familiar with the anatomy, the field of dissection and exposure can be reduced by at least 50% to obtain a true minimally invasive approach to the femur.

A. For this minimally invasive approach to the femur, two skin incisions that are 3 to 5 cm in length are made over the proximal and distal ends of the femur.

B. The subcutaneous fat and fascia are incised and retracted to expose the superficial leaf of the fascia lata. An incision is made through the fascia lata along the cranial border of the biceps femoris muscle.

PLATE 79

Minimally Invasive Approach to the Shaft of the Femur

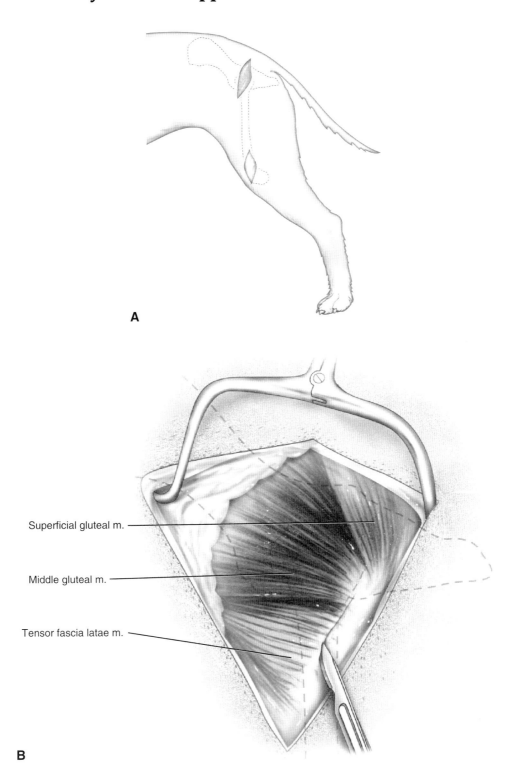

A

Superficial gluteal m.

Middle gluteal m.

Tensor fascia latae m.

B

Minimally Invasive Approach to the Shaft of the Femur *continued*

C. The borders of the superficial gluteal muscle are developed by dissection from the surrounding fascia, and the tendon of insertion of this muscle on the third trochanter is transected near the femur.

D. The superficial gluteal muscle is retracted proximally to expose the greater trochanter and middle gluteal muscle. An instrument is inserted caudal to the middle gluteal muscle and is used to palpate the medial surface of the greater trochanter and the trochanteric fossa. Location of the trochanteric fossa allows subsequent normograde insertion of an intramedullary pin or interlocking nail. The origin of the vastus lateralis is incised to expose the lateral aspect of the proximal region of the femur.

PLATE 79

Minimally Invasive Approach to the Shaft of the Femur *continued*

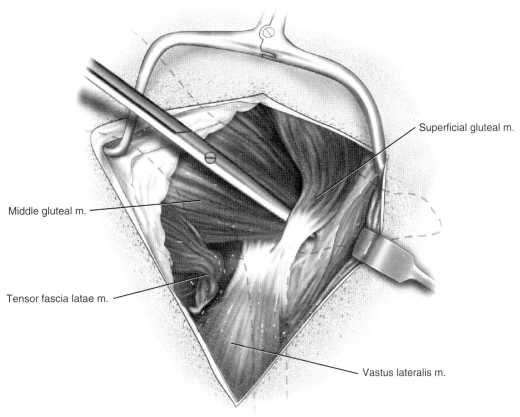

Superficial gluteal m.

Middle gluteal m.

Tensor fascia latae m.

Vastus lateralis m.

C

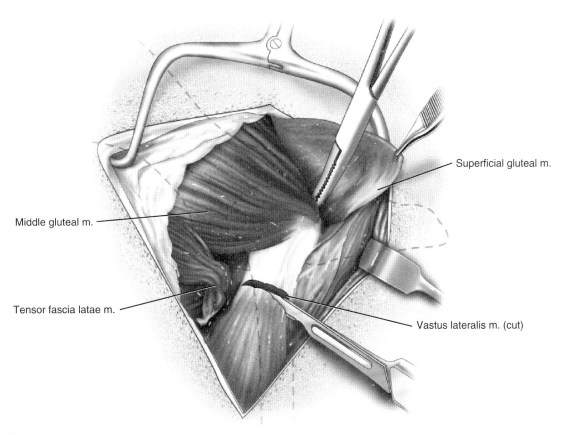

Superficial gluteal m.

Middle gluteal m.

Tensor fascia latae m.

Vastus lateralis m. (cut)

D

Minimally Invasive Approach to the Shaft of the Femur *continued*

E. After identification of the patella and lateral trochlear ridge by palpation, a 2- to 4-cm longitudinal skin incision is made (see Plate 80). The subcutaneous tissue is incised in the same line as the skin incision. An incision is made in the fascia lata along the cranial margin of the biceps femoris muscle.

F. Retraction of the biceps femoris muscle caudally and vastus lateralis muscle cranially provides exposure of the distal end of the femur. It may be necessary to ligate and transect the distal branch of the caudal femoral artery and vein. However, the capsule of the stifle joint should not be incised unless there is an indication to gain exposure of this joint.

PLATE 79

Minimally Invasive Approach to the Shaft of the Femur *continued*

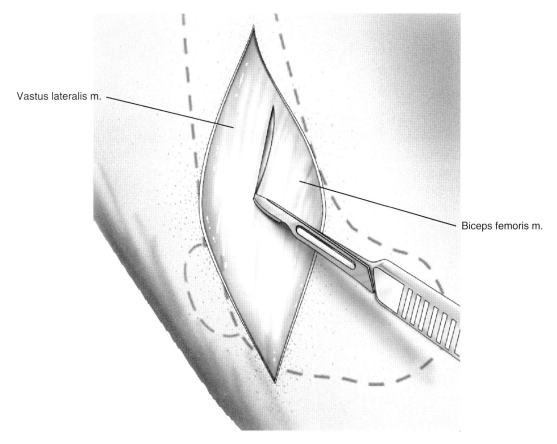

Vastus lateralis m.

Biceps femoris m.

E

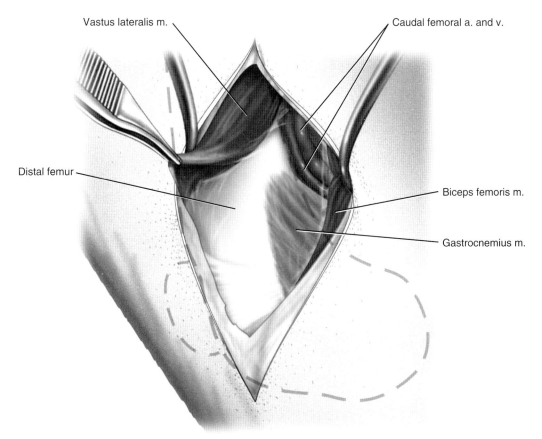

Vastus lateralis m.

Caudal femoral a. and v.

Distal femur

Biceps femoris m.

Gastrocnemius m.

F

Minimally Invasive Approach to the Shaft of the Femur *continued*

G. A blunt instrument, such as the soft-tissue retractor illustrated here, is passed along the lateral side of the femoral shaft to create an epiperiosteal tunnel.

CLOSURE

The vastus lateralis muscle is reattached to the deep or middle gluteal muscle. Interrupted mattress sutures are used in repair of the tendon of the superficial gluteal muscle. The fascia lata is sutured to the cranial border of the biceps muscle, followed by the subcutaneous fat and fascia in a second layer. Closure of the distal incision begins with suturing of the fascia lata to the biceps femoris muscle in a continuous pattern, followed by the subcutaneous fat and fascia in a second layer.

PLATE 79

Minimally Invasive Approach to the Shaft of the Femur *continued*

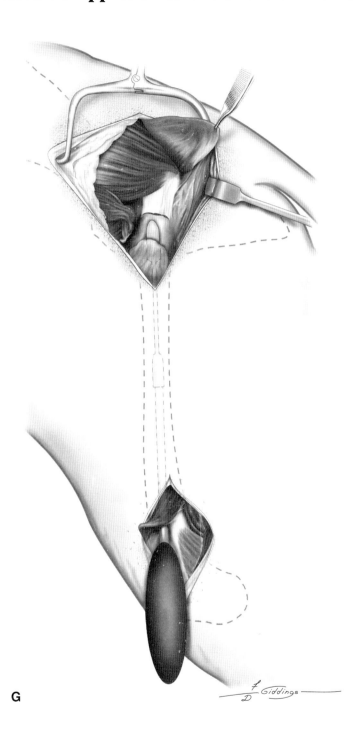

G

Approach to the Distal Femur and Stifle Joint Through a Lateral Incision

Based on a Procedure of Paatsama[34]

INDICATIONS

1. Open reduction of supracondylar, lateral condylar, intercondylar, and distal physeal fractures of the femur.
2. Exploration of the stifle joint.
3. Medial patellar luxation reconstructions.

ALTERNATIVE APPROACHES

Depending on the compartment of most surgical interest, approaches to the stifle can be made via a lateral incision (see Plate 81), medial incision (see Plate 82), bilateral exposure (see Plate 83), or osteotomy of the tibial tuberosity (see Plate 84).

PATIENT POSITIONING

Lateral recumbency with the hindlimb suspended for draping, or dorsal recumbency to allow for conversion to bilateral exposure of the joint (see Plate 83 or 84) when required.

DESCRIPTION OF THE PROCEDURE

A. After palpation of the patella and lateral trochlear ridge, a curved parapatellar skin incision is made extending from the tibial tuberosity to the level of the patella, and then an equal distance proximally. The subcutaneous fascia is incised in the same line as the skin incision. The fascia lata and lateral fascia of the stifle joint are exposed by undermining the subcutaneous fat and fascia, which are then retracted with the skin.
B. Another curved incision, similar to that in the skin, is made through the fascia lata along the cranial border of the biceps. The incision continues distally into the lateral fascia of the stifle joint. As it crosses the trochlear ridge, it curves to parallel the lateral border of the patella and the patellar ligament. Enough fascia is left on the lateral edge of the patella to receive sutures when the joint is closed.

PLATE 80

Approach to the Distal Femur and Stifle Joint Through a Lateral Incision

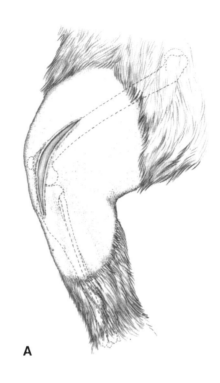

A

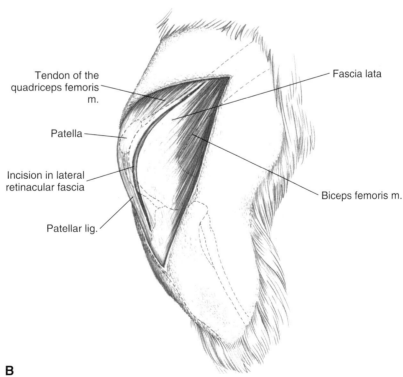

Tendon of the quadriceps femoris m.

Fascia lata

Patella

Incision in lateral retinacular fascia

Patellar lig.

Biceps femoris m.

B

Approach to the Distal Femur and Stifle Joint Through a Lateral Incision *continued*

    C. The biceps and attached lateral fascia are retracted caudally. In separating the biceps from the vastus lateralis, an intermuscular septum formed from the fascia lata is found attached to the femur. This fascia must be incised to allow mobilization of the quadriceps and biceps. Muscular branches of the distal caudal femoral vessels crossing the distal femur must be ligated in some cases. A parapatellar incision is now made through the joint capsule.

    D. With the joint extended, the patella and quadriceps can be luxated medially. Lateral retraction of the joint capsule with the biceps and lateral fascia fully exposes the interior of the joint. Incision and retraction of the infrapatellar fat pad may be necessary for inspection of the menisci and cruciate ligaments.

ADDITIONAL EXPOSURE

Proximally this approach can be extended by combining with the approach to the shaft of the femur (see Plate 77) to expose the entire bone. The muscular branch of the caudal femoral artery that crosses the distal femur to supply the vastus lateralis muscle will need to be ligated. The joint capsule usually need not be incised to expose supracondylar fractures, but it is always incised for exposure of physeal fractures, which are intracapsular.

CLOSURE

The joint capsule and lateral fascia of the stifle joint are closed in one layer with interrupted sutures. Sutures must only be placed in the outer fibrous layer of the joint capsule to prevent suture material from abrading articular cartilage. The fascia lata incision proximal to the patella can be closed with a continuous-pattern suture.

PLATE 80

Approach to the Distal Femur and Stifle Joint Through a Lateral Incision *continued*

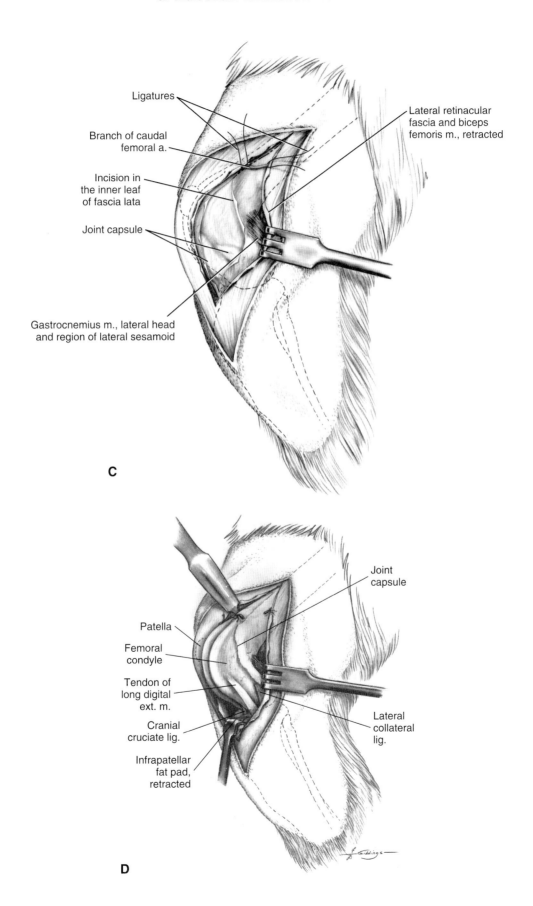

Ligatures

Branch of caudal femoral a.

Incision in the inner leaf of fascia lata

Joint capsule

Gastrocnemius m., lateral head and region of lateral sesamoid

Lateral retinacular fascia and biceps femoris m., retracted

C

Joint capsule

Patella

Femoral condyle

Tendon of long digital ext. m.

Cranial cruciate lig.

Infrapatellar fat pad, retracted

Lateral collateral lig.

D

Approach to the Stifle Joint Through a Lateral Incision

INDICATIONS

1. Cranial cruciate ligament reconstructions (see Comments).
2. Meniscectomy (see Comments).
3. Exploration of the stifle joint.

ALTERNATIVE APPROACHES

Depending on the compartment of most interest, approaches to the stifle can be made via a medial incision (see Plate 82), bilateral exposure (see Plate 83), or osteotomy of the tibial tuberosity (see Plate 84). For cranial cruciate ligament reconstruction the authors favor a medial approach (see Plate 82), particularly in chronic injuries.

PATIENT POSITIONING

Either lateral or dorsal recumbency with the hindlimb suspended for draping.

DESCRIPTION OF THE PROCEDURE

A. The skin incision starts over the tibial tuberosity lateral to the patellar ligament. It continues proximally to the level of the patella and then an equal distance proximally following the cranial border of the femur (see Comments).
B. The arthrotomy incision follows the same line as the skin. The distal portion is made in the lateral fascia first with the scalpel, starting opposite the distal pole of the patella and a few millimeters lateral to the patellar ligament and continuing distally to the tibia. A stab incision is made into the joint at the proximal end of this incision, which will allow entry into the joint with little danger of damaging articular cartilage of the femoral condyle. One blade of a scissor is inserted into the joint and the scissor is advanced proximally, cutting joint capsule, lateral parapatellar fibrocartilage, and fascia lata. As the proximal part of the incision is started, it is directed slightly laterally so as to cut through the vastus lateralis parallel to the muscle fibers and to leave enough tissue on the lateral side of the patella to permit suturing.

PLATE 81
Approach to the Stifle Joint Through a Lateral Incision

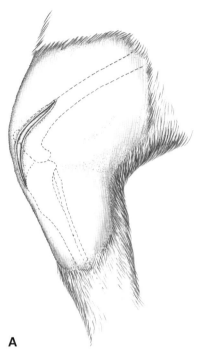

A

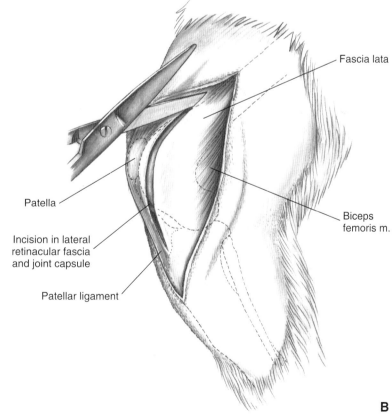

Fascia lata

Patella

Incision in lateral
retinacular fascia
and joint capsule

Patellar ligament

Biceps
femoris m.

B

Approach to the Stifle Joint Through a Lateral Incision *continued*

C. The patella can now be luxated medially. If the patella will not stay in position medially, the proximal end of the incision is lengthened. Distal retraction of the fat pad exposes the cruciate ligaments and menisci.

ADDITIONAL EXPOSURE

This exposure can be extended proximally for access to the supracondylar region by following the approach shown in Plate 80.

For exposure of the lateral fabella when performing extracapsular stabilization of a cranial cruciate ligament rupture, the approach can be extended caudolaterally as shown in Plate 85C.

CLOSURE

Distally, the joint capsule and lateral fascia of the stifle joint are closed in one layer with interrupted sutures. Sutures are placed in the outer fibrous layer of the joint capsule to prevent any suture material from penetrating the joint in a region where it could abrade articular cartilage. Proximal to the patella the fascia lata can be closed with a continuous-pattern suture. Subcutis and skin are closed routinely.

COMMENTS

For cosmetic reasons, this skin incision is often made medially, as in Plate 82. The skin can easily be undermined and retracted laterally to make the lateral arthrotomy.

PLATE 81

Approach to the Stifle Joint Through a Lateral Incision *continued*

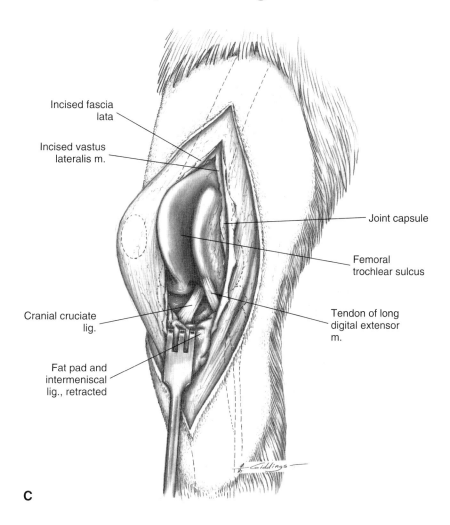

Incised fascia lata

Incised vastus lateralis m.

Joint capsule

Femoral trochlear sulcus

Cranial cruciate lig.

Tendon of long digital extensor m.

Fat pad and intermeniscal lig., retracted

C

Approach to the Stifle Joint Through a Medial Incision

INDICATIONS

1. Cranial cruciate ligament reconstructions (see Comments).
2. Exploration of the stifle joint.
3. Medial meniscectomy.

ALTERNATIVE APPROACHES

Depending on the compartment of most interest, approaches to the stifle can be made via a lateral incision (see Plate 81), bilateral exposure (see Plate 83), or osteotomy of the tibial tuberosity (see Plate 84). For cranial cruciate ligament reconstruction the authors favor the medial approach (see Plate 82). Chronic cases often have damage to the caudal horn of the medial meniscus, and medial meniscectomy is more easily performed from the medial approach.

PATIENT POSITIONING

Dorsal recumbency (as illustrated in Plate 82A) with the hindlimb suspended for draping.

DESCRIPTION OF THE PROCEDURE

A. The skin incision starts over the tibial tuberosity medial to the patellar ligament. It continues proximally to the level of the patella and then an equal distance proximally following the cranial border of the femur.
B. The arthrotomy incision follows the same line as the skin. The distal portion in the medial fascia is made first with the scalpel, starting opposite the distal pole of the patella and a few millimeters medial to the patellar ligament and continuing distally to the tibia. A stab incision is made into the joint at the proximal end of this incision, which will allow entry into the joint with little danger of damaging the articular cartilage of the femoral condyle. One blade of a scissor is inserted into the joint and the scissor is advanced proximally, cutting joint capsule, medial parapatellar fibrocartilage, medial fascia, and the vastus medialis muscle and cranial part of the sartorius muscle (also see Plate 81B). As the proximal part of the incision is started, it is directed medially so as to cut through the cranial sartorius and vastus medialis muscles parallel to their fibers and to leave enough tissue on the medial side of the patella to permit suturing.

PLATE 82
Approach to the Stifle Joint Through a Medial Incision

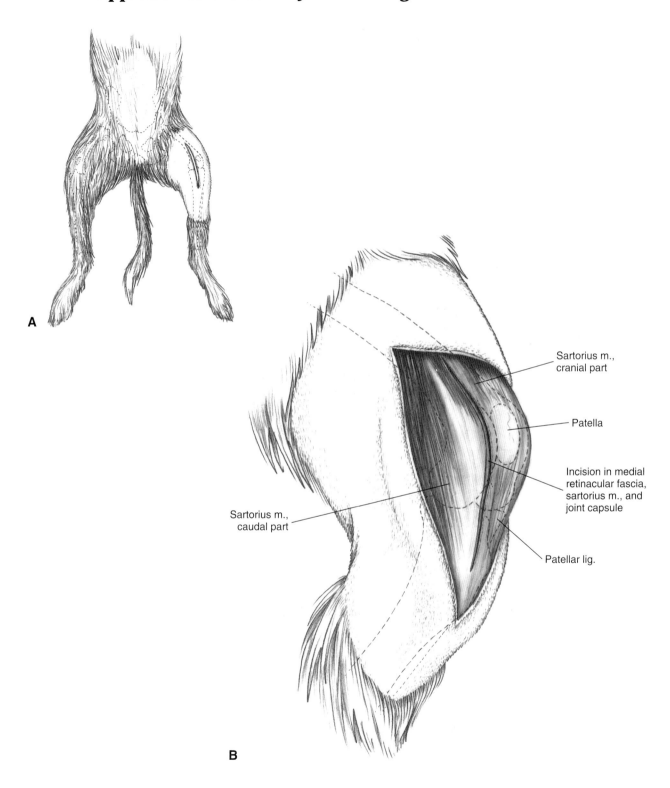

A

Sartorius m.,
cranial part

Patella

Incision in medial
retinacular fascia,
sartorius m., and
joint capsule

Sartorius m.,
caudal part

Patellar lig.

B

Approach to the Stifle Joint Through a Medial Incision *continued*

C. The patella can now be luxated laterally. If the patella will not stay in position laterally, the proximal end of the incision is lengthened. Distal retraction of the fat pad exposes the cruciate ligaments and menisci.

ADDITIONAL EXPOSURE

This exposure can be extended to the caudomedial compartment of the stifle joint, as shown in Plate 87C-E.

For extension of exposure more distally to the tibia, this approach can be combined with the approach to the proximal tibia (see Plate 89) or the shaft of the tibia (see Plate 90).

CLOSURE

Distally, the joint capsule and medial fascia of the stifle joint are closed in one layer with interrupted sutures. Sutures must be placed only in the outer fibrous layer of the joint capsule to prevent any suture material from penetrating the synovial membrane in a region where it could abrade articular cartilage. Proximal to the patella, the cranial part of the sartorius and the vastus medialis muscles can be closed with a continuous-pattern suture. Subcutis and skin are closed routinely.

COMMENTS

Medial exposure is preferred over the lateral approach whenever possible. Scar formation is hidden, the interior of the joint is more widely exposed, and medial meniscectomy is more readily performed through a medial incision.

PLATE 82

Approach to the Stifle Joint Through a Medial Incision *continued*

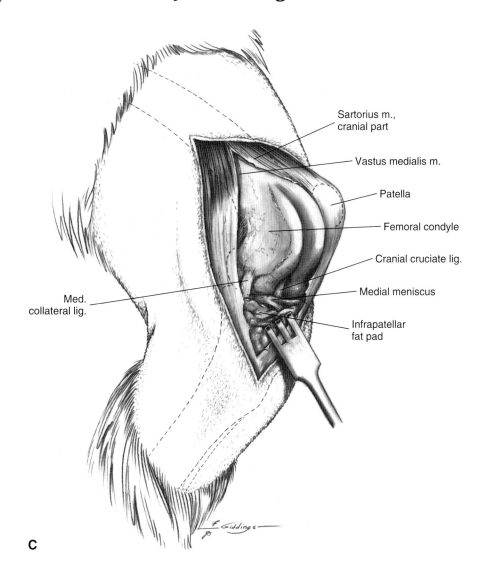

Sartorius m., cranial part

Vastus medialis m.

Patella

Femoral condyle

Cranial cruciate lig.

Medial meniscus

Infrapatellar fat pad

Med. collateral lig.

C

Approach to the Stifle Joint with Bilateral Exposure

INDICATIONS

1. Open reduction of fractures of the distal femur.
2. Double Rush pin or cross-pin fixation of the femur.

ALTERNATIVE APPROACHES

For more extensive exposure an alternative approach is by osteotomy of the tibial tuberosity (see Plate 84).

PATIENT POSITIONING

Dorsal recumbency with the hindlimb suspended for draping.

DESCRIPTION OF THE PROCEDURE

This procedure is a combination of the Approach to the Distal Femur and Stifle Joint Through a Lateral Incision and the Approach to the Stifle Joint Through a Medial Incision (see Plates 80 and 82).

A. The skin incision is as shown in Plate 80A, although slightly elongated proximally to allow for easier retraction to the medial side. The skin and subcutis are undermined and medially retracted sufficiently to allow access to the medial arthrotomy. If desired, the skin incision can be placed medially as in Plate 82A, again lengthened proximally to allow easier retraction to the lateral side.

B. Entrance to the lateral side is shown in Plate 80B-D.

PLATE 83

Approach to the Stifle Joint with Bilateral Exposure

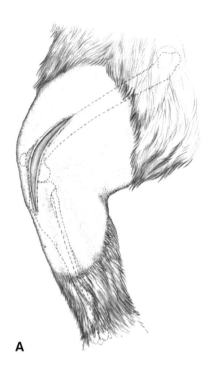

A

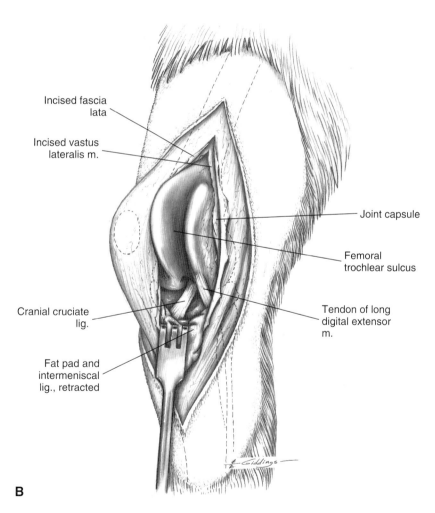

Incised fascia lata

Incised vastus lateralis m.

Joint capsule

Femoral trochlear sulcus

Cranial cruciate lig.

Tendon of long digital extensor m.

Fat pad and intermeniscal lig., retracted

B

Approach to the Stifle Joint with Bilateral Exposure *continued*

C. To expose the medial side, see Plate 82B and C.
D. The entire condylar and supracondylar portion of the femur and the cranial compartment of the stifle joint are now exposed.

ADDITIONAL EXPOSURE

To gain exposure of the entire femur, this approach can be combined with the approach to the shaft of the femur (see Plate 77).

CLOSURE

Suturing is done as previously explained for the medial and lateral approaches.

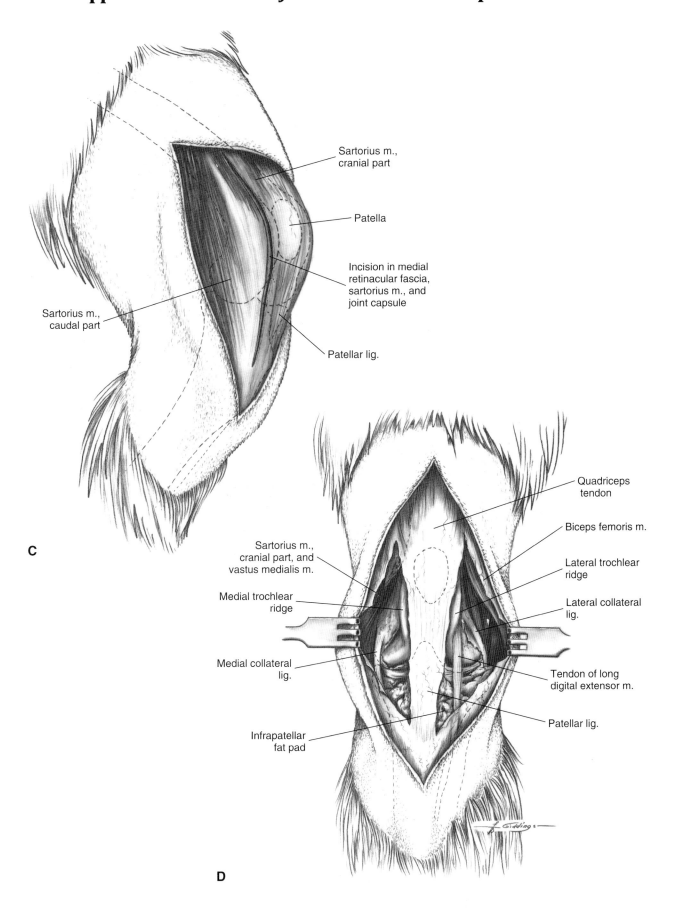

Sartorius m.,
cranial part

Patella

Incision in medial
retinacular fascia,
sartorius m., and
joint capsule

Sartorius m.,
caudal part

Patellar lig.

C

Quadriceps
tendon

Biceps femoris m.

Lateral trochlear
ridge

Lateral collateral
lig.

Sartorius m.,
cranial part, and
vastus medialis m.

Medial trochlear
ridge

Medial collateral
lig.

Tendon of long
digital extensor m.

Patellar lig.

Infrapatellar
fat pad

D

Approach to the Distal Femur and Stifle Joint by Osteotomy of the Tibial Tuberosity

Based on a Procedure of Nunamaker[32]

INDICATIONS

Open reduction of comminuted fractures of the femoral condyles or supracondylar region.

ALTERNATIVE APPROACHES

For procedures that require somewhat less exposure the alternative approach is via bilateral incisions (see Plate 83).

PATIENT POSITIONING

Dorsal recumbency with the hindlimb suspended for draping.

DESCRIPTION OF THE PROCEDURE

A. An osteotome or oscillating power saw is used to remove the tibial tuberosity from the tibia, containing the insertion of the patellar ligament. Care must be exercised so as to not damage the articular cartilage of the femoral condyles or the meniscal cartilages while performing this osteotomy.
B. The detached tibial tuberosity, patellar ligament, and patella are now reflected proximally to expose the femoral condyles, cruciate ligaments, and menisci. If the supracondylar area of the femur must also be exposed, the medial and lateral incisions can be extended proximally as needed.

ADDITIONAL EXPOSURE

To gain exposure of the entire femur, this approach can be combined with the approach to the shaft of the femur (see Plate 77).

CLOSURE

The tibial tuberosity is attached to the tibia with Kirschner wires and tension band wire (see Figure 23). Subcutaneous tissues and skin are closed in layers. The medial and lateral joint capsules and fascia are closed in one layer, using an interrupted pattern. Fasciae of the quadriceps and biceps muscles are sutured with a continuous pattern.

PLATE 84

Approach to the Distal Femur and Stifle Joint by Osteotomy of the Tibial Tuberosity

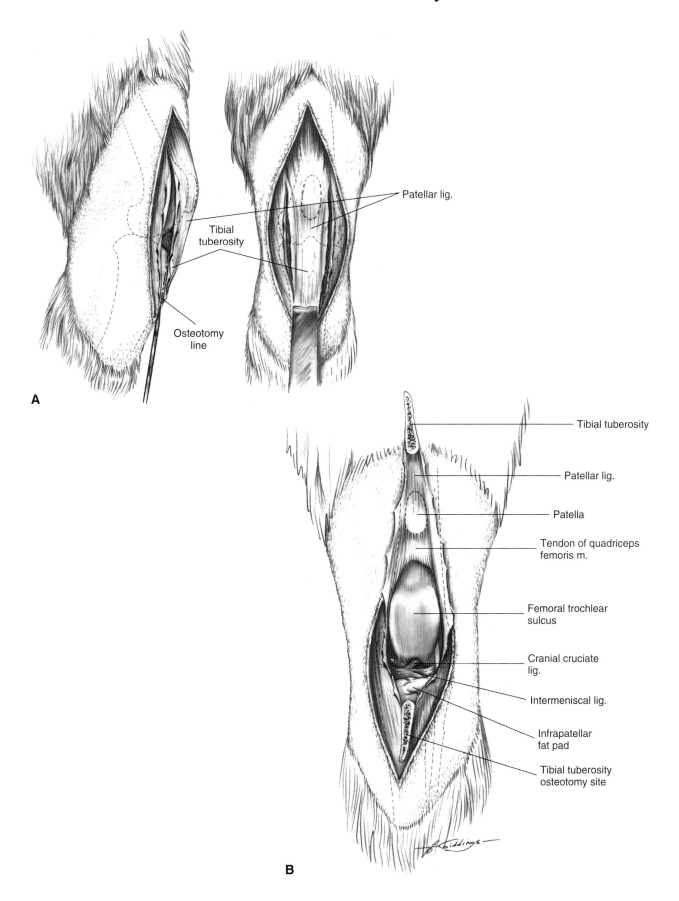

Patellar lig.

Tibial tuberosity

Osteotomy line

A

Tibial tuberosity

Patellar lig.

Patella

Tendon of quadriceps femoris m.

Femoral trochlear sulcus

Cranial cruciate lig.

Intermeniscal lig.

Infrapatellar fat pad

Tibial tuberosity osteotomy site

B

Approach to the Lateral Collateral Ligament and Caudolateral Part of the Stifle Joint

INDICATIONS

1. Removal of the caudal horn of the lateral meniscus.
2. Repair of the lateral collateral ligament or tendon of the popliteus muscle.
3. Open reduction of fractures of the caudal articular surface of the lateral femoral condyle.

ALTERNATIVE APPROACH

The approach to the stifle joint through a craniolateral arthrotomy provides access to the trochlear groove, the cranial poles of the menisci, and the cruciate ligaments (see Plate 80C and D and Plate 81B and C).

PATIENT POSITIONING

Lateral recumbency with the affected limb suspended for draping.

DESCRIPTION OF THE PROCEDURE

A. The skin incision is made directly over the distal femur and proximal tibia. The incision commences at the lower third of the femur and continues distally through the proximal fourth of the tibia.
B. Subcutaneous tissues are incised on the same line and retracted with the skin. An incision is made in the aponeurosis of the biceps femoris muscle just cranial to the muscle fibers. It is not necessary to penetrate the joint capsule, although this may be preferable in order to visualize the cranial compartment of the joint (see Plate 80C).

PLATE 85

Approach to the Lateral Collateral Ligament and Caudolateral Part of the Stifle Joint

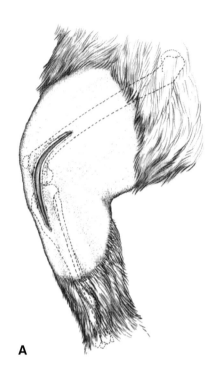

A

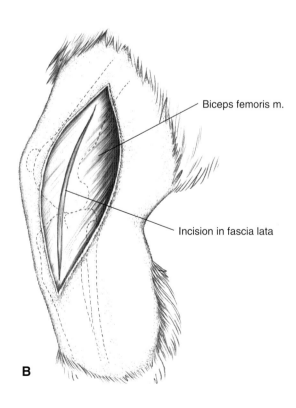

Biceps femoris m.

Incision in fascia lata

B

Approach to the Lateral Collateral Ligament and Caudolateral Part of the Stifle Joint *continued*

    C. As the biceps muscle and attached fascia lata are undermined and retracted caudally, the lateral collateral ligament and tendon of the popliteus muscle are exposed, although still covered by fascia. The lateral fabella can be palpated within the origin of the lateral head of the gastrocnemius muscle. Note the position of the peroneal nerve and protect it from excessive tension.

    D. The caudolateral compartment of the joint is exposed by incising the joint capsule caudally from the collateral ligament. The popliteal tendon and a portion of the joint capsule are elevated to increase exposure. Take care to not damage the meniscus while making this incision.

ADDITIONAL EXPOSURE

Greater exposure of comminuted fractures is gained by combining this approach with the bilateral approach (see Plate 83) or the approach with tibial tuberosity osteotomy (see Plate 84).

CLOSURE

Interrupted sutures are placed in the joint capsule. The aponeurosis of the biceps femoris and the rest of the lateral fascia are closed with continuous sutures. Closure of subcutaneous tissues and skin is routine.

PLATE 85

Approach to the Lateral Collateral Ligament and Caudolateral Part of the Stifle Joint *continued*

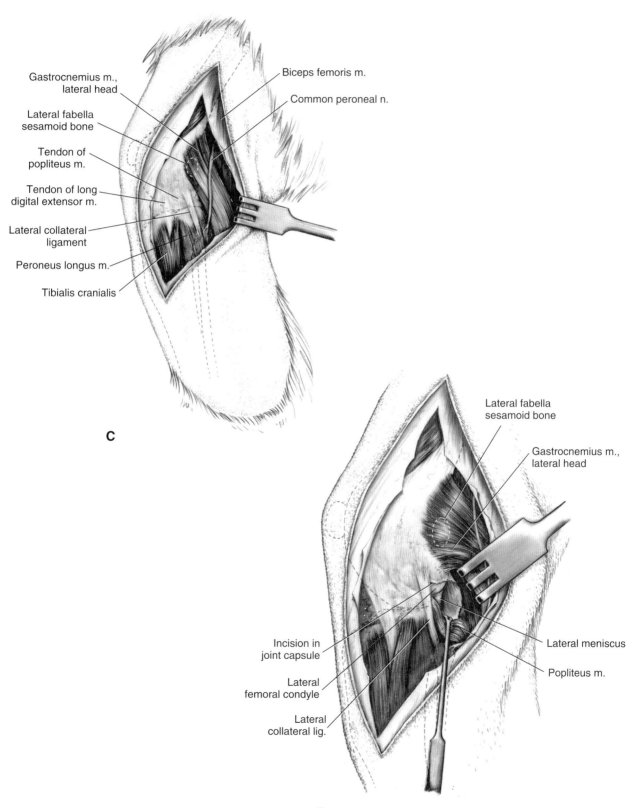

Gastrocnemius m., lateral head

Lateral fabella sesamoid bone

Tendon of popliteus m.

Tendon of long digital extensor m.

Lateral collateral ligament

Peroneus longus m.

Tibialis cranialis

Biceps femoris m.

Common peroneal n.

C

Lateral fabella sesamoid bone

Gastrocnemius m., lateral head

Incision in joint capsule

Lateral femoral condyle

Lateral collateral lig.

Lateral meniscus

Popliteus m.

D

Approach to the Stifle Joint by Osteotomy of the Origin of the Lateral Collateral Ligament

INDICATIONS

1. Reduction of fractures of the caudal part of the lateral femoral condyle.
2. Exploration of the caudolateral part of the stifle joint.
3. Avulsion of the insertion of the caudal cruciate ligament.

ALTERNATIVE APPROACH

The caudolateral approach (see Plate 85), which spares the lateral collateral ligament, provides more limited exposure but is adequate for most surgery of the lateral meniscus.

PATIENT POSITIONING

Lateral recumbency with the affected limb suspended for draping.

DESCRIPTION OF THE PROCEDURE

This procedure is a continuation of the Approach to the Lateral Collateral Ligament and Caudolateral Part of the Stifle Joint (see Plate 85).

A. Incision of the joint capsule is continued cranially after elevating the lateral collateral ligament from the joint capsule and lateral retinaculum. This will expose the tendon of the popliteus muscle and its insertion on the femoral condyle. An osteotome is used to outline a block of bone that contains the entire origin of the lateral collateral ligament.

B. The block of bone is freed from the underlying condyle. Be sure to take an adequate amount of bone because a block that is too small is difficult to fix securely in place. Note the wedge shape of the bone block; this will have some inherent stability when replaced. Adduction and internal rotation of the tibia will expose the interior of the joint.

CLOSURE

The bone block origin of the ligament is reattached to the femur by means of a lag screw (see Figure 24A). This can be simplified by predrilling before cutting the bone block. Interrupted sutures are placed in the joint capsule. The aponeurosis of the biceps femoris and the rest of the lateral fascia are closed with continuous sutures. Closure of the subcutaneous tissues and skin is routine.

PLATE 86

Approach to the Stifle Joint by Osteotomy of the Origin of the Lateral Collateral Ligament

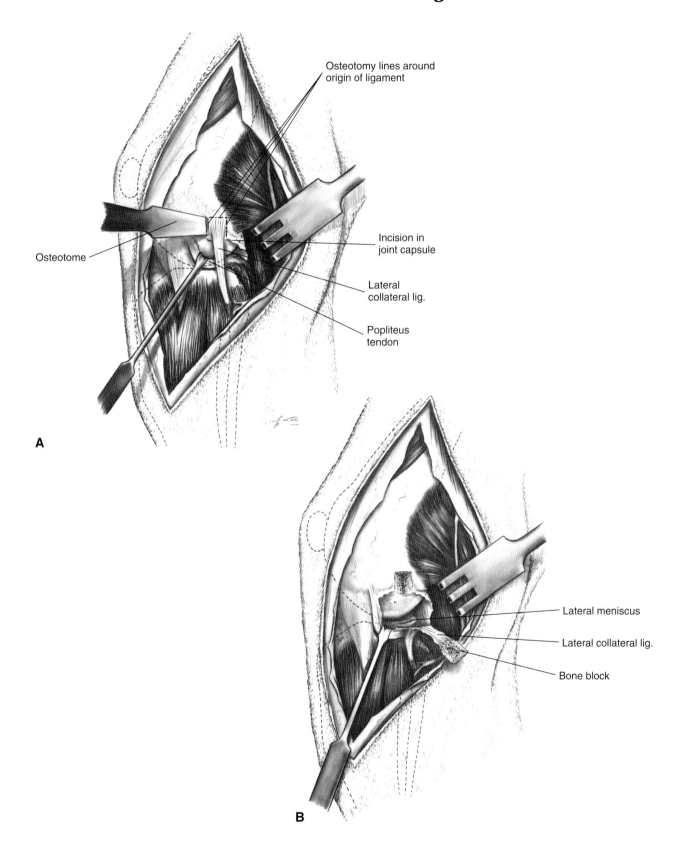

Osteotomy lines around origin of ligament

Incision in joint capsule

Lateral collateral lig.

Popliteus tendon

Osteotome

A

Lateral meniscus

Lateral collateral lig.

Bone block

B

Approach to the Medial Collateral Ligament and Caudomedial Part of the Stifle Joint

INDICATIONS

1. Removal of the caudal horn of the medial meniscus.
2. Repair of the medial collateral ligament.
3. Open reduction of fractures of the caudal part of the medial femoral condyle.

ALTERNATIVE APPROACH

More extensive exposure of the medial compartment of the stifle joint can gained by the osteotomy of the origin of the medial collateral ligament (see Plate 88).

PATIENT POSITIONING

Dorsal recumbency with the affected hindlimb suspended for draping.

DESCRIPTION OF THE PROCEDURE

A. The skin incision extends from the distal fourth of the femur distally to the proximal fourth of the tibia, crossing the joint between the medial tibial condyle and tibial tuberosity. Subcutaneous tissues are incised on the same line and mobilized with the skin.
B. An incision is made in the deep fascia along the cranial border of the caudal part of the sartorius muscle.

PLATE 87

Approach to the Medial Collateral Ligament and Caudomedial Part of the Stifle Joint

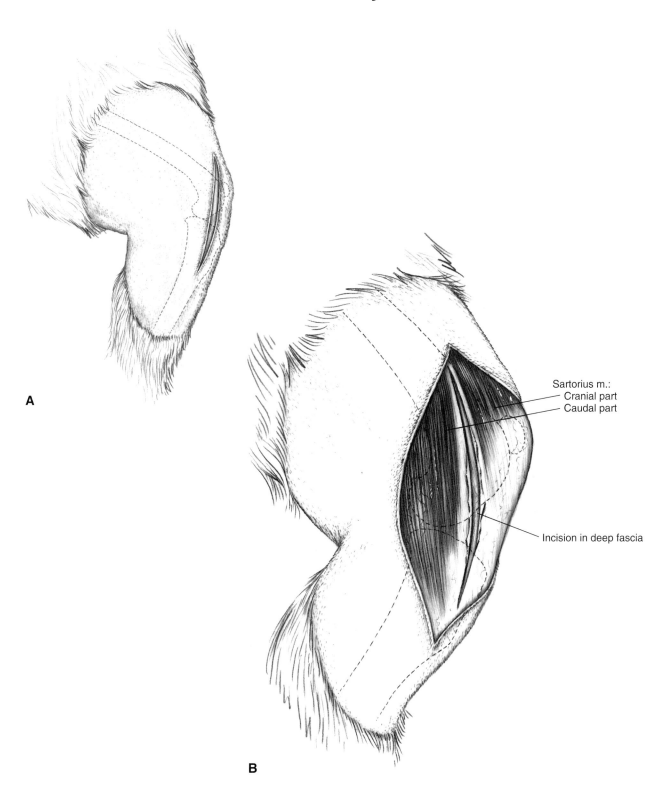

A

B

Sartorius m.:
Cranial part
Caudal part

Incision in deep fascia

Approach to the Medial Collateral Ligament and Caudomedial Part of the Stifle Joint *continued*

C. The caudal part of the sartorius muscle is retracted to expose the collateral ligaments.

PLATE 87

Approach to the Medial Collateral Ligament and Caudomedial Part of the Stifle Joint *continued*

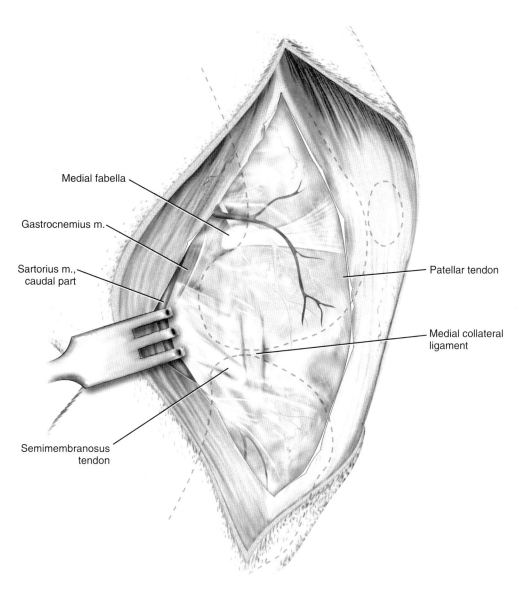

Medial fabella

Gastrocnemius m.

Sartorius m.,
caudal part

Semimembranosus
tendon

Patellar tendon

Medial collateral
ligament

C

Approach to the Medial Collateral Ligament and Caudomedial Part of the Stifle Joint *continued*

D. The joint capsule can be incised in a longitudinal direction, immediately caudal to the medial collateral ligament to expose the interior of the joint and the medial meniscus.

PLATE 87

Approach to the Medial Collateral Ligament and Caudomedial Part of the Stifle Joint *continued*

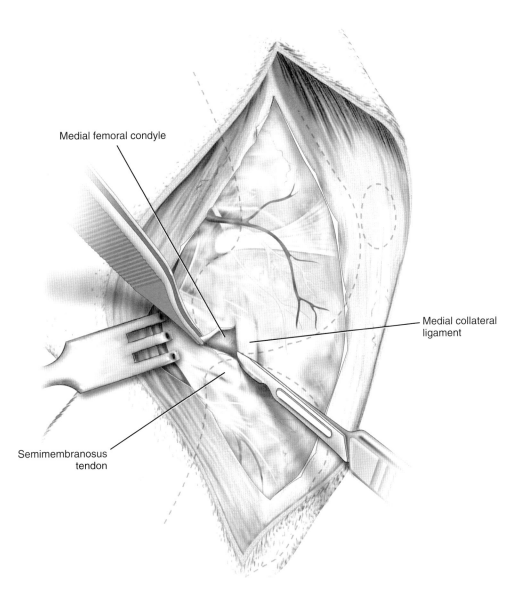

Medial femoral condyle

Medial collateral ligament

Semimembranosus tendon

D

Approach to the Medial Collateral Ligament and Caudomedial Part of the Stifle Joint *continued*

E. Additional exposure of the caudal horn of the medial meniscus is gained by extending the arthrotomy incision proximally toward the medial femorofabellar joint. Distally the arthrotomy is extended toward the tibial plateau. This will involve transection of the semimembranosus tendon, which has its insertion on the tibia, under the medial collateral ligament. The joint capsule can be sharply dissected from the medial meniscus caudally, as well as under the medial collateral ligament.

PLATE 87

Approach to the Medial Collateral Ligament and Caudomedial Part of the Stifle Joint *continued*

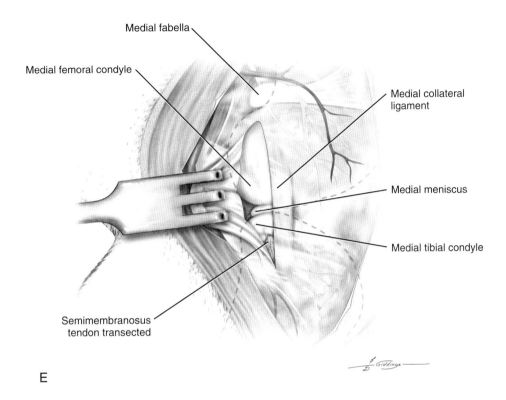

Medial fabella

Medial femoral condyle

Medial collateral ligament

Medial meniscus

Medial tibial condyle

Semimembranosus tendon transected

E

Approach to the Medial Collateral Ligament and Caudomedial Part of the Stifle Joint *continued*

F. The joint capsule can also be incised on the cranial side of the collateral ligament to expose the cranial pole of the medial meniscus.

ADDITIONAL EXPOSURE

This approach can be combined with the approach to proximal tibia (see Plate 89) when performing a tibial plateau rotational osteotomy for cranial cruciate rupture.

For total exposure of the stifle joint, this approach is usually combined with the standard medial approach to the stifle (see Plate 82). The transverse joint capsular incision is an extension of the incision shown in Plate 82C.

CLOSURE

Interrupted sutures are placed in the joint capsule and continuous interrupted sutures are used to close the deep fascial incision. Subcutaneous tissues and skin are closed routinely.

PLATE 87

Approach to the Medial Collateral Ligament and Caudomedial Part of the Stifle Joint *continued*

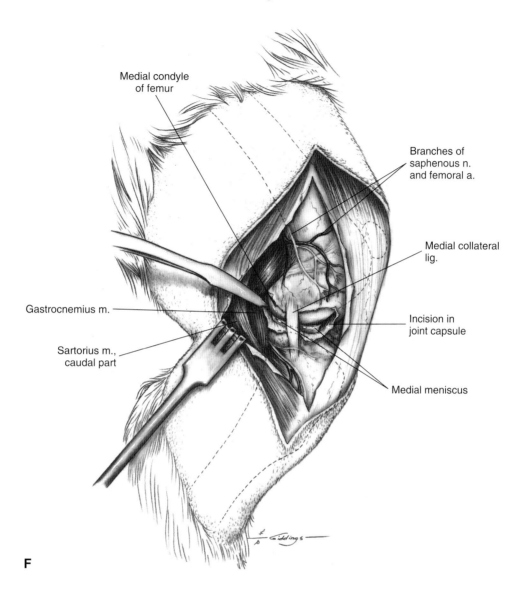

Medial condyle of femur

Branches of saphenous n. and femoral a.

Medial collateral lig.

Gastrocnemius m.

Incision in joint capsule

Sartorius m., caudal part

Medial meniscus

F

Approach to the Stifle Joint by Osteotomy of the Origin of the Medial Collateral Ligament

Based on a Procedure of Daly and Tarvin[9]

INDICATIONS

1. Reduction of fractures of the caudal part of the medial femoral condyle.
2. Exploration of the caudomedial part of the stifle joint.
3. Avulsion of the insertion of the caudal cruciate ligament.

ALTERNATIVE APPROACH

The caudomedial approach (see Plate 87), which spares the medial collateral ligament, provides more limited exposure but is adequate for most surgery of the medial meniscus.

PATIENT POSITIONING

Dorsal recumbency with the affected limb suspended for draping.

DESCRIPTION OF THE PROCEDURE

This procedure is a continuation of the Approach to the Medial Collateral Ligament and Caudomedial Part of the Stifle Joint (see Plate 87).

A. After completely freeing the ligament from the joint capsule, an osteotome is used to outline a block of bone that contains the entire origin of the medial collateral ligament.

B. The block of bone is freed from the underlying condyle. Be sure to take an adequate amount of bone because a block of bone that is too small is difficult to fix securely in place. Note the wedge shape of the bone block; this will have some inherent stability when replaced. Abduction and external rotation of the tibia will expose the interior of the joint.

CLOSURE

The bone block origin of the ligament is reattached to the femur by means of a lag screw (see Figure 24A). This can be simplified by predrilling before cutting the bone block. Interrupted sutures are placed in the joint capsule. The fascial incision is closed with either continuous or interrupted sutures. Closure of the subcutaneous tissues and skin is routine.

PLATE 88

Approach to the Stifle Joint by Osteotomy of the Origin of the Medial Collateral Ligament

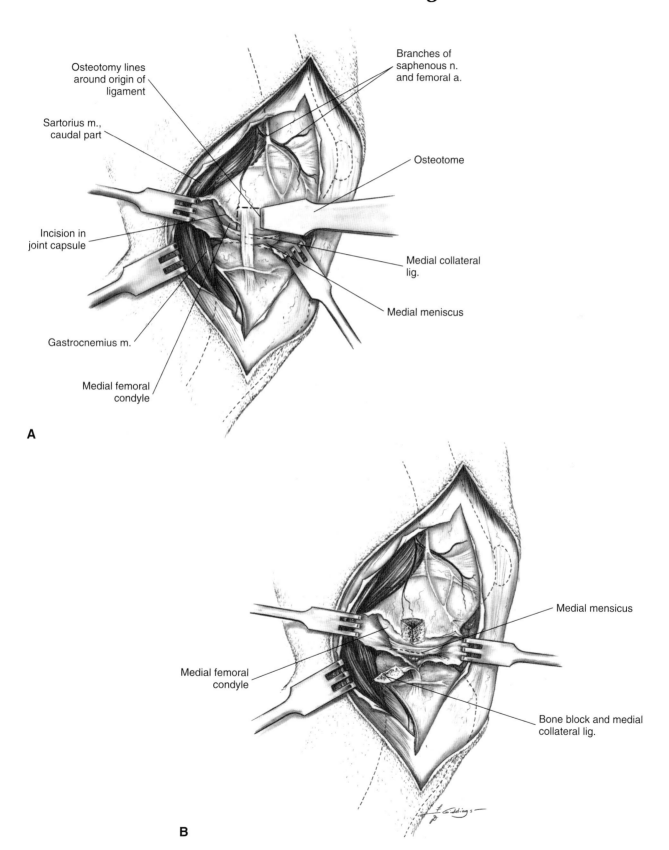

A

B

Approach to the Proximal Tibia Through a Medial Incision

Based on a Procedure of Slocum and Devine[44]

INDICATIONS

1. Open reduction and internal fixation of fractures of the proximal tibia.
2. Corrective osteotomy of proximal tibial deformity.
3. Rotational osteotomy of the tibial plateau for cranial cruciate ligament rupture.
4. Tibial tuberosity osteotomy and lateral transposition (steps F and G only).

PATIENT POSITIONING

Dorsal recumbency with the affected hindlimb suspended for draping.

DESCRIPTION OF THE PROCEDURE

A. The skin incision is made on the medial side of the proximal tibia. Commencing at the level of the patella, the incision extends distally over the medial collateral ligament to one third of the way down the tibial shaft. Take care to avoid incising the medial saphenous vein distally.
B. Incise the subcutaneous tissue and identify the cranial margin of the caudal belly of the sartorius muscle. Cut along the cranial edge of the sartorius with a scalpel and, continuing distally, transect the tendons of insertion of the sartorius, gracilis, and semitendinosus muscles on the tibia.
C. Undermine the sartorius muscle from the underlying joint capsule and medial collateral ligament. Incise and elevate the periosteum caudal and cranial to the medial collateral ligament to expose the medial cortex. Caudal to the medial collateral ligament, take care to avoid transecting the tendon of the semimembranosus muscle or branches of the medial genicular artery.
D. Incise the medial border of the insertion of the popliteus muscle and, working in a proximal-to-distal direction, elevate the origin of the popliteus muscle from the bone.

PLATE 89
Approach to the Proximal Tibia Through a Medial Incision

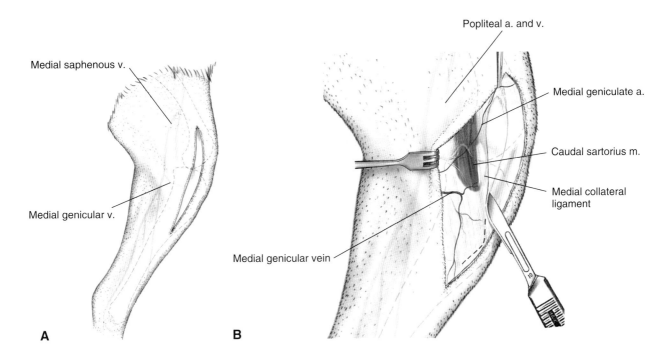

Medial saphenous v.

Medial genicular v.

A

Popliteal a. and v.

Medial geniculate a.

Caudal sartorius m.

Medial collateral ligament

Medial genicular vein

B

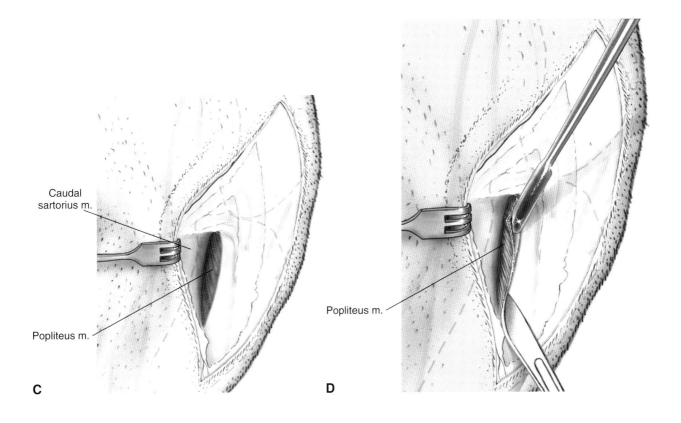

Caudal sartorius m.

Popliteus m.

C

Popliteus m.

D

Approach to the Proximal Tibia Through a Medial Incision *continued*

E. For complete exposure of bone caudally, elevate the flexor digitorum longus, caudal tibial, and flexor hallucis longus muscles from the caudal cortex of the tibia. Stay close to the bone to avoid severing the popliteal artery.

F. Incise along the cranial border of the cranial tibialis muscle, just lateral to the tibial tuberosity.

G. The cranial tibialis muscle is elevated from the lateral cortex of the tibia. The extent of muscle elevation necessary depends on the intended surgical procedure. Care is taken that the tendon of the long digital extensor muscle is not damaged.

ADDITIONAL EXPOSURE

Proximally this approach can be extended for inspection of the medial meniscus by combining with a caudomedial arthrotomy (see Plate 87C) or craniomedial arthrotomy (see Plate 82C).

CLOSURE

The cranial border of the sartorius muscle is sutured to the adjacent fascia with a continuous-pattern suture. The popliteus and cranial tibialis muscles are not sutured. These will reattach to the tibia by fibrosis. Subcutaneous tissues and skin are closed routinely.

PRECAUTIONS

The popliteal artery crosses the flexor surface of the stifle joint between the two heads of the gastrocnemius muscles. It deviates laterally under the popliteus muscle and on leaving it perforates the origin of the flexor hallucis longus muscle to reach the interosseous space.

PLATE 89

Approach to the Proximal Tibia Through a Medial Incision *continued*

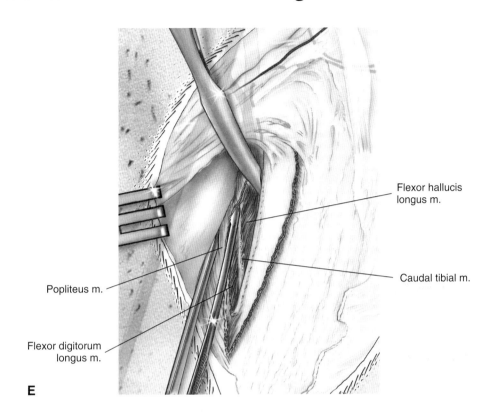

Flexor hallucis
longus m.

Caudal tibial m.

Popliteus m.

Flexor digitorum
longus m.

E

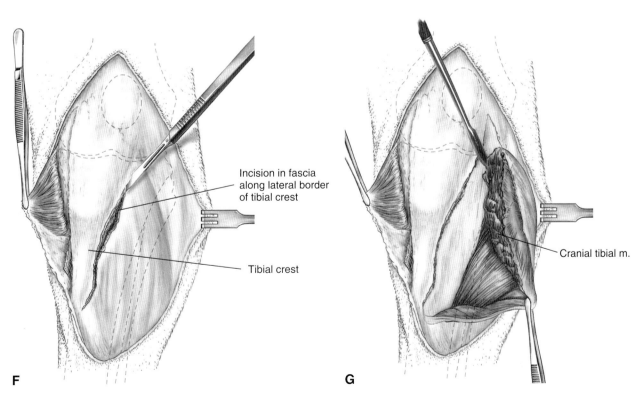

Incision in fascia
along lateral border
of tibial crest

Tibial crest

Cranial tibial m.

F

G

Approach to the Shaft of the Tibia

Based on Procedures of Brinker[4] and Wilson[52]

INDICATION

Open reduction of fractures of the shaft of the tibia.

PATIENT POSITIONING

Dorsal recumbency with the affected hindlimb suspended for draping.

DESCRIPTION OF THE PROCEDURE

A. The skin incision can be varied to suit the situation. For maximal exposure of both the medial and lateral cortices and for bone plate application, the curved incision shown provides the best approach. A straight medial incision can be used for intramedullary pinning but would result in the plate being directly under the skin incision with only scanty subcuticular tissue to cover it if used in plating procedures. A curved, laterally based incision can be used if a plate is to be applied laterally.

The medially based incision shown here starts proximally over the medial tibial condyle and curves cranially to the midline of the tibia at midshaft. It then curves caudally to end near the medial malleolus. The subcutis is incised on the same line. Although not essential, an effort is made to preserve the saphenous vessels and nerve crossing the tibia.

B. The bone is exposed by incision of the crural fascia over the medial shaft of the bone. Elevating the fascia exposes the muscles.

C. The cranial tibial and medial digital flexor muscles can be retracted by incising fascia along their borders to free them from the bone.

PLATE 90
Approach to the Shaft of the Tibia

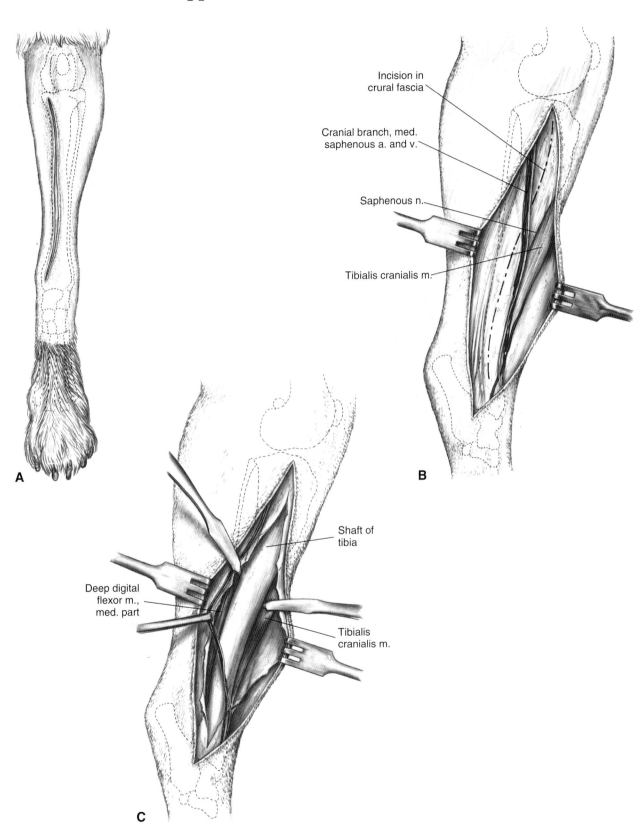

Incision in
crural fascia

Cranial branch, med.
saphenous a. and v.

Saphenous n.

Tibialis cranialis m.

Shaft of
tibia

Deep digital
flexor m.,
med. part

Tibialis
cranialis m.

A

B

C

Approach to the Shaft of the Tibia *continued*

D. To expose the lateral cortex, the crural fascia is incised along the cranial border of the cranial tibial muscle, starting at the tibial tuberosity and extending distally to the tendinous portion of the muscle.
E. The cranial tibial and long digital extensor muscles are retracted caudolaterally to expose the tibial shaft. The cranial tibial artery courses between the tibia and fibula and can be damaged by the tips of the Hohmann retractor if they are placed over the artery. Exposure of the distal lateral region of the tibia can be gained by incising fascia lateral to the tendons of the cranial tibial and long digital extensor muscles. Cranial retraction of these tendons provides visualization of the tibia.

ADDITIONAL EXPOSURE

Proximally this approach can be extended to expose the medial side of the proximal tibia as shown in Plate 89.

CLOSURE

The deep crural fascia must be closed securely. Continuous sutures are used here and in the subcutaneous tissues. Skin and subcutis are closed routinely.

PLATE 90

Approach to the Shaft of the Tibia *continued*

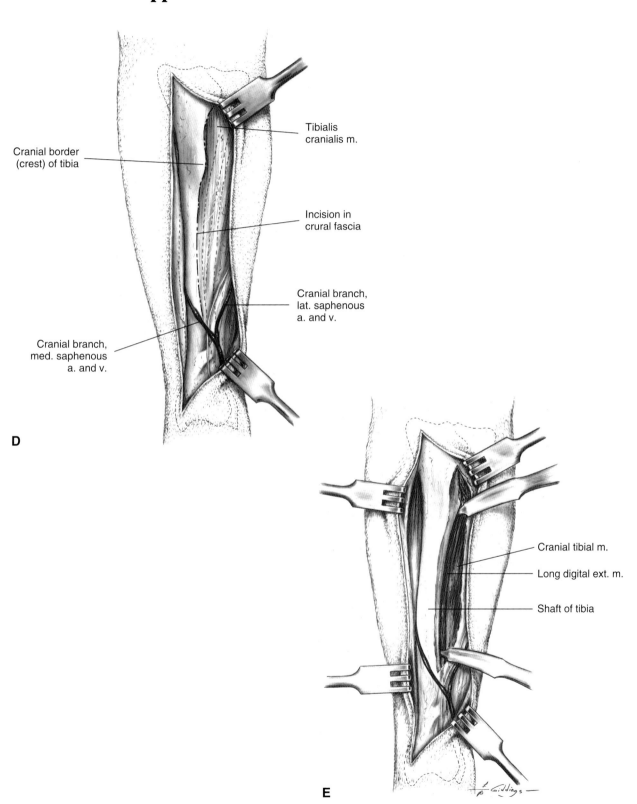

Tibialis
cranialis m.

Cranial border
(crest) of tibia

Incision in
crural fascia

Cranial branch,
lat. saphenous
a. and v.

Cranial branch,
med. saphenous
a. and v.

D

Cranial tibial m.

Long digital ext. m.

Shaft of tibia

E

Minimally Invasive Approach to the Shaft of the Tibia

INDICATION

Minimally invasive plate osteosynthesis or interlocking nailing of fractures involving the tibial shaft.

PATIENT POSITIONING

Dorsal recumbency with the affected hindlimb suspended for draping.

DESCRIPTION OF THE PROCEDURE

The magnitude of exposure has been intentionally enlarged in the following descriptive illustrations, to highlight the relevant features of the surgical anatomy. Once familiar with the anatomy, the field of dissection and exposure can be reduced by at least 50% to obtain a true minimally invasive approach to the tibia.

A. Proximal and distal incisions that are 2 to 4 cm in length are made on the medial side of the tibia.

B. Proximally the subcutaneous tissues are incised in the same line as the skin incision. The caudal portion the sartorius muscle is identified, and an incision is made in the fascia along the cranial border of this muscle. This incision is continued distally to transect the tendons of the sartorius, gracilis, and semitendinosus muscles.

PLATE 91
Minimally Invasive Approach to the Shaft of the Tibia

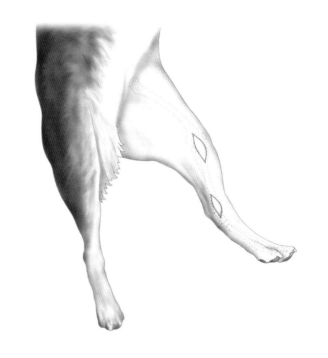

A

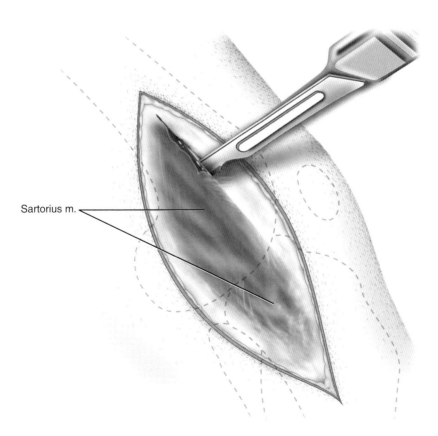

Sartorius m.

B

Minimally Invasive Approach to the Shaft of the Tibia *continued*

C. Caudal retraction of the caudal portion of the sartorius muscle allows identification of the patellar tendon, medial collateral ligament, and popliteus muscle. These structures serve as important landmarks for subsequent placement of a bone plate or intramedullary device.

PLATE 91

Minimally Invasive Approach to the Shaft of the Tibia *continued*

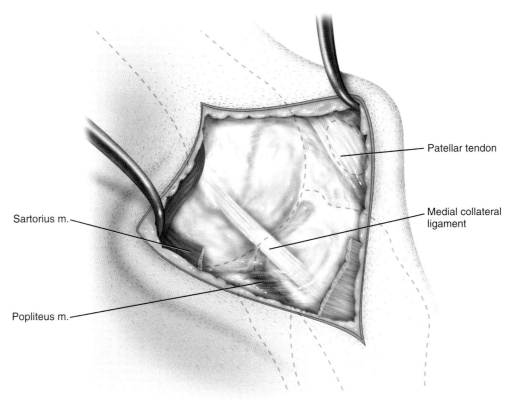

Patellar tendon

Medial collateral ligament

Sartorius m.

Popliteus m.

C

Minimally Invasive Approach to the Shaft of the Tibia *continued*

D. After incision of the skin and subcutaneous tissues on the medial side of the tibia, just proximal to the medial malleolus, a soft-tissue retractor as illustrated here is used to create an epiperiosteal tunnel on the medial side of the tibia. The tunnel connecting the proximal and distal incisions should pass deep to the medial saphenous artery and vein.

CLOSURE

Closure consists of suturing of the cranial margin of the sartorius muscle to adjacent fascia in a continuous pattern, followed by closure of the subcutaneous fat and fascia in a second layer. The distal incision is closed with a continuous suture in the subcutaneous tissues, followed by the skin closure.

PLATE 91
Minimally Invasive Approach to the Shaft of the Tibia *continued*

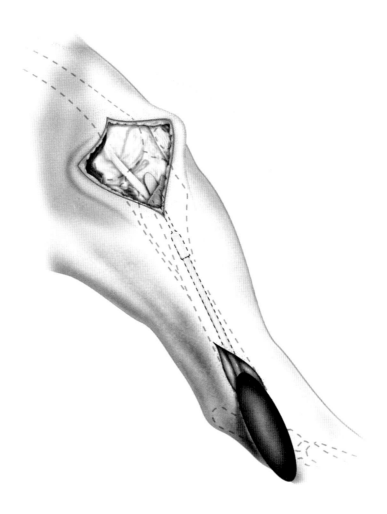

D

Approach to the Lateral Malleolus and Talocrural Joint

INDICATIONS

1. Open reduction of fractures of the lateral malleolus of the fibula.
2. Open reduction of supramalleolar fractures of the tibia.
3. Open reduction of luxation of the talocrural joint.
4. Repair of lateral collateral ligaments.
5. Osteochondroplasty for osteochondritis dissecans of the lateral trochlear ridge.

PATIENT POSITIONING

Lateral recumbency with the affected limb suspended for draping.

DESCRIPTION OF THE PROCEDURE

A. A curved skin incision is centered over the lateral surface of the talocrural joint. It commences proximally at the level of the lateral saphenous vein and continues distally to the level of the tarsometatarsal joint.
B. The subcutaneous and crural fascia is incised on the same line as the skin and is retracted with the skin. The extensor retinaculum overlying the lateral malleolus is incised parallel to the dorsal edge of the peroneus longus tendon, taking care to avoid cutting this small tendon. The tendon can now be retracted in any direction.
C. The lateral trochlear ridge of the talus is exposed by extending the joint and incising the joint capsule from the tibia distally, dorsal and parallel to the collateral ligament. This incision can be extended beyond what is shown here. The plantar aspect of the lateral talar ridge can be exposed by an incision in the joint capsule after retracting the tendons of the peroneus brevis and lateral digital extensor muscles and flexing the joint. A portion of the lateral extensor retinaculum must be elevated to make this incision, and care must be taken to preserve as much as possible of the short, deep part of the lateral collateral ligament.

CLOSURE

The extensor retinaculum and joint capsule are closed with interrupted sutures. The crural and subcutaneous fascia is closed with continuous-pattern sutures, followed by routine skin closure.

PLATE 92

Approach to the Lateral Malleolus and Talocrural Joint

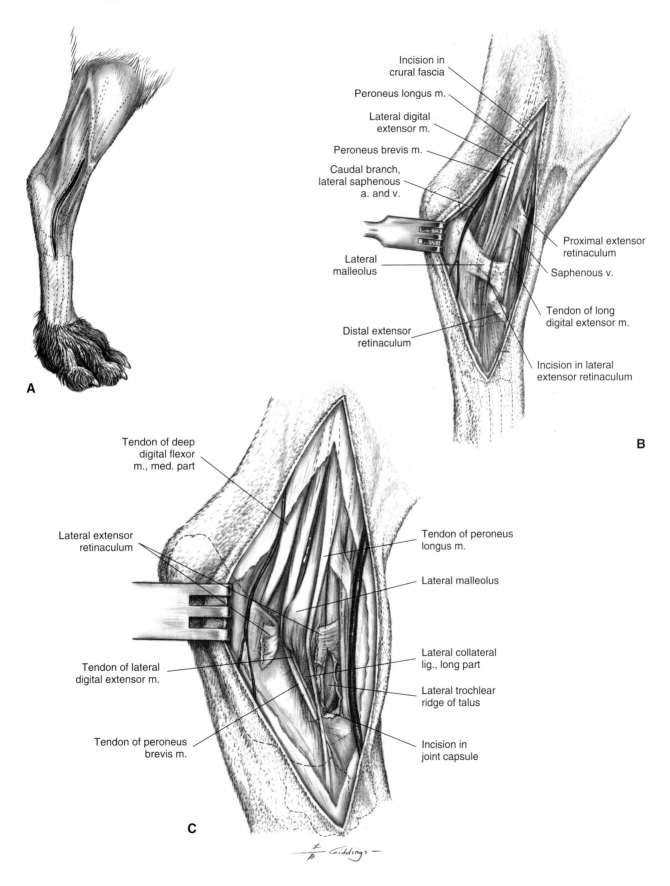

B

Incision in
crural fascia

Peroneus longus m.

Lateral digital
extensor m.

Peroneus brevis m.

Caudal branch,
lateral saphenous
a. and v.

Lateral
malleolus

Distal extensor
retinaculum

Proximal extensor
retinaculum

Saphenous v.

Tendon of long
digital extensor m.

Incision in lateral
extensor retinaculum

A

C

Tendon of deep
digital flexor
m., med. part

Lateral extensor
retinaculum

Tendon of lateral
digital extensor m.

Tendon of peroneus
brevis m.

Tendon of peroneus
longus m.

Lateral malleolus

Lateral collateral
lig., long part

Lateral trochlear
ridge of talus

Incision in
joint capsule

Giddings

Approach to the Medial Malleolus and Talocrural Joint

INDICATIONS

1. Open reduction of fractures of the medial malleolus of the tibia.
2. Open reduction of supramalleolar fractures of the tibia.
3. Open reduction of luxation of the talocrural joint.
4. Repair of medial collateral ligaments.
5. Osteochondroplasty for osteochondritis dissecans of the medial ridge of the talus.

PATIENT POSITIONING

Dorsal recumbency with the affected limb suspended for draping, or lateral recumbency with the affected hindlimb down.

DESCRIPTION OF THE PROCEDURE

A. A curved skin incision is centered over the medial surface of the talocrural joint. It commences proximally at the distal fourth of the tibia and continues distally to the level of the tarsometatarsal joint.
B. The subcutaneous and crural fasciae are incised on the same line as the skin and retracted with the skin. The medial ridge of the talus is exposed by a joint capsule incision that starts proximally on the tibia, continues parallel to the collateral ligament, and ends distally on the neck of the talus.
C. Retraction of the joint capsule and extension of the joint expose the dorsal aspect of the medial trochlear ridge of the talus. The plantar aspect of the ridge is accessed by a joint capsule incision plantar to the collateral ligament. The tendons of the tibialis caudalis and deep digital flexor muscles must be elevated and protected as this incision is made; this requires incising the overlying medial retinacular tissues parallel to the tendons. Varying degrees of flexion, extension, and rotation of the tarsus are required to visualize the talus.

PLATE 93

Approach to the Medial Malleolus and Talocrural Joint

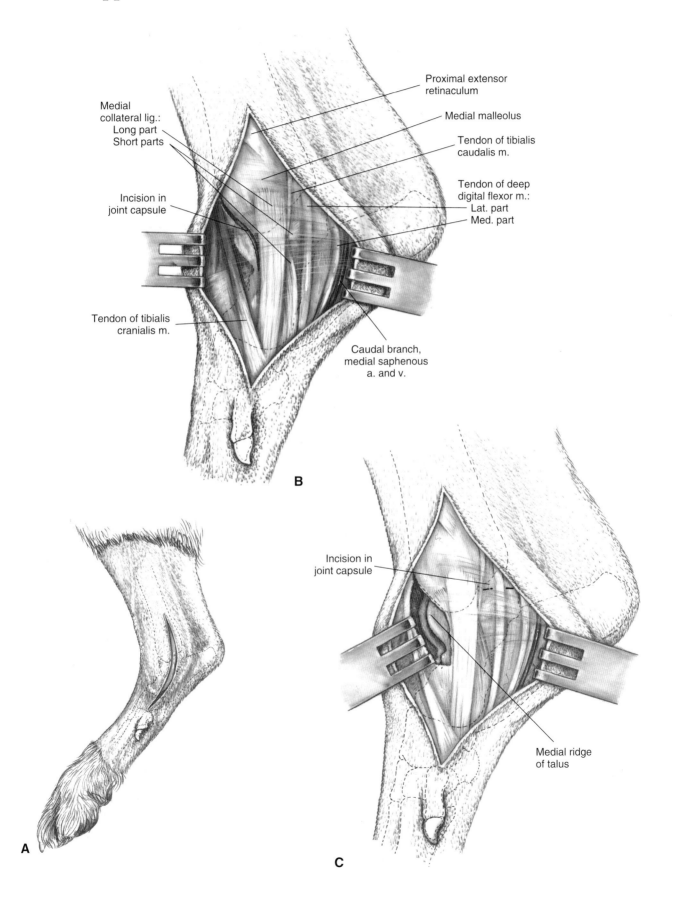

Proximal extensor retinaculum

Medial collateral lig.:
Long part
Short parts

Medial malleolus

Tendon of tibialis caudalis m.

Incision in joint capsule

Tendon of deep digital flexor m.:
Lat. part
Med. part

Tendon of tibialis cranialis m.

Caudal branch, medial saphenous a. and v.

B

Incision in joint capsule

Medial ridge of talus

A

C

Approach to the Medial Malleolus and Talocrural Joint *continued*

ADDITIONAL EXPOSURE

D. **Based on a Procedure of Dew and Martin.**[12] For additional exposure of the talocrural joint and caudal aspect of the distal end of the tibia, the skin incision is extended proximally along the caudomedial border of the tibia. The retinaculum overlying the tendon of the flexor hallucis longus (the lateral part of the tendon of the deep digital flexor) is incised longitudinally.
E. The flexor hallucis longus tendon can now be retracted caudally to improve visualization of the proximal articular surface of the talus. Extension of the tarsus while retracting the tendon provides exposure of the sustentaculum tali.

CLOSURE

The extensor joint capsule incisions are closed with interrupted sutures. The crural and subcutaneous fasciae are closed with continuous-pattern sutures, followed by routine skin closure.

PLATE 93

Approach to the Medial Malleolus and Talocrural Joint *continued*

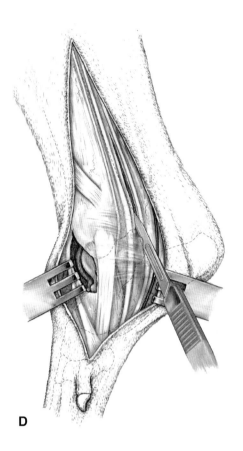

D

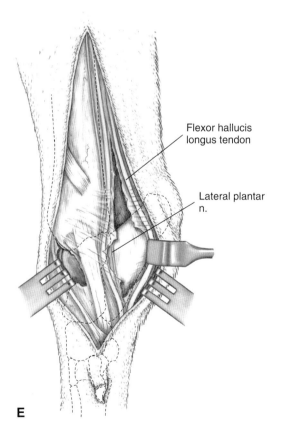

Flexor hallucis
longus tendon

Lateral plantar
n.

E

Approach to the Tarsocrural Joint by Osteotomy of the Medial Malleolus

Based on a Procedure of Sinibaldi[42]

INDICATION

Open reduction of fractures of the trochlea of the talus (see Comment).

ALTERNATIVE APPROACH

The medial (see Plate 93) and lateral (see Plate 92) approaches provide more limited, although adequate, exposure for osteochondroplasty for osteochondritis dissecans lesions of the talus.

PATIENT POSITIONING

Dorsal recumbency with the affected hindlimb suspended for draping.

DESCRIPTION OF THE PROCEDURE

This procedure is a continuation of Approach to the Medial Malleolus and Talocrural Joint (see Plate 93).

A, B. The medial collateral ligament is isolated from the joint capsule by incisions along the dorsal and plantar aspects of the ligament. These incisions should completely penetrate the joint capsule in order to allow sufficient visualization of the interior of the joint to judge the angle of the osteotomy, shown in Plate 94B.

PLATE 94

Approach to the Tarsocrural Joint by Osteotomy of the Medial Malleolus

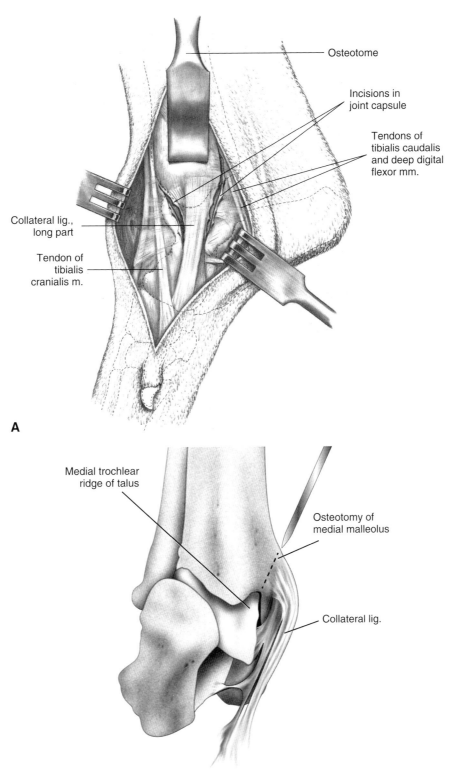

Osteotome

Incisions in joint capsule

Tendons of tibialis caudalis and deep digital flexor mm.

Collateral lig., long part

Tendon of tibialis cranialis m.

A

Medial trochlear ridge of talus

Osteotomy of medial malleolus

Collateral lig.

B

Approach to the Tarsocrural Joint by Osteotomy
of the Medial Malleolus *continued*

C. The medial malleolus is removed with an osteotome, placed as shown in Plate 94B. The osteotomy angle should encompass enough of the malleolus to include most of the origin of the collateral ligament but must not be so deep as to intrude on the weight-bearing articular surface of the tibial cochlea. Care also must be taken to avoid cutting into the medial ridge of the talus. It may be necessary to incise part of the proximal extensor retinaculum to obtain the proper angle of the osteotome. Retraction of the malleolus and attached ligaments and pronation of the tarsus allow visualization of the entire surface of the trochlea of the talus.

CLOSURE

The malleolus is reattached with pins and tension band wire (see Figure 23B) or a lag screw (see Figure 24A). Interrupted sutures are used in the joint capsule, and a continuous pattern is used in the crural and subcutaneous fascia.

COMMENT

Experience indicates that this approach is somewhat traumatic to the joint and should be reserved for trochlear fracture repair, where maximal exposure is necessary.

PLATE 94

Approach to the Tarsocrural Joint by Osteotomy of the Medial Malleolus *continued*

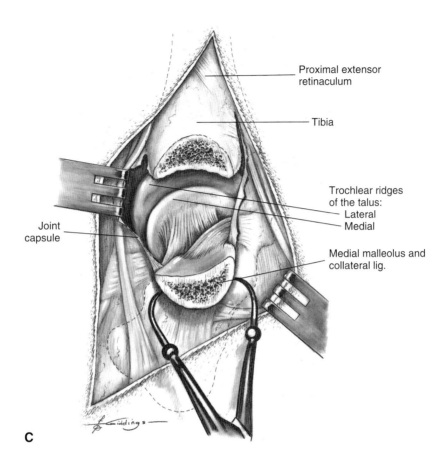

Proximal extensor retinaculum

Tibia

Trochlear ridges of the talus:
Lateral
Medial

Medial malleolus and collateral lig.

Joint capsule

C

Approach to the Calcaneus

INDICATIONS

1. Open reduction of fractures of the body and tuber calcanei of the calcaneus.
2. Avulsion of the gastrocnemius tendon from the tuber calcanei.

PATIENT POSITIONING

Lateral recumbency with the affected hindlimb suspended for draping.

DESCRIPTION OF THE PROCEDURE

A. The skin incision begins on the lateral side of the common calcanean tendon just proximal to the tuber calcanei. As it curves distally, it remains lateral to the plantar midline of the calcaneus and ends at the level of the fourth tarsal bone.
B. The skin and thin subcutaneous fascia are reflected to expose the deep fascia. The lateral border of the tendon of the superficial digital flexor muscle is located by palpation or visualization through the fascia. An incision is made parallel to the lateral border of the tendon, through deep fascia and the lateral retinacular attachment of the tendon to the calcaneus, and is continued proximally to allow separation of the tendon from the gastrocnemius tendon.
C. Medial retraction of the tendon of the superficial digital flexor muscle completes the exposure.

ADDITIONAL EXPOSURE

For the open reduction of fractures and arthrodeses, this approach can be extended for additional exposure of the plantar (see Plate 96) and distal (see Plate 98) regions of the tarsus.

CLOSURE

Interrupted, nonabsorbable sutures are used to approximate the deep fascial and retinacular incision. This part of the closure must be very secure to prevent the tendon from slipping medially over the calcaneus. Subcutis and skin are closed routinely.

PRECAUTIONS

During exposure of the lateral surface of the calcaneus, take care not to disrupt the short part of the lateral collateral ligament. This is very important in the cat because the long part of the lateral collateral ligament is absent in the cat.

PLATE 95
Approach to the Calcaneus

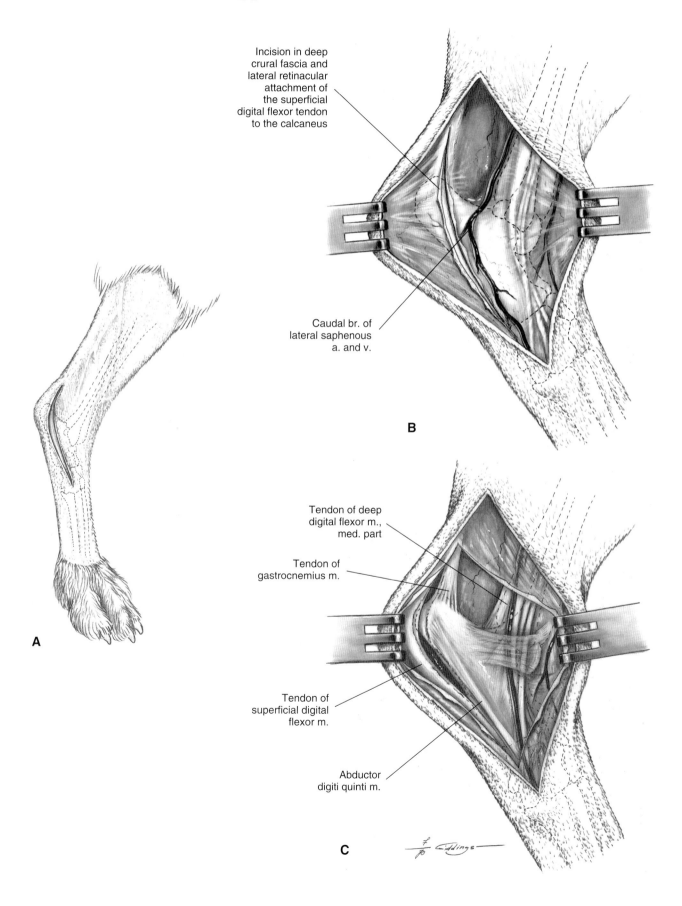

Incision in deep crural fascia and lateral retinacular attachment of the superficial digital flexor tendon to the calcaneus

Caudal br. of lateral saphenous a. and v.

B

Tendon of deep digital flexor m., med. part

Tendon of gastrocnemius m.

Tendon of superficial digital flexor m.

Abductor digiti quinti m.

A

C

Approach to the Calcaneus and Plantar Aspects of the Tarsal Bones

INDICATION

Arthrodesis of the calcaneoquartile or tarsometatarsal joints.

PATIENT POSITIONING

Lateral recumbency with the affected hindlimb suspended for draping.

DESCRIPTION OF THE PROCEDURE

This approach is based on the Approach to the Calcaneus (see Plate 95).
A. Beginning on the lateral side of the common calcanean tendon, the skin incision curves ventrally along the calcaneus and then turns medially to cross the ventral midline at the level of the proximal metatarsal bones.
B. Elevation of the superficial digital flexor tendon is depicted in Plate 95B and C. The tendon is elevated distally to just beyond its bifurcation. A small branch of the plantar nerve will be found medial to the plantar midline in the fascia covering the deep digital flexor tendon. Incising this fascia lateral to the nerve will expose the deep digital flexor tendon.
C. The tendon of the deep digital flexor is elevated and retracted medially with the superficial tendon. The plantar ligament structure and tarsal bones come into view, but individual tarsal bones are difficult to discern visually. Probing with a needle will allow individual joint spaces to be located and incised.

CLOSURE

Interrupted, nonabsorbable sutures are used to approximate the deep fascial and retinacular incisions and bring both digital flexor tendons back to their normal positions.

PLATE 96

Approach to the Calcaneus and Plantar Aspects of the Tarsal Bones

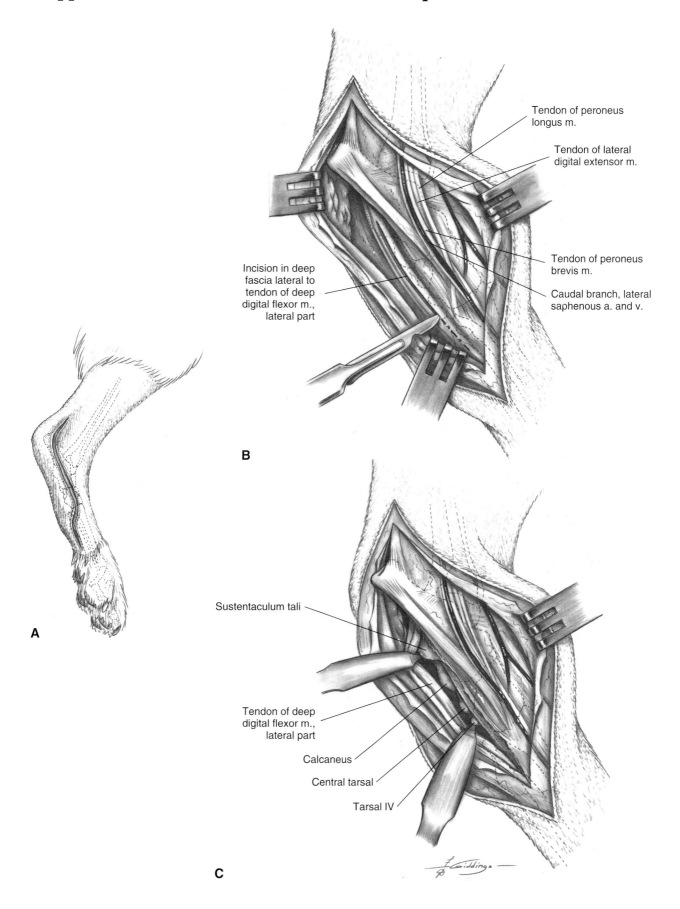

Tendon of peroneus longus m.

Tendon of lateral digital extensor m.

Tendon of peroneus brevis m.

Caudal branch, lateral saphenous a. and v.

Incision in deep fascia lateral to tendon of deep digital flexor m., lateral part

B

A

Sustentaculum tali

Tendon of deep digital flexor m., lateral part

Calcaneus

Central tarsal

Tarsal IV

C

Approach to the Lateral Bones of the Tarsus

INDICATIONS

1. Open reduction of fractures or luxations of the base of the calcaneus or fourth tarsal bones.
2. Arthrodesis of the calcaneoquartile joint or lateral part of the tarsometatarsal joint.
3. Repair of injuries of the lateral ligaments of the calcaneoquartile joint or lateral part of the tarsometatarsal joint.

PATIENT POSITIONING

Lateral recumbency with the affected hindlimb suspended for draping.

DESCRIPTION OF THE PROCEDURE

A. A lateral incision is made from midcalcaneus to the base of the fifth metatarsal bone.
B. The plantar metatarsal vessels can be seen in the deep fascia and are positioned either superficial or plantar to the collateral ligaments of the tarsocrural joint. The deep fascia is incised dorsal to these vessels.
C. Retraction and elevation of the fascia reveal the underlying bones, tendons, and ligaments.

ADDITIONAL EXPOSURE

For the open reduction of fractures and arthrodeses, this approach can be extended proximally for additional exposure of the lateral (see Plate 95) and plantar (see Plate 96) aspects of the calcaneus.

CLOSURE

Deep fascia is closed with interrupted sutures, followed by closure of the skin. There is usually insufficient subcutaneous tissue to close as a separate layer. A padded bandage should be used for several days to prevent serum accumulation in the subcutis.

PLATE 97

Approach to the Lateral Bones of the Tarsus

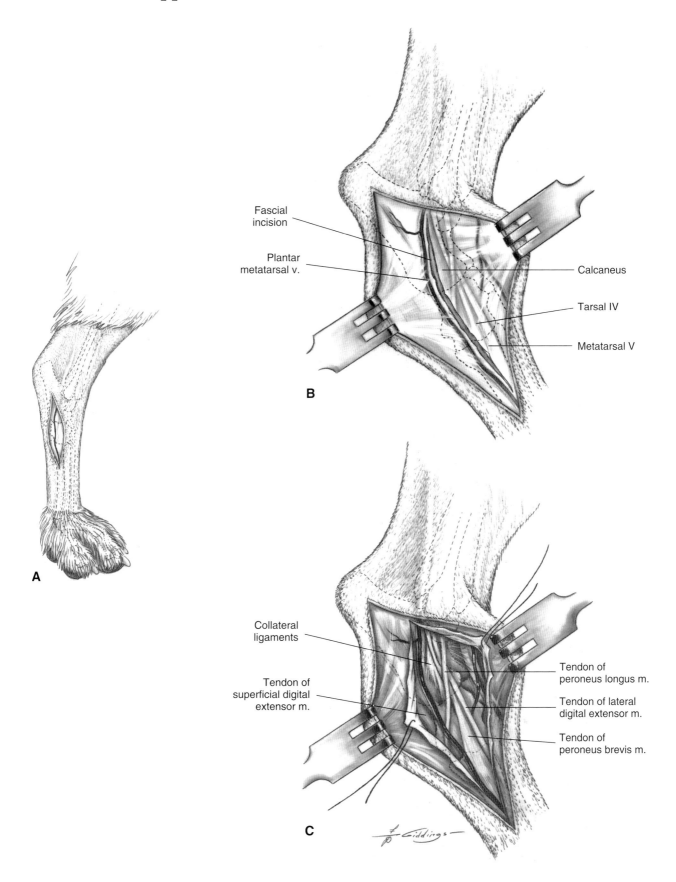

B

Fascial incision

Plantar metatarsal v.

Calcaneus

Tarsal IV

Metatarsal V

A

C

Collateral ligaments

Tendon of superficial digital extensor m.

Tendon of peroneus longus m.

Tendon of lateral digital extensor m.

Tendon of peroneus brevis m.

Approach to the Medial Bones of the Tarsus

INDICATIONS

Open reduction of fractures or luxations of the neck and head of the talus, the central tarsal, or the second and third tarsal bones.

PATIENT POSITIONING

Dorsal recumbency with the affected hindlimb suspended for draping.

DESCRIPTION OF THE PROCEDURE

A. A longitudinal incision is made starting near the medial malleolus and extending to the base of metatarsal II. The length of the incision can be adjusted to fit the specific area of interest.
B. The subcutaneous fascia and skin are undermined and retracted. The deep fascia is incised between the tendon of the cranial tibial muscle and the branching metatarsal vessel from the saphenous vein. The metatarsal vein crossing the tendon is ligated.
C. The fascia lying on the surface of the tarsal bones is incised after retracting the cranial tibial tendon.
D. Elevation of the fascia reveals the tarsal bones and ligaments. A small Hohmann retractor can be placed under the fascia to expose the dorsal surface of the central tarsal. By keeping the elevation close to the bone, structures such as the dorsal pedal artery can be avoided.

CLOSURE

The deep fascia is joined by one row of interrupted sutures, followed by the skin. The subcutaneous tissues are usually too scant to require a separate layer. A padded bandage is used postoperatively for 5 to 7 days to prevent serum accumulation in the subcutis.

PLATE 98

Approach to the Medial Bones of the Tarsus

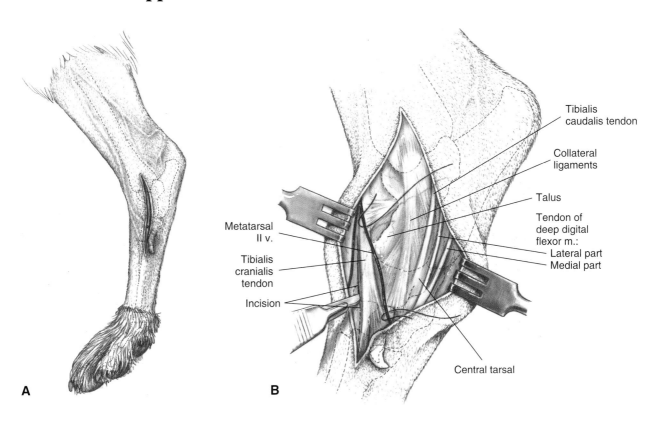

Tibialis caudalis tendon

Collateral ligaments

Talus

Tendon of deep digital flexor m.:
Lateral part
Medial part

Metatarsal II v.

Tibialis cranialis tendon

Incision

Central tarsal

A

B

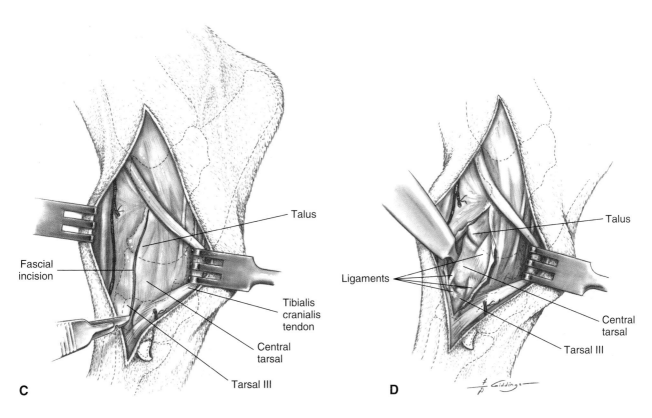

Talus

Fascial incision

Tibialis cranialis tendon

Central tarsal

Tarsal III

Talus

Ligaments

Central tarsal

Tarsal III

C

D

Approaches to the Metatarsal Bones

INDICATION

Open reduction of fractures.

DESCRIPTION OF THE PROCEDURE

A. The anatomy shown here is considerably simplified compared with that in the live animal. Only important structures are shown; other elements such as small tendons and blood vessels have been omitted. In an average-sized dog, these vestigial structures are so small that their identification and preservation are not practical during surgery.

B. The incisional technique varies according to the bone or bones to be exposed. A single bone is approached by an incision directly over the bone and two adjoining bones by an incision between them. If more than two bones need to be exposed, two parallel longitudinal incisions (Plate 60B) or a single curved incision (Plate 99B) can be used. The curved incision commences at the proximal end of metatarsal V, runs medially to the midshaft of metatarsal II, and then curves laterally again to end over the distal end of metatarsal V. The crescent-shaped skin flap can be elevated and retracted to expose a large part of all four bones. Metatarsals II and V can be approached directly, without elevation of any important tendons or vessels. The deep fascia is incised and elevated to allow visualization of these bones. Exposure of metatarsal bones III and IV requires the undermining and retraction of the tendon of the long digital extensor muscle and the accompanying blood vessels.

CLOSURE

Deep fascia is closed to ensure that tendons and vessels are securely held in their proper positions.

COMMENTS

A deep layer of small metatarsal blood vessels is found on and between the bones. These vessels are too small to avoid in most animals, and the resulting hemorrhage must be controlled by tamponade. Apply a snug bandage for 72 hours postoperatively to control oozing hemorrhage at the operative site.

PLATE 99
Approaches to the Metatarsal Bones

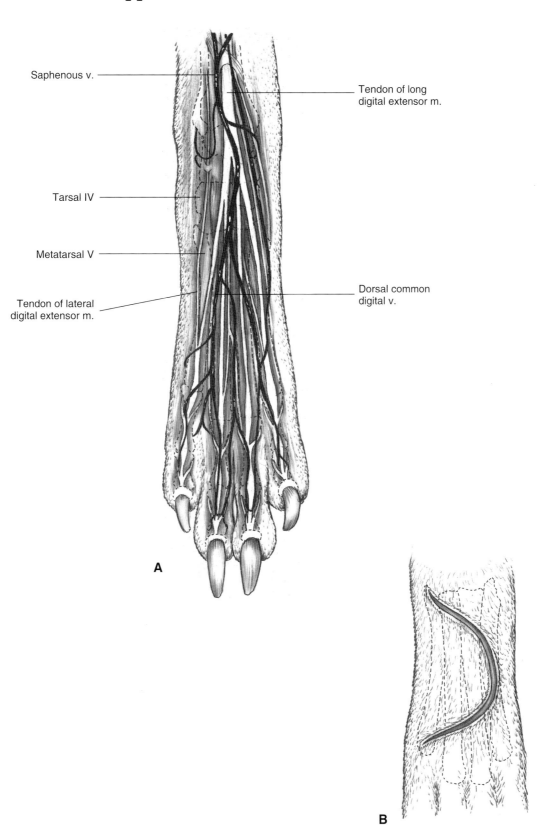

Saphenous v.

Tendon of long
digital extensor m.

Tarsal IV

Metatarsal V

Dorsal common
digital v.

Tendon of lateral
digital extensor m.

A

B

Approach to the Proximal Sesamoid Bones

This procedure is identical to Approach to the Proximal Sesamoid Bones illustrated in Plate 61 of Section 5, The Forelimb.

Approaches to the Phalanges and Interphalangeal Joints

This procedure is identical to the procedure illustrated in Plate 62 of Section 5, The Forelimb.

References

1. Alexander JE: Open reduction and fixation of a shoulder luxation, *Small Anim Clin* 2:379, 1962.
2. Alexander JE, Archibald J, Cawley AJ: Pelvic fractures and their reduction in small animals, *Mod Vet Pract* 43:41, 1962.
3. Archibald J, Brown NM, Nasti E, Medway WM: Open reduction for correction of coxofemoral dislocation, *Vet Med* 48:273, 1953.
4. Brinker WO: Fractures. In Mayer K, Lacroix JV, Hoskins HP, editors: *Canine surgery*, ed 4, Santa Barbara, Calif, 1957, American Veterinary Publications.
5. Brown RE: A surgical approach to the coxo-femoral joint of dogs, *North Am Vet* 34:420, 1953.
6. Brown SG, Rosen H: Craniolateral approach to the canine hip: a modified Watson-Jones approach, *J Am Vet Med Assoc* 159:1117, 1971.
7. Carozzo C, Cachon T, Genevois J-P, Fau D, Remy D, Daniaux L, Collard F, Viguier E: Transiliac approach for exposure of lumbosacral intervertebral disk and foramen: technique description, *Vet Surg* 37:27, 2008.
8. Chalman JA, Slocum B: The caudolateral approach to the canine elbow joint, *J Am Anim Hosp Assoc* 19:637, 1983.
9. Daly WR, Tarvin GB: Medial condyle osteotomy as an approach to repair of medial condyle fractures in dogs, *Vet Surg* 10:119, 1981.
10. De Angelis M, Schwartz A: Surgical correction of a cranial dislocation of the scapulohumeral joint in a dog, *J Am Vet Med Assoc* 156:435, 1970.
11. Déjardin LM, Guiot LP: *Procedure presented at the First AOVET Master Course on Small Animal Minimally Invasive Osteosynthesis, Las Vegas, Nev,* December 15-18, 2011.
12. Dew TL, Martin RA: A caudal approach to the tibiotarsal joint, *J Am Anim Hosp Assoc* 29:117, 1993.
13. Dueland R: Triceps tenotomy approach for distal fractures of the canine humerus, *J Am Vet Med Assoc* 165:82, 1974.
14. Flo GL, Brinker WO: Lateral fenestration of thoracolumbar disc, *J Am Anim Hosp Assoc* 11:619, 1975.
15. Funkquist B: Decompression laminectomy for cervical disk protrusion in the dog, *Acta Vet Scand* 3:88, 1962.
16. Gahring DR: A modified caudal approach to the canine shoulder joint, *J Am Anim Hosp Assoc* 21:613, 1985.
17. Gorman HA: Hip joint prostheses, *Vet Scope* 7(2):3, 1962.
18. Hoerlein BF, Few AB, Petty MF: Brain surgery in the dog: preliminary studies, *J Am Vet Med Assoc* 143:21, 1963.
19. Hohn RB: Surgical approaches to the canine hip, *Anim Hosp* 1:48, 1965.
20. Hohn RB: Osteochondritis dissecans of the humeral head, *J Am Vet Med Assoc* 163:69, 1973.
21. Hohn RB: *Unpublished paper read at Fifth Annual Course on Internal Fixation of Fractures,* Ohio State University, Mar 27-30, 1974.
22. Hohn RB, Janes JM: Lateral approach to the canine ilium, *Anim Hosp* 2:111, 1966.
23. Hohn RB et al: Surgical stabilization of recurrent shoulder luxation, *Vet Clin North Am* 1:537, 1971.
24. Hurov LI, Lumb WV, Hankes GH, Smith KW: Wedge grafting of the canine carpus, *J Am Vet Med Assoc* 148:260, 1966.
25. Lenehan TM, Nunamaker DM: Lateral approach to the canine elbow by proximal ulnar diaphyseal osteotomy, *J Am Vet Med Assoc* 180:523, 1982.
26. Lipsitz D, Bailey CS: Lateral approach for cervical spinal cord decompression, *Prog Vet Neurol* 3:39, 1992.
27. Montavon PM, Boudrieau RJ, Hohn RB: Ventrolateral approach for repair of sacroiliac fracture-dislocation in the dog and cat, *J Am Vet Med Assoc* 186:1198, 1985.
28. Montavon PM, Damur D: *Personal communication,* 2002.
29. Montgomery RD, Milton JL, Mann FA: Medial approach to the humeral diaphysis, *J Am Anim Hosp Assoc* 24:433, 1988.
30. Mostosky UV, Cholvin NR, Brinker WO: Transolecranon approach to the elbow joint, *Vet Med* 54:560, 1959.
31. Newton GT: Craniolateral approach to the humerus with transection of the brachialis muscle, *Vet Surg* 20:281, 1991.
32. Nunamaker DM: Personal communication, 1975.
33. Olsson SE: On disk protrusion in the dog, *Acta Orthop Scand Suppl* VIII, 1951.
34. Paatsama S: *Ligament injuries in the canine stifle joint: a clinical and experimental study,* Thesis, Stockholm, 1952, Royal Veterinary College.
35. Parker A: Surgical approach to the cervicothoracic junction, *J Am Anim Hosp Assoc* 9:374, 1973.
36. Pozzi A, Lewis DD: Surgical approaches for minimally invasive plate osteosynthesis in dogs, *Vet Comp Orthop Traumatol* 22:316, 2009.

37. Probst CW, Flo GL, McLoughlin MA, DeCamp CE: A simple medial approach to the canine elbow for treatment of fragmented coronoid process and osteochondritis dissecans, *J Am Anim Hosp Assoc* 25:331, 1989.

38. Redding RW: Laminectomy in the dog, *Am J Vet Res* 12:123, 1951.

39. Rossmeisl JH, Lanz OI, Inzana KD, Bergman RL: A modified lateral approach to the canine cervical spine; Procedural description and clinical application in 16 dogs with lateralized compressive myelopathy or radiculopathy, *Vet Surg* 34:436, 2005.

40. Rudy RL: Fractures of the maxilla and mandible. In Bojrab J, editor: *Current techniques in small animal surgery*, Philadelphia, 1975, Lea & Febiger, p 369.

41. Seeman CW: A lateral approach for thoracolumbar disc fenestration, *Mod Vet Pract* 49:73, 1968.

42. Sinibaldi K: *Unpublished paper read at the Fourth Annual Conference of the Veterinary Orthopedic Society, Vail, Colo*, Feb 21-24, 1977.

43. Slocum B, Devine T: Pelvic osteotomy technique for axial rotation of the acetabular segment in dogs, *J Am Anim Hosp Assoc* 22:331, 1986.

44. Slocum B, Devine T: Tibial plateau leveling osteotomy for repair of cranial cruciate ligament rupture in the canine, *Vet Clin North Am Small Anim Pract* 23(4):787, 1993.

45. Slocum B, Hohn RB: A surgical approach to the caudal aspect of the acetabulum and body of the ischium in the dog, *J Am Vet Med Assoc* 167:65, 1975.

46. Snavely DA, Hohn RB: A modified lateral surgical approach to the elbow of the dog, *J Am Vet Med Assoc* 169:826, 1977.

47. Sorjonen DC, Shires PK: Atlantoaxial instability: a ventral surgical technique for decompression, fixation, and fusion, *J Am Coll Vet Surg* 10:22, 1981.

48. Stoll SG: *Unpublished paper read at the Fifth Annual Conference of the Veterinary Orthopedic Society, Snowmass, Colo*, Feb 11-18, 1978.

49. Turner TM, Hohn RB: Craniolateral approach for repair of condylar fractures or joint exploration, *J Am Vet Med Assoc* 176:1264, 1980.

50. Wadsworth PL, Henry WB: Dorsal surgical approach to acetabular fractures in the dog, *J Am Vet Med Assoc* 165:908, 1974.

51. Wallace MK, Berg J: Craniolateral approach to the humerus with transection of the brachialis muscle, *Vet Surg* 20:97, 1991.

52. Wilson JW: An anterior approach to the tibia, *J Am Anim Hosp Assoc* 10:67, 1974.

53. Yturraspe DJ, Lumb WV: Dorsolateral muscle separating approach for thoraco-lumbar intervertebral disk fenestration in the dog, *J Am Vet Med Assoc* 162:1037, 1973.

Index

Note: Page number followed by "f" indicate figures.